Advance Praise for *Undo It!*

"If you want to see what medicine will be like ten years from now, read this book today."
—Rita F. Redberg, M.D., editor in chief, *JAMA Internal Medicine*

"The Ornishes' work is elegant and simple and deserving of a Nobel Prize since it can change the world!"
—Richard Carmona, M.D., M.P.H., F.A.C.S.,
seventeenth Surgeon General of the United States,
distinguished professor, University of Arizona

"This is one of the most important books on health ever written."
—John Mackey, CEO, Whole Foods Market

"Dr. Dean Ornish pioneered the revolutionary field of lifestyle medicine: using lifestyle changes to prevent and reverse—UNDO!—heart disease, type 2 diabetes, prostate cancer, high blood pressure, depression, weight gain, high cholesterol, and other chronic diseases. His new unifying hypothesis is truly game-changing and can save your health and your life."
—Kim A. Williams, M.D., President Emeritus,
American College of Cardiology

"Once again, Dr. Dean Ornish, this time in a very productive collaboration with his wife, Anne Ornish, gives us clear mind and body recommendations to make our lives longer, healthier, more productive, and more joyful. Our research together showed that intensive lifestyle changes can slow, stop, or even reverse the progression of very early-stage prostate cancer."
—Peter Carroll, M.D., M.P.H., distinguished professor and chair,
Department of Urology, University of California, San Francisco

"This book will change your life. After forty years of research, the Ornishes have distilled their findings and the medical literature into a fact-based, simple recipe for longer, healthier life. Every day people ask me how they can activate their longevity genes to reverse aging and stave off age-associated diseases. Now I can say, 'Go read *Undo It!*'"
—David A. Sinclair, Ph.D., A.O., professor of genetics,
Harvard Medical School

"My friend Dean Ornish has dedicated his life to making the world a better place by directing over forty years of pioneering research to prove that real foods and other lifestyle changes—including loving and supporting one another—can reverse most chronic diseases and global warming, as well as free up significant resources to feed the hungry. These findings are empowering and inspiring millions of people with new hope and new choices. Highly recommended!"
—Marc Benioff, CEO, Salesforce.com; owner, *Time* magazine

"Dean Ornish is from the future!"
—Jack Hidary, senior adviser and quantumagician, Google X

"A century after Einstein, physics is still looking for its unified field theory, but we now have a unified theory for lifestyle medicine with Dean and Anne Ornish's profound program. They provide a beautiful virtuous circle that combines the latest scientific evidence on health with deep insights into human psychology and well-being."
—Ray Kurzweil, inventor and author of *New York Times* bestsellers
The Singularity Is Near and *How to Create a Mind*

"In their brilliant new book, Dr. Dean Ornish and Anne Ornish help us see that relatively simple ingredients—real food, physical activity, and loving relationships—hold the key to better health. They offer a refreshing and remarkably clear prescription for how we can reverse chronic disease and live healthier, more fulfilling lives."
—Vivek Murthy, M.D., M.B.A., nineteenth Surgeon General of
the United States

"This book is a life saver! Dr. Dean Ornish and Anne Ornish provide simple, important steps anyone can follow to live a healthier life and assure personal happiness. The best part is that we can all use this gift as a guide to correct some bad eating and lifestyle habits and get a fresh, new start. We just have to commit, act on it, and live."

—Beyoncé Knowles-Carter

"My good friends Dean and Anne Ornish have written the definitive, scientifically proven book on how to actually *reverse* most chronic diseases by changing your lifestyle. If you read only one book on health and healing this year, this is it."

—Tony Robbins

"With the cost of chronic disease care placing a major burden on our society, the Ornishes' easy, evidence-based program couldn't be more welcome. It combines the most advanced findings of medical science with practical guidelines that anyone can follow to lead a longer, happier, and healthier life. Everyone needs to read this book and follow its good advice."

—Delos M. (Toby) Cosgrove, M.D., CEO, The Cleveland Clinic

"If people follow the revolutionary program outlined in this brilliant and game-changing book, we can undo most chronic diseases, reverse global warming, and feed the hungry. Side effects to watch for include more energy, inner peace, and better sex. What are you waiting for?"

—James Cameron, director, *Avatar, The Terminator,* and *Titanic,* and
Suzy Cameron, author, *OMD*

"Dr. Dean Ornish's forty years of revolutionary scientific research proving that comprehensive lifestyle changes can often reverse most chronic diseases essentially created the field of lifestyle medicine, which is the most exciting movement in medicine today. His new unifying theory is elegantly simple, profound, and life-transforming."

—Michael Greger, M.D., F.A.C.L.M., author, *How Not to Die;*
founder, NutritionFacts.org

"As knowledgeable and experienced practitioners in lifestyle medicine, Dean and Anne Ornish provide readers with not only their valuable perspective on health but also immediately practical guidance for lifestyle changes, including user-friendly (and delicious!) recipes."
—Elizabeth Blackburn, Ph.D., Nobel laureate in
Physiology or Medicine

"Dean Ornish's inspired research has revolutionized the world of medicine, proving that even our most difficult illnesses can be reversed. This ground-breaking book may be the most practical and helpful book you will ever read."
—Neal D. Barnard, M.D., F.A.C.C., George Washington University
School of Medicine

"*Undo It!* is a magnificent book. You will be deeply grateful for its wisdom, and your body will thank you for the rest of your life."
—John Robbins, #1 *New York Times* bestselling author; president,
Food Revolution Network

"Dr. Ornish's pioneering research used high-tech scientific measures to prove, for the first time, the power of low-tech lifestyle changes to reverse the most common chronic diseases. In this book, he and Anne clearly show you why and how. Highly recommended!"
—Eric Schmidt, CEO, Google/Alphabet

"Because of Dean and Anne's amazing work, my father pursued a plant-based diet combined with daily exercise and lots of time with family and friends, resulting in a turnaround in his health. We're thankful for Dean's work and care, and you will be too when you feel more able to live out loud. Run, don't walk, to buy this generous, practical, lively book. It will change your life."
—Jacqueline Novogratz, CEO, Acumen

"This is the only book you need to buy to change the way you eat and to add ten good years to your life. Buy this book, read the book, and then buy another copy of the book and give it to someone you love. This book is both a treasure trove and a treasure."
—George Halvorson, CEO, Kaiser Permanente

"I was fortunate to have Dean Ornish come into my life when I needed his guidance the most. After suffering a heart attack and going into cardiac arrest, I was in uncharted territory and Dean was my beacon of light. All the things in *Undo It!* are the guidelines that he gave me to get me back on course, for which I am forever grateful. I encourage everyone to listen to and *do* everything Dr. Ornish has to say."
—Bob Harper, #1 *New York Times* bestselling author

"No one has done as much as Dean Ornish to define, study, and prove the lifestyle formula for reversing chronic disease and cultivating vitality. Here, he and Anne share the clear, simple, empowering, and complete details of that formula with you. This book is a gift you give yourself and the people you love."
—David L. Katz, M.D., M.P.H., director, Yale-Griffin Prevention Research Center; president, American College of Lifestyle Medicine

"Dr. Dean Ornish and Anne Ornish have written a breakthrough, evidence-based book that provides a clear guide for living a longer, better life. From the team who first proved that lifestyle changes can reverse heart disease and other chronic illnesses, they now reveal how social connectedness and even love are the next blockbuster drugs."
—Dan Buettner, National Geographic Fellow and *New York Times* bestselling author of *The Blue Zones*

"*Undo It!* is the key to transforming your life in every good way—your health, your love life, and your sense of aliveness. Immerse yourself in the healing that this book promises to unleash. You are in the hands of experts here; I know of no greater authorities than Dean and Anne Ornish, and I heartily recommend giving yourself over to their wisdom."
—Kathy Freston, *New York Times* bestselling author of *The Lean, Quantum Wellness,* and *Clean Protein*

"If a book has the name Ornish on it you can be assured that reading it will be rewarding. Highly recommended!"
—William C. Roberts M.D., editor in chief, *The American Journal of Cardiology*

"*Undo It!* is a masterful book that provides a pathway to achieve the transformative benefits of the authors' lifestyle approaches to improving health and well-being. This is a must read."
   —Ralph Snyderman, M.D., chancellor emeritus, Duke University

"This book by Dean and Anne Ornish is an excellent summary of what people can do to live healthier, happier lives—eat well, move more, stress less, love more—what an inspiring message from a husband-and-wife team!"
   —Patrick Conway, M.D., C.M.O., Centers for Medicare & Medicaid
         Services; CEO, Blue Cross and Blue Shield of North Carolina

"As usual my friend and mentor (this time with his wife, Anne) leads the way with practical science-backed advice that will help you lead a long, healthy, fulfilling, and joyful life. Every human should read this book, and it should be mandatory reading for everyone in educational institutions."
                                        —Deepak Chopra, M.D.

ALSO BY DEAN ORNISH, M.D.

The Spectrum
Love and Survival
Everyday Cooking with Dr. Dean Ornish
Eat More, Weigh Less
Dr. Dean Ornish's Program for Reversing Heart Disease
Stress, Diet, and Your Heart

For more information and to find a certified lifestyle medicine program near you or to attend one of our residential retreats, please go to www.ornish.com.

Undo It!

Undo It!

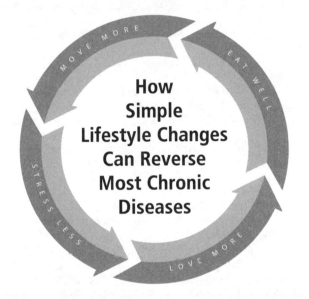

How
Simple
Lifestyle Changes
Can Reverse
Most Chronic
Diseases

MOVE MORE

EAT WELL

STRESS LESS

LOVE MORE

Dean Ornish, M.D., and Anne Ornish

BALLANTINE BOOKS

NEW YORK

No book can replace the diagnostic expertise and medical advice of a trusted physician. Please be certain to consult with your doctor before making any decisions that affect your health, primarily if you suffer from any medical condition or have any symptom that may require treatment.

Published in the United States by Ballantine Books, an imprint of Random House, a division of Penguin Random House LLC, New York.

BALLANTINE and the HOUSE colophon are registered trademarks of Penguin Random House LLC.

LIBRARY OF CONGRESS CATALOGING-IN-PUBLICATION DATA
Names: Ornish, Dean, author. | Ornish, Anne, author.
Title: Undo it! : how simple lifestyle changes can reverse most chronic diseases / Dean Ornish, MD, and Anne Ornish.
Description: New York: Ballantine Books, [2019] | Includes bibliographical references and index.
Identifiers: LCCN 2018038262 (print) | LCCN 2018049526 (ebook) | ISBN 9780525480013 (Ebook) | ISBN 9780525479970 (hardcover:alk. paper)
Subjects: LCSH: Chronic diseases—Alternative treatment. | Chronic diseases—Diet therapy. | Health behavior. | Self-care, Health.
Classification: LCC RC108 (ebook) | LCC RC108 .O76 2019 (print) | DDC 616/.044—dc23
LC record available at https://lccn.loc.gov/2018038262

Printed in the United States of America on acid-free paper

randomhousebooks.com

246897531

First Edition

Book design by Diane Hobbing

To Luke and Jazz, who always inspire us to love more.

Contents

Preface

For more than twenty years, I have had the honor and privilege of collaborating with Anne Pearce Ornish—my wife and partner, best friend, co-parent, co-conspirator, and agent provocateur. We've worked closely together and continued to evolve and refine our lifestyle medicine program during this time.

This book represents the distilled essence of what we've learned about the power of lifestyle medicine. In this process, a radically simple yet transformative vision became increasingly clear; we appreciate the opportunity to share it with you here.

Anne is the director of program development and our digital platform at the nonprofit Preventive Medicine Research Institute. This includes creating www.ornish.com and Empower, the learning management system that all of our sites use to train their patients in our lifestyle medicine program in hospitals, clinics, health systems, and physician groups around the country—which Medicare and many insurance companies are now covering nationwide.

Her contributions to the evolution and refinement of this lifestyle medicine program are too many to count. Anne is highly trained and experienced in lifestyle medicine, yoga therapy, mobile applications, and web design, with over two decades of successful innovation in the health and wellness world.

Our collaboration appears in these pages as well. We thought it would be useful for each of us to share our complementary voices, perspectives, and experiences with you. The yin and the yang. In Chapters 1–3 and 4–7, I describe *why* our program works—the scientific evidence. In Chapters 4–7, as well as in the recipes, exercise, and stress management sections, Anne then describes the *how*.

This also reflects what we do in our work training people worldwide. I discuss the science and direct the research studies documenting the power of our lifestyle medicine program, and then she guides people in how to incorporate it into their lives.

It is fitting that Anne and I—husband and wife—bring you our lifestyle medicine program together. We know that a lack of love and intimacy are at the root of what makes us sick and their presence is what makes us healthy and happy. We've learned that people who feel loved and supported are much more likely to make and maintain lifestyle choices that are life-enhancing than self-destructive.

This is a science-based, love-based program. That's why it works so well. With it, we hope to entice and empower you to experience even greater happiness and pleasure, healing and meaning. And to rediscover inner sources of peace, joy, and well-being.

In that spirit, please accept this book as our love offering to you, our co-creation, love made manifest. We hope you find it to be useful.

Dean Ornish, M.D.

Founder and President, Preventive Medicine Research Institute

Clinical Professor of Medicine, University of California, San Francisco

Sausalito, California, June 21, 2018 (summer solstice)

Undo It!

CHAPTER 1

It Works!

If you can't explain it simply, you don't understand it well enough.
—attributed to Albert Einstein

Our favorite key on the computer is the undo button. Click!—a fresh start.

We've often thought, "Wouldn't it be nice if there were an undo button for our health as well?"

Well, now there is!

This is the era of lifestyle medicine: that is, using simple yet powerful lifestyle changes to reverse—undo!—the progression of the most common chronic diseases as well as to help prevent them.

For more than four decades, one of us (Dean) has directed a series of randomized controlled trials and demonstration projects proving, for the first time, that the radically simple lifestyle medicine program described in this book can often reverse the progression of many of the most common chronic diseases. It can be undertaken in combination with drugs and surgery, or sometimes as an alternative to them.

We continue to be amazed and inspired that the more diseases we study, and the more underlying biological mechanisms we research, the more new reasons and scientific evidence we have to explain why these simple lifestyle changes are so powerful, how transformative and far-ranging their effects can be, and how quickly people can show significant and measurable improvements—often in just a few weeks or even less.

We are excited that our research and the studies of other investigators are proving that many of the most common and debilitating chronic diseases and even much of the damage of aging at a cellular level can often be slowed, stopped, or even reversed by this lifestyle medicine program. These include:

- Reversing even severe coronary heart disease
- Reversing type 2 diabetes
- Reversing, slowing, or stopping the progression of early-stage non-aggressive prostate cancer
- Reversing high blood pressure
- Reversing elevated cholesterol levels
- Reversing obesity
- Reversing some types of early-stage dementia
- Reversing some autoimmune conditions
- Reversing emotional depression and anxiety

Our studies have been published in the leading peer-reviewed medical and scientific journals and presented at the most well-respected physician conferences. No other lifestyle program has this level of scientific evidence on reversing these chronic diseases. This is one reason why a panel of independent experts from *U.S. News & World Report* rated "The Ornish Diet" as "#1 for Heart Health" in 2011, 2012, 2013, 2014, 2015, 2016, and 2017.

Awareness is the first step in healing, and science is a powerful tool for raising awareness. Our peer-reviewed research findings provide the credibility to help overcome what is often the biggest obstacle: skepticism that such simple lifestyle changes can have such powerful, far-reaching measurable improvements—and how fast you can feel better.

In that spirit, we are including this information not to boast but (hopefully) to inspire and empower, to rise above the noise and misinformation that are so prevalent.

We've used high-tech, state-of-the-art scientific measures to prove the power of this low-tech lifestyle medicine intervention. The science may motivate you to get started; the extraordinary benefits you are likely to quickly experience are what make it sustainable.

Radically Simple, Yet Powerfully Proven

We learned from Steve Jobs that people who have spent their lives deeply understanding something complex can make it really simple for others to learn. When you really know a subject, you can reduce it down to the essence of what's most important.

For example, Steve said that he was more proud of what he left out of the iPhone than what he included. Although the underlying technology is highly complex, there is an elegant Zen simplicity in its design that makes it extraordinarily powerful and intuitively easy to use because it is based on a deep understanding of what is most important and what really matters—and what doesn't. You don't even need a user manual. He and Jony Ive applied this same ethos to the ecosystem of all Apple products they created, which made it the most valuable and emulated company in the world.

In that spirit, this book represents the quintessence of what we've learned about the power of lifestyle medicine. We emphasize the research that we have conducted rather than a comprehensive review of the scientific literature. We've included only what's most essential, and we hope you find it to be useful.

We have shown, time and time again, that this lifestyle medicine program often works to reverse and help prevent many of the most common chronic diseases for most people.

We've consistently achieved bigger changes in lifestyle, better clinical outcomes, larger cost savings, and greater adherence than have ever been reported. If you carefully follow the lifestyle changes we describe in this book, there's a good chance it may be effective for you as well.

Here It Is, Why It Works, and How You Can Do It

Our program has four major components, each a healing modality on its own and synergistic when done together:

- A *whole-foods plant-based diet,* naturally low in animal protein, fat, sugar, and refined carbohydrates and high in flavor—primarily fruits, vegetables, whole grains, legumes, and soy products in their natural, unprocessed forms. The principles of eating this way are simple and clear. We outline these in Chapter 4 and offer amazingly delicious recipes in Chapter 8.
- *Moderate exercise,* such as walking and strength training. Do what you enjoy—if you like it, you'll do it. Chapter 5 shows why and how a little exercise goes a very long way.
- *Stress management.* Chapter 6 introduces you to techniques (including meditation and gentle yoga) that can enable you to do more and stress less.
- *Love, social support, and intimacy.* People who feel lonely, depressed, and isolated are three to ten times more likely to get sick and die prematurely from virtually all causes when compared to those who have strong feelings of love, connection and community. Chapter 7 describes how we can transform isolation into healing.

In short: eat well, move more, stress less, love more. That's it. Boom!

This book is based directly on the scientifically proven nine-week lifestyle medicine program that we have implemented in hospitals, physician groups, health systems, and clinics across the country.

We've proven this lifestyle medicine program works exceptionally well in the real world. We have clinical outcomes data from tens of thousands of diverse patients who have gone through this program at a continually growing number of sites throughout the country and from millions of people who have made these lifestyle changes from my earlier books. It is both effective and achievable. The lessons we've learned from this extensive experience form the basis and structure of this book.

In 2010, after sixteen years of comprehensive review, I appreciate that the Centers for Medicare and Medicaid Services (CMS) created a new benefit category, "intensive cardiac rehabilitation," to begin providing

Medicare coverage for "Dr. Ornish's Program for Reversing Heart Disease." This was the first time that CMS provided Medicare coverage for a lifestyle medicine intervention to reverse heart disease.

This had the strong bipartisan personal support of both Bill Clinton when he was president of the United States and Newt Gingrich when he was Speaker of the House, as well as leading members of the U.S. Senate and House of Representatives across the political spectrum. Other supporters included the director of the National Heart, Lung, and Blood Institute of the National Institutes of Health, the head of the AARP, and leading physicians and scientists across the country.

This was an important recognition of the value of lifestyle medicine as one of the few areas that transcend our increasingly polarized and dysfunctional political environment.

Many commercial insurance companies are now also covering our lifestyle medicine program. Some of these are covering it not only for reversing heart disease but also for reversing type 2 diabetes, high blood pressure, obesity, and elevated cholesterol levels.

This was a game-changer, as reimbursement directly affects medical practice and even medical education. Now it is sustainable for physicians and other healthcare professionals to offer our lifestyle medicine program. We're helping to create a new paradigm of healthcare at a time when it is so badly needed by providing better care to more people at lower cost.

Most physicians spend only about ten minutes with a patient at an office visit. This is often frustrating for both doctors and patients, since there is insufficient time to talk about what matters most: what's going on in their lives with respect to their diet, exercise, sources of stress, their marriage, their kids, their work, their friends, their finances, their home, and their spiritual life.

In our new lifestyle medicine paradigm, Medicare and insurance companies are paying for seventy-two hours of training each patient rather than only ten minutes. This new paradigm of lifestyle medicine allows physicians to leverage their time in meaningful ways by using a multidisciplinary team approach. The physician acts as "quarterback" and he or she provides oversight for the intervention, divided into eighteen four-hour sessions offered twice per week for nine weeks or for a twelve-day immersion retreat with six hours of classes per day. Each session is as follows:

- One hour of supervised exercise, led by an exercise physiologist
- One hour of stress management, led by a certified yoga/meditation teacher
- One hour of a support group, led by a licensed clinical psychologist or social worker
- One hour of a group meal and a lecture by a registered dietitian and nurse

In addition to being medically effective, our approach is also cost-effective. It turns out that only 5 percent of patients account for 50–80 percent of all healthcare costs. These are people who have chronic diseases—and heart disease is the most expensive condition in terms of total healthcare spending.

In a demonstration project, Mutual of Omaha found that almost 80 percent of people who were eligible for bypass surgery or a stent were able to safely avoid it by going through our lifestyle medicine program instead—saving almost $30,000 per patient in the first year.

In a second demonstration project, Highmark Blue Cross Blue Shield found that our lifestyle medicine program cut overall healthcare costs by 50 percent in the first year, and these cost savings were sustained for at least three years. And only 1 percent of these patients who went through our program incurred claims costs in excess of $25,000 after the first year, compared to 4 percent of control group patients—a threefold difference in costs.

For more information and to find a program near you or to attend an immersion retreat, please go to www.ornish.com.

Here's an especially dramatic example of how powerful this lifestyle medicine program can be. Robert Treuherz, M.D., is a specialist in internal medicine who had such a massive heart attack that he was told the damage to his heart was so great that he needed a heart transplant to survive.

While waiting for a donor heart to become available, he went through our lifestyle medicine program at the UCLA Medical Center to get in better shape for this surgery. Nine weeks later, he improved so dramatically that he no longer needs a heart transplant! Here's his story, along with the perspective of his wife, Claudia:

Dr. Robert Treuherz: I'm a sixty-one-year-old internal medicine doctor who was also trained in critical care medicine at one of the most well-respected medical centers in New York. Yet I never received any training in nutrition or other lifestyle changes.

I thought meditation and yoga were woo-woo—I didn't take them seriously. Also, I had a very male-oriented perception of what love and affection meant, without a more mature outlook like one eventually develops.

I was enjoying robust good health, living and practicing medicine in Lake Arrowhead at 6,000 feet. I was a ski instructor and was in the ski patrol in college. When my wife, Claudia, and I would ski, we'd have four kids between us and I could ski them into the ground without running out of breath.

Then on October 29, 2015, I had a massive heart attack. I had severe blockages in my coronary arteries which resulted in a drop in my ejection fraction to only 11 percent. [*The ejection fraction is the percentage of blood that the heart pumps with each beat. Normally, this is at least 50 percent—i.e., a healthy heart pumps half of its volume or more with each beat.*] They put in a stent to try to open one of the main arteries that was 100 percent clogged.

The first two weeks after that happened, I was given no prognosis. I mean that in the most literal, concrete way possible. I was told, my wife was told, my mom was told, my family was told, "Say goodbye. That's it! You're done. You're not going to get out of here alive."

It was a violent paradigm change. All of a sudden, my whole reality was altered.

I managed to survive the first two weeks, then got transferred to another facility, where an angiogram was repeated. They found a complete occlusion of the stent.

About twelve hours later, I had a full cardiac arrest. When I came to, ten to twelve hours later, I was intubated because I had literally died.

I came out of this dark void, which was so unsettling. My love for my wife and family pulled me out of it. Maybe it's to be here to help other people get an opportunity to go through this program. My vital capacity when I came out of this was close to zero. I was having chest pain anytime I walked more than a few steps. I couldn't go up the stairs to my bedroom unless one of my sons carried me upstairs.

When I look at pictures of me after the heart attack when I came home, frankly, I've seen many dead people who look better than I did, way better. That's not being dramatic, it really isn't. That's absolutely a fact. I was just gray, washed out.

I couldn't manage my weight, couldn't manage my diuretics, couldn't compensate for my heart failure even with many powerful medications.

I entered a traditional cardiac rehab program at Providence St. Joseph's Hospital. They wouldn't let me continue because every time I started to exercise, I'd have a paradoxical response to the exercise. My blood pressure would drop and I would become sweaty and pass out because my heart was pumping so badly that I couldn't tolerate even the minimum amount of cardiac rehab I was being offered.

The fall in my health from where I had been before my heart attack to this led to a catastrophic emotional depression. I was told over and over again, "You're going to die. You're going to die." The kind of depression that puts you in is hard even to describe.

One of my cardiologists later said that my heart disease was so advanced that only a heart transplant would help.

I was afraid to move, afraid to exercise because everything I did caused chest pain. While waiting for a heart transplant, I came into the Ornish Lifestyle Medicine Program at the UCLA Medical Center. When they first evaluated me, they said, "You know, this guy's too sick for the program. We're scared to take him because he's going to drop dead on the exercise court." They were afraid I wouldn't make it.

After only nine weeks on this program, my ejection fraction increased from only 11 percent to over 30 percent (now 35 percent), so I no longer needed to have a heart transplant! The difference is like science fiction. My cholesterol levels have dropped more than 50 percent, and my angina is gone.

The outcome is difficult to describe. I can't believe I'm even standing here, let alone that I'm working again four days a week as a doctor in Lake Arrowhead. Yesterday I took a long walk in the Big Bear area at an altitude of 7,500 feet for forty-five minutes with no chest pain.

My relationship with my wife, Claudia, is what we both want it to be, so much closer. I can enjoy my kids, enjoy everything so much more.

Claudia: After his heart attack, I did not think he was going to live the rest of the year. When I called the children, the prognosis was very grim. The doctors said, "Call the kids. Doesn't look good." Mom was there. When we brought him home, he couldn't go up the stairs. He couldn't walk from the couch to the kitchen or from the kitchen to the bedroom. He was having chest pain almost all the time. We were both constantly living in fear.

Robert: When I went into this program, I really didn't have that much faith in it. I went into it because I just didn't know what else to do, and the science impressed me.

I whined about the food. It seemed like the end of the world that I couldn't eat everything. It wasn't. After only a few weeks, my palate changed and I began enjoying the meals.

The paradox is that what seems to be the hardest path turns out to be the easiest one, the path of least resistance. Once you've made that commitment, then you start to feel better so rapidly, you experience that it's clearly worth doing.

Claudia asked me today, "Well, what are you going to say if you're asked what's the difference between this program and another program?" The difference I would say is eighteen inches, the distance from your brain to your heart. Once your brain decides to change your behavior, your heart follows.

That's what the constellation of all of the four components of Dr. Ornish's program does working in concert. It's an absolute game changer. And we're teaching our kids so that this doesn't happen to them.

I came out of that void to do something more. Maybe if I can empower and inspire some people to make these lifestyle changes, maybe that's why I got a second chance.

Claudia: You don't just come back from the brink of death to squander it away. There is a purpose. There is a meaning to all of this. If it is to help other people change and transform, it's a beautiful thing. I think that's why he is still here. We are both feeling humbled and very grateful. I'm still in awe. I have my husband back, which is incredible!

We've heard many thousands of stories like this over the years (several are on video at ornish.com.) They still move us to tears and continue to inspire us to do this work. Empowering people to relieve suffering brings meaning and purpose to our lives, for which we remain grateful.

If It's Pleasurable and Meaningful, It's Sustainable

During the past decades, we've learned what enables people to make sustainable changes in their lives.

For example, 94 percent of the people who enroll in our nine-week lifestyle medicine program at all of our sites completed the seventy-two hours of training, and 85–90 percent are still following it one year later.

To put this in context, most physicians believe their patients will take cholesterol-lowering drugs like statins or blood pressure medications that they prescribe but think their patients are unlikely to make sustainable lifestyle changes. In fact, though, only about half of patients are still taking these drugs just six months after they have been prescribed even though they are of proven benefit in those with heart disease. One-third of these prescriptions are not even filled.

The reason for this is that cholesterol-lowering drugs and blood pressure medications don't make you feel better, but lifestyle changes usually do.

When most doctors prescribe statins or drugs to lower blood pressure, it usually goes something like this: "Take these pills every day for the rest of your life. They won't make you feel better—and they may even make you feel worse. But they will help prevent something really bad like a heart attack or stroke from happening years down the road that you don't want to think about." So you don't.

A central theme of this book is that fear is not a successful motivator over the long term. It's often very effective in the short run—for about a month after someone has a heart attack, for example, they'll do just about anything that their doctor or nurse prescribes—but it usually doesn't last. It's just too scary to continue believing that something bad may happen.

For lifestyle changes to be sustainable, they have to be pleasurable and meaningful, fun and joyful, loving and feeling good, as well as effective—and freely chosen. What you gain has to be much more than what you give up—and quickly!

With our lifestyle medicine program, it is. Life is to be enjoyed and savored.

Because the underlying biological mechanisms that affect our health are so dynamic, when you make the lifestyle changes described in this book, you're likely to feel so much better so quickly that it makes these choices worth doing—not just to live longer, but also to feel better in ways that matter most. After all, what's the point of living longer if you're not enjoying life?

The old saying about an ounce of prevention and a pound of cure is true. It usually takes a lot more changes in diet and lifestyle to reverse a disease than to prevent it.

If you don't have a chronic disease and are otherwise healthy, then what matters most is your *overall* way of eating. So if you indulge yourself one day, just eat healthier the next. By contrast, if you go on a diet, chances are you'll go off the diet sooner or later, and then you may feel shame and guilt, which truly are toxic emotions. Our earlier book, *The Spectrum*, describes this approach in more detail.

But it takes bigger lifestyle changes to *reverse*—undo—many chronic diseases. I'd love to be able to tell you that moderate lifestyle changes can often reverse chronic diseases, but that wouldn't be true.

Thus, this book is specific and prescriptive because it is intended to reverse a wide variety of chronic diseases. It outlines in simple terms how to change your diet and lifestyle in ways that are based on decades of experience. You get to be the beneficiary of what we've learned from doing this for so long—a lot of wisdom comes from making mistakes along the way and learning from them. And the studies cited here are referenced in the back of this book for those who want to go to their primary sources.

Paradoxically, big changes in lifestyle made all at once are often easier to make than moderate, gradual ones when reversing a disease. We know that's counterintuitive, but here's why it's often true: when you make only moderate lifestyle changes, you're not able to eat and do everything you want but you're not making changes big enough to feel that much better or for your clinical measures to improve very much. In a real sense, you get the worst of both worlds.

The more you change your lifestyle, the more you improve in how you feel and in everything you measure. So when you make really big changes in your diet and lifestyle, you are likely to feel so much better (usually within days) that it reframes the reason for making these changes from fear of dying (which is not sustainable) to joy in living (which is).

Then these benefits come from your own experience, which you learn to trust. You connect the dots between what you do and how you feel: "When I eat well, move more, stress less, and love more, I feel really good to the degree I make these lifestyle changes. When I don't, I don't feel as well. So I'll do more of this and less of that."

Here's one of many examples of how lifestyle medicine quickly and meaningfully improves the *quality* of our lives.

The effects of lifestyle are systemic, the same process manifesting in organs throughout your body. For example, the same biological mechanisms that control blood flow to your brain and to your heart also control blood flow to your sexual organs.

Blood vessel problems are the leading cause of erectile dysfunction. That's why Harvard's Dr. Michael P. O'Leary writes that erections "serve as a barometer for overall health" and that erectile dysfunction (impotence) can be an early warning sign of trouble in the heart or elsewhere. Erectile dysfunction affects at least 18 million men, probably many more. Over half of men with type 2 diabetes also have erectile dysfunction.

It's why men who have erectile dysfunction are at much higher risk of having heart disease, memory loss, dementia, or stroke as their arteries are often clogged throughout their body.

We've been writing for many years that even a single meal high in animal protein and fat can significantly decrease blood flow to your brain and to your heart (more on this in Chapter 2).

But for many people, an even more motivating example than increasing blood flow to your brain and your heart can be found in *The Game Changers,* a powerful new documentary film produced by legendary filmmaker James Cameron with James Wilks and Joseph Pace and directed by Academy Award winner Louie Psihoyos.

This movie addresses the most common misconceptions about eating a whole-foods plant-based diet—that meat is necessary for protein, strength, and optimal health. It tells powerful stories about world-class elite athletes who dramatically improved their performance after changing to a whole-foods plant-based diet.

One scene was so impactful that most of the film crew changed to a plant-based diet after shooting it! A leading urologist, Dr. Aaron Spitz, gave three elite athletes in their twenties a single high-quality meat-based dinner (organic chicken, grass-fed beef, or organic pork) and then measured how many erections they had and how hard these were while they slept during that night. The next evening, he gave them a single plant-based dinner and repeated the studies.

He documented that these three men had 300–500 percent more frequent erections during the night after a plant-based meal than a meat-based meal. These erections were, on average, four times longer in duration (almost forty-five minutes versus eleven minutes), and they were harder and had a wider circumference. After just one meal!

As Dr. Spitz said in the film, "I think this is going to wake a lot of people up. I think it's going to wake up people who have penises and I think it's going to wake up people who like people who have penises."

Or as Robin Williams once quipped, "God gave men both a penis and a brain, but unfortunately not enough blood supply to run both at the same time." Now, maybe we can!

This explodes the most common myths about living healthier—such as "Am I going to live longer or is it just going to *seem* longer?" or "The only way to live to one hundred is by not doing all the things that make you want to live to one hundred," and other variations on this theme.

Again, what you gain in the most meaningful ways is so much more than what you give up—and how fast you can experience these benefits.

Food can be good for you *and* fun for you.

If you go on our lifestyle medicine program, under your doctor's supervision you may be able to reduce or even wean off many medications to lower cholesterol, blood pressure, or blood sugar that you were probably told you'd have to take forever, because you're directly addressing many of their underlying *causes*. For this reason, it's important that you include your doctor if you are going on this program to reverse a chronic disease so they can monitor your progress and adjust your medications and other treatments as needed.

Chapter 2 describes how and why this program works so well.

CHAPTER **2**

Why It Works

A New Unified Theory of Health and Healing

Like all revolutionary new ideas, the subject has had to pass through three stages, which may be summed up by these reactions: (1) "It's crazy—don't waste my time." (2) "It's possible, but it's not worth doing." (3) "I always said it was a good idea."
—Arthur C. Clarke

Like most physicians, I was trained to view heart disease, diabetes, prostate cancer, and other chronic illnesses as being fundamentally different from each other. Different diagnoses, different diseases, different treatments.

But they're really not as different as they seem because they share many common origins and pathways.

Why These Same Lifestyle Changes Have So Many Powerful and Far-Reaching Benefits

One of the most surprising findings in our research was that the same lifestyle medicine program described in this book has such far-reaching impacts on undoing such a wide range of diverse chronic illnesses.

This flies in the face of the latest trends in personalized medicine. Many books, new lines of food, and healthcare companies are promising to tailor a diet and lifestyle program based on your genome, blood test results, and clinical status.

But this is largely a myth. In our research, there wasn't one set of lifestyle recommendations for reversing heart disease and different ones for reversing prostate cancer, diabetes, and other chronic illnesses. It was the same lifestyle medicine program for reversing all of these.

We found that these same lifestyle changes described in this book can reverse and thus help prevent the progression of a wide variety of the most common, costly, and disabling chronic diseases. Also, the more closely people adhered to this program, the more they improved in every way we measured and the better they felt—at any age! These findings are giving many people new hope and new choices.

Why is this true?

The reason these same lifestyle changes are beneficial in reversing so many chronic diseases is that they each affect and share so many common underlying biological causes, mechanisms, and pathways.

One of the important implications of this new unifying theory is to stop seeing chronic diseases as being fundamentally different from each other and to begin viewing them as diverse manifestations and expressions of similar underlying mechanisms, all of which are powerfully affected by the lifestyle choices we make every day—for better and for worse. That is why the effects of lifestyle changes are not disease-specific—because they affect all of these mechanisms.

These biological mechanisms include changes in, among others:

- Chronic inflammation and immune system dysfunction
- Chronic emotional stress, depression, overstimulation of the sympathetic nervous system, stress hormones, and lack of sleep
- Gene expression and sirtuins
- Telomeres

- The microbiome
- Oxidative stress, cellular metabolism, and apoptosis
- Angiogenesis
- Stasis

And others.

Although this may seem like a radical theory, on further reflection it's not really that surprising. We know, for example, that regular exercise will help prevent and improve a wide variety of conditions—it's not disease-specific—whereas a sedentary lifestyle significantly increases the risk of many chronic diseases—also not disease-specific.

It's not as though you need to do one type of exercise to help prevent or reverse heart disease and a different one to help prevent or reverse prostate cancer or type 2 diabetes. More important is to find a way of exercising that you're likely to maintain—if you like it, you'll do it.

For the same reason, the same whole-foods plant-based diet described in this book enhances our well-being in just about every aspect we can measure and helps prevent and even reverse the progression of so many different chronic diseases because this way of eating beneficially affects all of these mechanisms. Conversely, an unhealthy diet greatly increases the risk of a myriad of chronic illnesses via the same mechanisms.

Similarly, stress management techniques such as meditation and yoga improve our health in multiple ways, whereas sustained emotional stress significantly increases the risk of numerous chronic diseases via these same mechanisms.

Love and intimacy help keep us healthy, but people who are lonely and depressed are three to ten times more likely to get sick and die prematurely from virtually all causes.

Seen from this perspective—that is, the same mechanisms affect a wide variety of chronic illnesses—also provides additional scientific evidence to explain why people often have several chronic diseases (called co-morbidities) at the same time and why they share so many common risk factors. For example, many people with heart disease also have high blood pressure, type 2 diabetes, elevated cholesterol levels, obesity, and other chronic illnesses.

It also makes clear why these same lifestyle medicine changes can help prevent and improve all of these co-morbidities simultaneously since they beneficially affect the same mechanisms that are underlying causes of these conditions. They all interrelate.

For example, this widespread effect was found in the European Prospective Investigation into Cancer and Nutrition (EPIC) study of almost 25,000 men and women. The same lifestyle choices had a large impact on a *variety* of conditions.

Those with four healthy lifestyle factors—moderate exercise of at least 30 minutes per day; not smoking; normal weight; and a high intake of fruits, vegetables, and whole grains and low meat consumption—had a 78 percent lower risk of developing *any* chronic disease, including a 93 percent lower risk of getting type 2 diabetes, an 81 percent reduced risk of a heart attack, a 50 percent lower risk of a stroke, and a 36 percent reduction in all forms of cancer!

That's worth repeating: although the majority of Americans have type 2 diabetes or pre-diabetes, this study showed that at least 93 percent of diabetes is completely preventable—today! And if people made the bigger lifestyle changes described in this book, it's probably closer to 100 percent preventable and often even reversible.

Also, a 2018 large-scale study of more than 100,000 patients by the Harvard School of Public Health found that those adopting just five healthy lifestyle habits had an 82 percent lower risk for dying from cardiovascular disease, a 65 percent lower chance of dying from cancer, and a 74 percent lower risk of dying from all causes during follow-up. These same lifestyle habits had a major impact on all of these chronic diseases.

Each component of an unhealthy lifestyle that they studied—diet, smoking, physical activity, alcohol consumption, and weight—showed a significant association with increased premature death from all causes, from cancer, and from heart disease. Those who were not overweight, never smoked, exercised an average of 30 minutes per day, didn't drink to excess, and ate a healthy diet lived an average of *twelve to fourteen years longer*.

We just need to put into practice what we already know.

The guiding principle of our lifestyle medicine program has always been based on addressing the underlying *causes* of illnesses on many levels simultaneously. By analogy, if you have a rock in your shoe, don't blame the stone, use painkillers or surgery to cut the affected nerves, or wear thicker socks—just take out the rock!

Each of the program's four components—eat well, move more, stress less, and love more—has profound and dynamic beneficial effects on all of these shared mechanisms that cause us to get sick and enable us to heal. Because of this, we can often begin to undo what has been a lifetime of damage relatively quickly. Our bodies often have a remarkable capacity to begin healing, and much more quickly than we had once believed, when we work at this causal level.

Too Much of a Good Thing

All of these lifestyle factors and mechanisms interrelate, which is why our program involves a variety of comprehensive lifestyle changes.

A recurring theme of our program is that mechanisms that have evolved to heal us can actually become harmful or even lethal when chronically overstimulated by harmful lifestyle factors—and this is often the case in modern times.

Your mind and body have not yet had time to evolve to deal with the excesses and disruptions of twenty-first-century life: a diet high in animal protein, fat, and sugar; a sedentary lifestyle; often chronic and unrelenting emotional stress; and the widespread breakdown of social networks that used to give people a strong sense of connection, community, and love, often leading to chronic emotional depression. The result of this disruption is that many people are not healthy and not happy and are often emotionally depressed and chronically ill.

The Pound of Cure

It takes bigger lifestyle changes to reverse disease than to prevent it—the pound of cure instead of the ounce of prevention. But it's the same idea—since these same mechanisms affect so many different diseases, this makes it radically simple. And it's achievable—we can help prevent these diseases in the first place by making the lifestyle changes described in this book.

There is definitely a place for personalized medicine for certain conditions. For example, specific immune therapies tailored to a particular cell type of a pancreatic tumor or a specific melanoma cell line may be effective. Even then, lifestyle changes may be beneficial in helping to augment the body's immune system. But for the most common chronic diseases, this same lifestyle medicine program may slow, stop, and even reverse their progression.

Let's examine these biological mechanisms in more detail. You can skip the rest of this chapter if you find it to be too technical for your level of interest. We included this information because you may find it empowering to know why the more mechanisms we study, the more science we have to explain why the lifestyle medicine program described in this book is so powerful in undoing such a wide variety of chronic diseases.

Chronic Inflammation/Immune Function

An unhealthy diet (especially one high in animal protein, fat, and refined carbohydrates), a sedentary lifestyle, chronic stress, and social isolation each increase chronic inflammation, whereas a healthy diet, moderate exercise, stress management techniques, and love and intimacy each decrease it.

Inflammation is a powerful immune mechanism in your body for healing when tissues are injured by bacteria, trauma, toxins, heat, or any other causes. It helps infections and wounds to heal and toxins to be eliminated.

Inflammation can be healing when it's acute but can be deadly when it's chronically activated and stays on high alert due to these same lifestyle factors—another example of too much of a good thing.

Hallmarks of acute ("good") inflammation include:

- *Enhanced immune function.* This results from the release of white blood cells and other mediators of immunity, which neutralize and remove invading organisms.
- *Pain.* Chemicals that stimulate nerve endings are released, making the area more sensitive so you don't touch it and allow the area to repair itself.
- *Redness and heat.* To enhance healing, your blood vessels dilate, bringing more blood to the affected area, which feels warm to the touch.
- *Swelling and immobility.* This also encourages you to allow the affected part of your body to rest and heal. The damaged cells release

chemicals including histamine, bradykinin, and prostaglandins, allowing blood vessels to leak fluid into the tissues, causing swelling. This helps isolate the foreign substance from further contact with body tissues.

- *Phagocytosis.* The chemicals released by damaged cells also attract white blood cells called phagocytes that "eat" germs and dead or damaged cells. This process is called phagocytosis. Phagocytes eventually die. Pus is formed from a collection of dead tissue, dead bacteria, and live and dead phagocytes, which are eliminated via your lymphatic system (more on this later).

Acute inflammation comes on quickly and resolves rapidly, usually lasting for only a few days or so until healing occurs.

In contrast, chronic inflammation tends to occur more slowly but may last for months or even years. It plays an important role in almost every major chronic disease, including cancer, heart disease, diabetes, depression, and dementia, among others.

- *Arteries.* Chronic inflammation injures the lining of your arteries. Your body's attempt to heal these recurrent injuries is like putting a Band-Aid on the damage to the lining of an artery—and then, as the injuries continue, more and more Band-Aids get piled on top of each other, progressively obstructing the flow of blood. This can lead to the buildup of plaque (atherosclerosis) in your arteries, which reduces blood flow to your heart and brain, causing angina (chest pain), a heart attack, or a stroke. Inflammation also makes these plaques more unstable, which can cause them to rupture or a blood clot to form that closes off blood flow downstream, leading to a heart attack or stroke.
- *Brain.* In your brain, chronic inflammation and oxidative stress can lead to emotional depression and also to buildup of plaque (amyloid) and neurofibrillary tangles (tau) in your brain. Over time, this can lead to Alzheimer's disease by short-circuiting the neurons and causing neural degeneration and progressive dementia. Blockages of arteries reducing blood flow to your brain can lead to vascular dementia.
- *Joints.* In your joints, chronic inflammation can lead to arthritis.

- *Pancreas.* Chronic inflammation of the pancreas can lead to insulin resistance, type 2 diabetes, pancreatitis, and obesity. And too much insulin promotes chronic inflammation in a vicious cycle.
- *Cancer.* Oncogenes that promote prostate cancer, breast cancer, and colon cancer do so in part by causing inflammation at every stage in a cancer's growth. Some researchers believe that an inflammatory microenvironment is essential for all cancers. Smoking also promotes lung cancer by causing chronic inflammation.

A sedentary lifestyle increases inflammation, whereas exercise decreases it. Only twenty minutes of walking significantly reduces markers of inflammation.

A typical American diet is high in animal protein, which increases production of interleukins, blood chemicals that promote chronic inflammation. In contrast, plant-based proteins are low in inflammatory stimulants and contain literally thousands of protective substances such as phytochemicals, bioflavonoids, retinols, isoflavones, and others that actively decrease rather than increase chronic inflammation—providing a double benefit (protective rather than harmful).

Reducing animal protein intake is known to reduce levels of a growth factor called IGF-1, which promotes chronic inflammation, and lower IGF-1 levels are linked to longer life span and reductions in the risk of cancer and diabetes.

Most fruits and vegetables are anti-inflammatory, especially blueberries, strawberries, tomatoes, nuts, cruciferous vegetables such as broccoli, and green leafy vegetables.

Animal protein dramatically increases the risk of premature death independent of fat and carbohydrates. In a study of over 6,000 people, those ages fifty to sixty-five who reported eating diets high in animal protein had a 75 percent increase in overall mortality, a 400 percent increase in cancer deaths, and a 500 percent increase in type 2 diabetes during the following eighteen years, whereas plant-based proteins reduced the risk of premature death in all of these categories—again, a double benefit.

Intake of dietary cholesterol (which is only found in animal products) and harmful fats such as most saturated fats, hydrogenated fats, and trans fats increase chronic inflammation. In contrast, beneficial fats in moderate amounts such as omega-3 fatty acids (3 grams per day) and nuts in moderation decrease it. So do tea, coffee, magnesium, curcumin (a substance found in turmeric), and ginger, among others.

The American Heart Association diet includes fish, chicken, and beef in moderate amounts. While it's a step in the right direction, a recent study provided more evidence to explain why this diet doesn't go far enough to reverse heart disease in most people.

In this study, 100 patients with coronary heart disease were placed on a whole-foods vegan diet or an American Heart Association–recommended diet. After only eight weeks, inflammation was significantly lower in the vegan group compared with those on the American Heart Association recommended diet, as measured by highly sensitive C-reactive protein assays, even though weight loss was the same in both groups.

Naturally occurring sugars, when found in unprocessed fruits and vegetables, decrease inflammation. However, added sugar, high-fructose corn syrup, and refined carbohydrates such as white flour can cause chronic inflammation.

In one study, for example, consuming just one can of soda per day led to an increase in inflammatory markers. Consuming less than 2 ounces of high-fructose corn syrup causes a spike in measures of inflammation such as C-reactive protein (CRP) just thirty minutes later, and these markers remain elevated for several hours. In another study, eating just one slice of white bread resulted in higher blood sugar levels and an increase in another inflammatory marker (Nf-kBf).

Processing whole-wheat flour into white flour or brown rice into white rice removes the fiber and bran. This turns healthy carbohydrates into unhealthy ones that promote inflammation.

Fiber and bran fill you up before you get too many calories. Also, they slow the rate of absorption from your gut into your blood, so your blood sugar rises slowly and not too high. When fiber and bran are removed, your food gets rapidly absorbed, causing your blood sugar to spike to high levels, which in turn causes your pancreas to secrete insulin to bring your blood sugar back down.

After a while, it's as if these repeated surges of insulin cause your insulin receptors to say, "Oh, no, not more insulin!" so they downregulate and become less sensitive. Because of this, your body needs to make more and more insulin to lower your blood sugar an equivalent amount. This is called insulin resistance.

Insulin resistance also causes inflammation by increasing secretion of what are called cytokines from immune function cells. A vicious cycle results in which more insulin causes more inflammation, which causes more insulin resistance, often leading to metabolic syndrome and type 2 diabetes.

Another study found that microscopic toxins causing chronic inflammation were present mainly in meat products, fatty foods, dairy, and processed foods but were minimal or undetectable in fresh fruit and vegetables.

New research is showing that reducing chronic inflammation with drugs also reduces the risk of heart attacks, strokes, and premature death from heart disease, which provides even more evidence of the important role of inflammation. These new drugs are very expensive and, like all drugs, have side effects. Clearly, it's better to reduce inflammation with lifestyle medicine.

Chronic emotional stress also causes chronic inflammation. This occurs via changes in stress hormones and direct connections between your brain and nerves all over your body, as described below.

Chronic Emotional Stress and Depression Overstimulate the Sympathetic Nervous System

Chronic emotional stress is a common risk factor for 75–90 percent of chronic diseases, including the illnesses that cause the foremost morbidity and mortality.

The fight-or-flight response is a series of physiological responses that are activated in our body during times of stress and danger. These help us to fight or to run in order to survive.

If someone pulls a knife on you in a robbery, your sympathetic nervous system goes into overdrive. There are direct nerve connections between your brain and every organ in your body. Also, the brain secretes hormones during times of stress that travel through your blood and affect all of your organs and every cell in your body as well.

During emotional stress, part of your brain called the amygdala causes your heart to pump faster and your kidneys to secrete stress hormones such as adrenaline, so you have more energy; your muscles to tense up, to provide more "body armor" in case you get hit; and the arteries in your arms and leg to constrict and your blood to clot faster so that you don't bleed as much in case you are injured.

These mechanisms help you to survive acute stresses—you give up your wallet and the robber leaves, or you fight back and win, or you run away. However it turns out, it's an acute stress and the danger is over.

In modern times, though, stresses can feel relentless. You don't have a chance to recover from one stress because two or three more are right behind. Because of this, the fight-or-flight response causes your sympathetic nervous system to become *chronically* activated. Paradoxically, what has evolved to help you survive can harm or even kill you.

If your muscles are chronically tensed, that can lead to chronic back or neck pain. Chronic stress may cause your arteries to constrict and blood to clot in your heart or brain, not just in your arms and legs, leading to a heart attack or stroke.

A recent study proved that chronic stress or depression increases inflammation as well. Researchers at Harvard used positron emission tomography (PET) scans to measure activity in the amygdala, the part of your brain that controls the fight-or-flight stress response as well as depression.

The researchers found that perceived chronic stress or depression in the people they studied caused markedly increased ongoing activity in their amygdala, which in turn caused their bone marrow to produce cells that cause inflammation. This, in turn, caused their coronary arteries to become inflamed and clogged—causing marked increases in cardiac events such as heart attacks and strokes.

Gene Expression

Another powerful mechanism affected by your lifestyle is the expression of your genes. When I was in medical school, I was taught that the only way to change your genes is to change your parents—i.e., impossible. Because of this, many people believe that they have "bad genes" and there's nothing they can do about it.

In fact, though, there is a lot we can do about our genes—and I say this not to blame but to empower. We're not merely victims of our genes; we have more control than we may realize.

My colleagues and I conducted research showing that changing lifestyle actually changes your genes—turning on (upregulating) genes that facilitate health and turning off (downregulating) genes that cause chronic inflammation, oxidative stress, and other mechanisms causing disease. For example, the selectin E gene, which promotes inflammation, was downregulated in our study.

Molecular switches (including methylation and proteins such as histones that turn genes off and on) are very responsive to lifestyle changes.

We found that more than 500 genes were favorably changed in study participants after only three months on our lifestyle medicine program! Hundreds of oncogenes that promote prostate cancer, breast cancer, colon cancer, and other conditions were switched off in only three months. We published this research with Dr. J. Craig Venter (the first person to sequence a human genome) in the *Proceedings of the National Academy of Sciences*.

In another study, researchers examined changes in gene expression in patients who went through our reversing heart disease program in Johnstown, a small steel-manufacturing town in rural Pennsylvania.

After twelve weeks, these lifestyle medicine changes "downregulated [turned off] genes important in the pathogenesis of atherosclerosis," including numerous genes involved in causing coronary artery blockages, chronic inflammation, oxidative stress, angiogenesis, and cholesterol metabolism. These improvements continued throughout the following year, and over five times as many genes were beneficially changed during this time.

Sirtuins are enzymes that wrap your DNA around these histone proteins as a way of turning off harmful genes—the first three letters of the word sirtuin, SIR, are an acronym for "silencing information regulator." Think of sirtuins as anti-aging proteins.

A lot of promising research is being conducted on sirtuins because of their important role in the aging process and in many chronic diseases, including cardiovascular disease, type 2 diabetes, and Alzheimer's disease. Again, research keeps discovering new ways to explain why lifestyle medicine is so healing.

Glycation is a natural process in which the sugar in your bloodstream attaches to proteins or fats, forming new, harmful, highly oxidant molecules called advanced glycation end products (AGEs).

Poetically, "AGE" makes you age.

AGEs suppress sirtuin activity—in other words, they turn off the switches (sirtuins) that turn off the harmful genes that cause us to age. Since sirtuins are anti-aging, suppressing them makes you age faster and increases your risk of getting a wide range of chronic diseases. AGEs also occur in your diet, especially in meat.

AGEs crosslink proteins together and contribute to increased oxidative stress, tissue stiffness, and inflammation—another example of how all of the mechanisms described in this chapter interrelate.

In the brain, AGE molecules may contribute to dementia; in the eye, they may be involved in cataracts and macular degeneration. In the arteries and heart, they are associated with hypertension, atherosclerosis, heart failure, and stroke. They are also linked to anemia, kidney disease, osteoporosis, and muscle loss, among others.

The traditional Western diet is high in AGE molecules, which suppress sirtuins and, in turn, accelerate aging. Because of this, sirtuin deficiency is both preventable and reversible by reducing AGEs in your diet.

Both the type of food and the way it's cooked affect the amount of AGE. Animal-derived foods that are high in fat and protein are generally AGE-rich and prone to new AGE formation during cooking. In contrast, carbohydrate-rich whole foods such as vegetables, fruits, and whole grains in their natural forms contain relatively few AGEs, even after cooking. (Is this pattern starting to sound familiar?)

For example, a soy burger cooked in a microwave has only 20 AGE units. Cooking it in a pan with a little vegetable oil spray increases it to only 30 AGE units. Adding 1 teaspoon olive oil to the pan increases it to 131 AGE units.

In contrast, a turkey burger cooked in a pan with a little vegetable oil spray has 7,171 AGE units. One serving of beefsteak, cooked in a pan with olive oil, has 9,052 AGE units. Two strips of bacon fried for five minutes with no added oil have 11,905 AGE units. One roasted chicken thigh with skin has 10,034 AGE units. Barbecuing the chicken thigh increases that to 16,668 AGE units—almost three orders of magnitude higher than the microwaved soy burger!

New companies are offering supplements that are intended to increase sirtuin levels, but human data are lacking. Time will tell whether or not these are beneficial.

In the meantime, it's clear that changing your diet in the ways outlined in this book will reduce AGEs and increase sirtuins, providing yet another mechanism to explain why a whole-foods plant-based way of eating is so beneficial.

In anti-aging research, caloric restriction has been shown to slow the aging process in animals, in part by reducing AGE. It also increases what is called autophagy, in which your body detoxifies and cleans out damaged cells, especially those involving your brain, and reduces chronic inflammation.

But it's hard to sustain because most people don't like to feel hungry all the time. One way to accomplish this is to have an early dinner and a late breakfast so that you have at least twelve hours between meals, sometimes called intermittent fasting, which may cause you to feel better, well, *fast*.

One of the easiest ways to restrict calories without feeling hungry is to change the *type* of food rather than the *amount* of it; that is, eat less sugar and refined carbohydrates and consume less fat.

You can eat virtually unlimited amounts of sugar without getting full, so it's easy to take in too many calories. Eating sugar doesn't curb your appetite, it increases it. In contrast, when you eat good carbs such as whole grains, the fiber fills you up before you get too many calories.

Also, fat has nine calories per gram, whereas protein and carbohydrates have only four calories per gram. Because of this, when you eat less fat, you consume fewer calories even though you're eating the same amount of food—because the food is less dense in calories. This was the premise of my book *Eat More, Weigh Less*. We found the average patient in our study lost 24 pounds in the first year even though they were eating more food and eating more frequently than before. Equally important, they kept off more than half that weight five years later.

Also, sugar causes your body to produce more insulin, which then blocks leptin, a hormone that reduces appetite and induces fat burning—so when you eat a lot of sugar, it actually increases your appetite rather than making you feel satiated.

In addition to this, the latest studies are showing, at least in mice, that calorie restriction works to extend life not only because it reduces total calories but, specifically, because it also reduces animal protein, which is more important in longevity. Again, the *type* of food is important, not just the amount. The researchers wrote, "Longevity and health were optimized when [animal] protein was replaced with [complex] carbohydrate. . . . Calorie restriction achieved by high-protein diets or dietary dilution [eating less] had no beneficial effects on lifespan." They lived 30 percent longer when replacing animal protein with good carbohydrates.

Why?

These researchers found that limiting animal protein intake reduces levels of a protein enzyme called TOR, and lowering TOR extends life. Another study also found that a plant-based diet downregulates TOR, prolonging life.

TOR controls cell growth and metabolism in response to nutrients, growth factors, cellular energy, and stress. It regulates how quickly your cells grow and proliferate.

Earlier in this chapter, we discussed why a recurring theme of our program is that *mechanisms that have evolved to heal us can actually become harmful or even lethal in modern times.* TOR is another example of this.

When you're young, you're more likely to survive if you grow fast. That's what TOR does—it regulates your cells, allowing them to grow and reproduce quickly. One scientist described it as a "speeding car without brakes."

Unfortunately, what's good at one stage of our life can become a problem at another. As we get older, we want TOR to slow down the rate at which our cells are growing. Cancer results when there is unrestrained cell growth and proliferation. For example, TOR levels are upregulated (turned on) in prostate cancer and breast cancer.

During our childhood, TOR is an engine of growth, but in adulthood it can be thought of as an engine of aging. Therefore, downregulating TOR—putting on the brakes—helps prevent chronic diseases and premature aging.

Until relatively recently (when viewed from an evolutionary timeline), most people died before they were old enough to develop chronic diseases. For example, just four hundred years ago, half or more of children in London didn't even survive to age fifteen. So those who grew quickly had an evolutionary advantage, as they were more likely to have children.

In modern times, public health advances such as clean water, better sanitation, and antibiotics extended life spans for most people well beyond what they had been in prior generations.

Now that people are living so much longer, it's important to find ways to downregulate TOR in order to slow down the rate at which you age. As described earlier, limiting intake of animal protein downregulates TOR.

Plants, especially cruciferous vegetables such as broccoli and cauliflower and fruits such as blueberries and strawberries, inhibit TOR. So do beverages such as green tea and soy milk and spices such as turmeric. Substances called flavonols, present in vegetables and fruits, possess antioxidant and anti-inflammatory properties as well as downregulating TOR. They also enhance autophagy, allowing your body to detoxify itself.

One of the amino acids found in protein, leucine, has an especially powerful impact on upregulating TOR. Not surprisingly, leucine is found primarily in animal foods, including meat, chicken, fish, and dairy—yet another mechanism to explain why a whole-foods plant-based diet is so beneficial. Avoiding these foods helps to downregulate TOR.

There is room for fine-tuning based on your genes—for example, some people are less efficient than others at metabolizing dietary sugar and refined carbohydrates. But since the diet we recommend is low in these anyway, those individual differences are much less important.

In other words, it doesn't matter if you're not very efficient at metabolizing sugar or refined carbohydrates in your diet if you're not eating too much of these in the first place.

As another example of this, prostate cancer often starts when a protective gene, PTEN, shuts down. But the tumors in men that lose only this gene don't usually spread beyond the prostate and rarely become lethal. The cancers change, though, if a second gene, called PML, also shuts down. When this happens, these quiescent cells are more likely to spread and kill.

Investigators were puzzled that prostate cancer didn't spread even when they intentionally turned off both of these genes in mice.

They had a moment of insight at a scientific meeting when they realized that the mice had been fed a low-fat vegetarian diet, which might have protected them. They wondered if putting these mice on a high-fat, meat-based Western diet would cause the cancer to spread.

It did—the Western diet caused them to quickly develop tumors that grew rapidly and spread.

The point is this: even when there is a known genetic predisposition to developing metastatic (lethal) cancer and other chronic diseases, the lifestyle medicine program outlined in this book may help prevent this from happening.

Similarly, our genes play a role in obesity, but they do not determine whether or not we gain weight by eating or not eating certain types of foods. For example, a 2018 study from Stanford set out to prove that some people are genetically able to metabolize carbohydrates better than fats, or vice versa—and that personalized diets based on these genes would result in greater weight loss.

It didn't. The authors concluded, "Neither genotype pattern [i.e., type of genes] nor baseline insulin secretion was associated with the dietary effects on weight loss."

In our Lifestyle Heart Trial, there was an average weight loss of 24 pounds in the first year. The primary determinant of the amount of weight lost was the degree of adherence to our lifestyle medicine program, not age or genetics. The more participants changed their lifestyle, the more weight they lost and the more they improved in all measures. In our study of almost 3,000 people who went through our lifestyle medicine program across twenty-four sites, participants lost an average of 8 percent of their body weight in the first year. From someone who weighed 200 pounds, that would be an average weight loss of 16 pounds.

So often, I hear people say, "Oh, it's all in my genes, and I've got bad genes, so there's nothing I can do about it." Fortunately, there is.

I have had the privilege of being one of President Bill Clinton's consulting physicians since 1993, when Hillary Clinton asked me to advise the chefs who cooked for them at the White House, at Camp David, and on Air Force One to make healthier meals.

The president initially did well and lost 26 pounds, but later, with the stresses of what he was going through politically, he understandably paid less attention to his diet and lifestyle choices at the time. In 2004, he underwent bypass surgery on four of his clogged coronary arteries.

In February 2010, he learned that one of his four bypass surgery grafts had clogged up since his operation almost six years earlier, and he had two stents placed to open it up. At a press conference then, one of his doctors said, "This was not a result of either his lifestyle or his diet," implying that it was because of his genes.

After watching this press conference, I sent an email to President Clinton saying, in effect, that it wasn't all in his genes—and if he would be willing to make bigger changes in his diet and lifestyle, there was a good chance that he could reverse his coronary heart disease.

"Our genes are a predisposition, but our genes are not our fate," I wrote to him. "If they were, then you'd be a victim, but you're not— you're one of the most powerful people on the planet. You're genetically predisposed to having heart disease because it runs in your family, but this just means that you need to make bigger changes to prevent or reverse it than someone else might. Our DNA is not our destiny."

We met together soon after, and he began following the lifestyle medicine program described in this book. He's remained on it since then and has talked publicly about how he continues to follow this program and is doing very well.

Whatever your politics are in our increasingly polarized nation, when a former president of the United States—especially one known for not eating in a healthy way—is successfully able to make and maintain these beneficial lifestyle changes and it improves his health so much over a period of many years, this sets a great example for everyone. These are human issues that transcend politics.

Again, even though our genes may vary, those differences are much less important if we lead a healthy lifestyle.

This is one of the reasons that until about fifty years ago, Japanese people living in Japan had a fraction of the heart disease, type 2 diabetes, and cancer that we have in the United States. Their population has a wide spectrum of different genes, just as we do in this country—but because their national diet and lifestyle were high in whole, plant-based foods and low in meat, most people didn't get chronic diseases even if they were genetically predisposed to doing so.

However, those Japanese who moved to Hawaii had a significantly higher rate of developing these diseases, and those who migrated to San Francisco suffered even more illnesses. Why? They began eating more animal protein, dietary fat, cholesterol, and refined carbohydrates in

Honolulu than in Japan, and even more when they moved to the U.S. mainland. Also, their social networks became progressively more disrupted as they moved closer to the mainland.

Similar data are available from China in T. Colin Campbell's landmark China Study. In rural China, fat intake was less than half that in the United States, and fiber intake was three times higher. Animal protein intake was very low, only about 10 percent of the U.S. intake. Mean serum total cholesterol was 127 mg/dL in rural China versus 203 mg/dL for adults aged twenty to seventy-four years in the United States.

Coronary artery disease mortality was *sixteen times higher* for American men and almost *six times higher* for U.S. women than for their Chinese counterparts. Unfortunately, this is now changing as many people in Asia are beginning to eat like us, live like us, and all too often die like us.

Telomeres

We also conducted the first controlled study showing that these lifestyle changes lengthen telomeres, the ends of our chromosomes that regulate aging. We conducted this research with Dr. Elizabeth Blackburn, who shared the Nobel Prize in Physiology or Medicine for her pioneering discoveries of telomeres.

Telomeres are like the plastic tips that keep your shoelaces from unraveling. They are located at the ends of your chromosomes and protect those DNA from damage. As you get older, your telomeres tend to get shorter and their structural integrity weakens, causing cells to malfunction and die more quickly.

In brief, as your telomeres get shorter, your life tends to get shorter.

Why? Shorter telomeres are associated with an increased risk of premature death from a wide variety of common chronic diseases—again, because these illnesses share common underlying mechanisms, including shorter telomeres. These include an increased risk of heart disease, prostate cancer, breast cancer, colon cancer, Alzheimer's disease, type 2 diabetes, and many others.

After only three months on our lifestyle medicine program, we measured, for the first time, a 30 percent increase in telomerase, the enzyme that repairs and lengthens telomeres.

After five years, average telomere length decreased in the control group by about 3 percent. This is what usually happens to most people over time. However, for those in the lifestyle medicine group, telomere length actually *increased* by 10 percent. The *Lancet Oncology* editors described this as "reversing aging at a cellular level," the first controlled study documenting that any intervention could lengthen telomeres.

Also, as we had previously found in other measures, those findings gave us the first indication of a dose-response correlation between the degree of adherence to our lifestyle medicine program and the increases in telomere length. The more people changed their lifestyle, the longer their telomeres grew.

Of course, lengthening and protecting telomeres doesn't mean we'll live forever. But these studies show that we can usually live healthy, long, and meaningful lives until just before we die instead of dwindling away with chronic diseases over a span of many years—in other words, to die young as old as possible.

Our Microbiome

We are mostly microbes. I was a little startled the first time I learned that we have over *100 trillion* organisms growing inside our bodies—what is now known as the microbiome.

And these microbes are mostly not our own. Most of these organisms come from somewhere else; only about 10 percent of the resident microbes in our bodies are intrinsically ours.

Instead of viewing these bacteria, viruses, and fungi as invaders that need to be killed with antibiotics and other drugs—what doctors often call the "therapeutic armamentarium," using the language of warfare—scientists learned that these diverse organisms live in a symbiotic relationship with us and, when in balance, keep us healthy in a multitude of ways. Some of our best friends are germs.

Humans, said Dr. David Relman, a Stanford microbiologist, are like coral, "an assemblage of life-forms living together." They have co-evolved with us over millennia. The dynamic balance of these different organisms that grow in our skin, mouth, nose, gut, and genitals has a profound impact on our health—for better and for worse. And this balance is influenced by (you guessed it) what we eat, how we respond to stress, how much exercise we get, and how much love and support we have.

The microbiome is another important mechanism to explain why these simple lifestyle changes have such widespread and powerful impacts on a wide variety of chronic diseases.

Scientists are just beginning to understand how widespread the microbiome's effects are. I predict that as we learn more, evidence will show that the microbiome plays a role in virtually all diseases and in keeping us healthy.

Your microbiome contains more than one hundred times as many genes as you have in your own genes. These microbiome genes can generate a variety of proteins such as neurotransmitters and hormones affecting a wide range of conditions—for better and for worse.

Your microbiome is malleable. When you follow the lifestyle medicine program in this book, you allow your body's microbiome to come back into balance, restoring homeostasis and improving your health in so many different ways. This is another example of why a single set of lifestyle changes has such far-reaching benefits.

We are now conducting research with Dr. Rob Knight at the University of California, San Diego, a leading microbiome scientist, to understand how the four components of our lifestyle medicine program—eat well, move more, stress less, love more—interact with our microbiome in healing ways.

Our preliminary findings are revealing how quickly these lifestyle changes beneficially affect the relative proportion of healing microbes to harmful ones—another example of the dynamism of these mechanisms that affect our health and well-being.

Just as making several healthy lifestyle changes is especially beneficial and even synergistic via many different mechanisms, so are the effects of unhealthy lifestyle changes. The microbiome also provides new dimensions of understanding about why unhealthy lifestyle changes are harmful—for example, eating meat.

One study compared the microbiome of those eating a vegan diet, vegetarian diet, and typical omnivorous American diet. Those eating a typical American diet had a higher proportion of microbes associated with chronic inflammation, insulin resistance, and cardiovascular disease. They also had blood tests showing increases in inflammatory markers such as C-reactive protein and TNF-α, higher LDL-cholesterol, and higher insulin levels.

Overuse of antibiotics causes harmful changes in your microbiome (since antibiotics kill good microbes as well as harmful ones) as well as increasing drug resistance. Just a single weeklong course of antibiotics can change your gut microbiome for up to a year.

Because of widespread antibiotic overuse, "superbugs" are beginning to emerge for which there are not yet effective drug treatments.

Almost 80 percent of antibiotics sold in this country are fed to livestock to make them grow faster so they can be slaughtered sooner. They're given to cows, pigs, and chickens to make them grow more quickly or as a cheap alternative to keeping them healthy.

This causes drug-resistant bacteria to emerge, and these bacteria can remain on meat and spread to humans. The Centers for Disease Control and Prevention (CDC) estimate that more than 400,000 U.S. residents become ill with infections caused by antibiotic-resistant food-borne bacteria every year, and that about one in five resistant infections are caused by germs from food and animals.

In 2013, researchers showed that people living near pig farms or crop fields fertilized with pig manure are 30 percent more likely to become infected with methicillin-resistant *Staphylococcus aureus* bacteria.

In addition, residues of the antibiotics fed to animals are frequently found in meat that you buy at the grocery, further contributing to antibiotic resistance. (Other residues found in meat include cancer-causing pesticides like dioxin and toxic heavy metals such as arsenic.) In 2010, the U.S. Department of Agriculture's own inspector general criticized the USDA for not providing better oversight about these toxic residues:

> One of the public food safety issues facing the United States is the contamination of meat with residual veterinary [antibiotic] drugs, pesticides, and heavy metals. "Residue" of this sort finds its way into the food supply when producers bring animals to slaughter plants while they have these residual contaminants in their system. When the animals are slaughtered, traces of the drugs or pesticides contained in these animals' meat is shipped to meat processors and retail supermarkets, and eventually purchased by consumers. . . .

Based on our review, we found that the national residue program is not accomplishing its mission of monitoring the food supply for harmful residues . . . which has resulted in meat with these substances being distributed in commerce. . . . Additionally, [the USDA Food Safety and Inspection Service] does not attempt to recall meat, even when its tests have confirmed the excessive presence of veterinary drugs.

If you want to avoid these toxic residues, this is one more very good reason not to eat meat.

Your microbiome is also playing an important role in weight loss beyond just the number of calories you consume. For example, not only are high-fat diets more dense in calories, they also alter the microbes in your gut in ways that makes you more likely to gain weight: they both affect the type of microbes and cause a decrease in their diversity.

It's not just the calories that you eat; more important are the calories you absorb from your gut into your blood—and this is influenced by your microbiome. A high-fat diet causes the growth of microbes that harvest energy more efficiently—in other words, you gain more weight eating the same amount of calories when they come from excessive fat. A high-fat diet also modulates genes associated with fat storage, making them more efficient at storing calories as fat in your body.

Diets high in sugar and refined carbohydrates also cause similar dysfunction of the microbiome. When we eat a lot of sugar, harmful bacteria thrive and start to grow out of control, while our beneficial bacteria decrease.

High-fat and high-sugar diets also can affect your microbiome in another way, by causing the lining of your intestines to become more permeable—a condition sometimes known as "leaky gut syndrome." Microbes leaking through the gut into the bloodstream can provoke a chronic inflammatory response, a tumor-inducing response, an autoimmune response, and/or increases in coronary artery blockages. They also affect insulin sensitivity and so can contribute to type 2 diabetes as well.

Inflammation increases permeability in the gut, and a more permeable gut causes more inflammation, in a vicious cycle. This can lead to weight gain and other chronic diseases.

In mice, when researchers transplanted the organisms in the gut of an obese mouse to one with a normal weight, the second mouse began to gain weight even though it was on the same diet.

Your microbiome also affects your mood. Gut microbiota can communicate with the central nervous system, which influences brain function and behavior. (This gives a new dimension to the term "gut feeling.")

These microbes manufacture neurotransmitters like serotonin and norepinephrine, which can help keep you from feeling anxious, depressed, and tired. In humans, over 90 percent of serotonin is produced in the gastrointestinal tract. Emotional stress affects your microbiome in harmful ways that increase your risk of getting sick.

Exercise increases the number of beneficial bacteria in your gut. In one study, six weeks of moderate exercise caused widespread increases in certain microbes that can help to produce substances called short-chain fatty acids, which reduce inflammation in your gut and in the rest of your body. They also work to help prevent insulin resistance, a precursor to diabetes, and to bolster our metabolism.

Emotional stress changes the relative proportion of microbes in your body in ways that increase the production of substances called interleukins, which increase inflammation and activate your immune system. Also, inflammation increases depression, and depression increases inflammation, in another vicious cycle. The stress management techniques and ways of enhancing love and intimacy described in this book help restore a healthy balance in your microbiome.

As described earlier, inflammation is an important underlying cause of Alzheimer's disease: it causes amyloid deposition in the brain, which damages its neurons and causes the tau protein to misfold and clump, causing brain neurons to get tangled, called neurofibrillary tangles. Alzheimer's disease patients have a lower abundance in their gut of bacteria that have anti-inflammatory activity and a greater amount of pro-inflammatory bacteria. Some clinical studies have shown that probiotics containing beneficial bacteria such as lactobacilli and bifidobacteria may improve patients' cognitive function.

Fermented foods such as tofu and tempeh help seed your microbiome with healthier organisms. You may also want to consider taking a probiotic supplement, especially after a course of antibiotics, to restore a dynamic equilibrium of normal gut flora.

Oxidative Stress, Cellular Metabolism, and Apoptosis

Electricity is the movement of electrons through wires. Electrons also provide energy for your mind and body.

When you eat and digest food, the electrons stored in its fat, protein, and carbohydrates are converted by a part of your cells called mitochondria to provide energy for you. Mitochondria are the powerhouses of your cells. Here, the electrons are combined with oxygen in your blood to make its energy available to you.

These electrons travel in pairs, which keeps them stable. Unfortunately, this process is not perfect. Sometimes, one of these electrons becomes isolated from the other one and becomes what is called a free radical (not to be confused with Patty Hearst in her early days . . .). These are unstable molecules that need another electron to become stable and will do just about anything to get it, regardless of how much damage is done in the process. It appears that even electrons don't like to be lonely!

When unstable molecules "steal" electrons from other molecules throughout your body in order to stabilize themselves, this is called oxidation. This creates instability in these molecules and damages these cells in a process called oxidative stress.

When iron rusts, this is another type of oxidative stress. In a real sense, our bodies tend to rust as we age.

Damage to your cells from oxidative stress, in turn, can lead to a wide range of chronic diseases and other problems:

- When your DNA is damaged, it can lead to many types of cancer by causing mutations that interfere with the mechanisms that keep your cells from growing uncontrollably (which is what cancer is) and that keep it from spreading—such as reducing apoptosis (programmed cell death to remove damaged cells from your body).
- When your arteries are damaged, it can lead to high blood pressure, blood clots, heart attacks, heart failure, impotence, and strokes.
- When your cell membranes are damaged, it can lead to premature aging and wrinkles.
- When the cells in your pancreas are damaged, it can lead to diabetes.

- When the cells in your brain are damaged, it can lead to dementia, including Alzheimer's disease, Parkinson's disease, ALS, multiple sclerosis, and depression.
- When proteins in your body are damaged, it can cause your immune system to stop recognizing them as being part of you and begin attacking them, causing many autoimmune diseases. For example, data from eight countries showed that dietary intake of meat and fat were associated with a highly significant increase in rheumatoid arthritis.

In short, a diet high in fat, animal protein, and refined carbohydrates increases oxidative stress. So do emotional stress, being sedentary, and being socially isolated.

Since the lifestyle medicine program described in this book addresses each of these components, understanding the important role of oxidative stress helps to explain why these lifestyle changes are so powerfully healing in both preventing and reversing a wide variety of chronic diseases.

Methionine is one of the essential amino acids in protein. It enhances oxidation, worsening oxidative stress. Whole plant-based foods are low in methionine, whereas beef, lamb, cheese, turkey, pork, fish, shellfish, eggs, and dairy are high in it. This provides another reason why a whole-foods plant-based diet reduces oxidative stress, whereas a meat-based diet increases it.

Antioxidants, as their name indicates, help to prevent oxidative stress. Many studies have shown that antioxidants that are naturally occurring in certain foods are much more effective than those found in vitamins and supplements.

Antioxidant-rich foods originate mostly from the plant kingdom, while meat, fish, and other foods from the animal kingdom are usually low in antioxidants and often high in oxidants.

A comprehensive listing that ranks the antioxidant content of over 3,000 different foods can be found at http://bit.ly/antioxidantfoods. The concentration of antioxidants in foods varies several thousandfold. The authors who prepared that listing wrote, "Comparing the mean value of the meat and meat products category with plant based categories, fruits, nuts, chocolate and berries have from *5 to 33 times higher* mean antioxidant content than the mean of meat products . . . due to the thousands of bioactive antioxidant phytochemicals found in plants."

Many common spices are also high in antioxidants. Some that are packed with antioxidants include cinnamon, cloves, curcumin, juniper berries, meadowsweet, mint, nutmeg, oregano, peppermint leaves, rosemary, St. John's wort, summer savory, thyme, and marjoram. A little cinnamon and blueberries on steel-cut oatmeal with low-sugar soy milk in the morning is a good way to start the day.

Angiogenesis

When tumors reach a certain size, they grow so quickly that they outgrow the blood supply of the organ they're invading. Because of this, tumors often secrete substances that stimulate new blood vessels to grow to feed the tumor. This process is called "angiogenesis," which means "growing new blood vessels."

Cancer cells frequently occur in just about everyone. Most of the time, these remain microscopic, don't spread, and are eradicated by your immune system, so they are of no clinical significance. Another mechanism that keeps cancers from growing is your body's ability to keep tumors from growing new blood vessels, which blocks their growth and keeps them from becoming harmful. This process is called anti-angiogenesis.

There are anti-angiogenesis drugs like Avastin that can kill some tumors by disrupting their blood supply and starving the tumor. Unfortunately, they are very expensive—often more than $100,000 per year—and may not work as well as lifestyle changes.

My colleagues and I conducted a randomized controlled trial of men with early-stage prostate cancer who went through our lifestyle medicine program. As described earlier, we found that these lifestyle changes slowed, stopped, and even reversed the progression of their prostate cancer.

One of the mechanisms for this improvement was a downregulation (decrease) of angiogenesis in these patients. In collaboration with Dr. Will Li and his colleagues at the Angiogenesis Foundation, we found that VEGF, a substance produced by tumors to grow new blood vessels to feed the tumor, was decreased substantially in these patients—

comparable to what can be achieved with drugs like Avastin, but at a fraction of the cost. We also measured an increase in two substances (platelet factor 4 and heparanase) that inhibit angiogenesis.

Angiogenesis also enhances chronic inflammation. When more blood is brought to a part of your body, it also brings with it the cells and inflammatory substances that increase inflammation.

Most of the foods that beneficially affect angiogenesis are in the whole-foods plant-based category. These include berries, cruciferous vegetables, green tea, and spices. In other words, angiogenesis is yet another mechanism to explain why these same foods are so powerful in preventing and reversing so many chronic diseases.

Blood Flow and Stasis

When a river flows, the water is often clean, delicious, and pure. When it stagnates, the water can become foul, brackish, and polluted.

The same is true for the flow of blood in your body—the river of life. Stasis occurs when your blood and other fluids are not flowing properly. This can lead to stagnation and illness.

The biological mechanisms that regulate blood flow—and our health in general—are so much more dynamic than once were thought. The latest research shows that you can get better or worse from eating just one meal, depending on what you consume.

Even a single meal high in animal protein and fat reduces blood flow. For example, Dr. Robert Vogel and his colleagues published a study comparing blood flow after a meal high in fat and animal protein (a McDonald's Egg McMuffin, Sausage McMuffin, and two hash brown patties) with a plant-based low-fat meal containing the same number of calories.

After only four hours, blood flow decreased by more than 50 percent in those having the McDonald's meal but not in those consuming a plant-based low-fat meal. Many plant-based foods increase nitric oxide formation, which dilates your blood vessels and increases blood flow.

In another study comparing diets, investigators found that patients eating the diet described in this book had significantly greater blood flow than those on an Atkins diet. Also, the more saturated fat these people consumed, the lower their blood flow.

A 2018 study documented that a single high-fat meal not only reduces blood flow but also induces pathological changes in your red blood cells. These changes cause these cells to enter blood vessel walls, triggering oxidative stress and inflammation; they also destabilize vulnerable plaques that clog up arteries (more on this in Chapter 3), making these plaques much more likely to cause a heart attack and stroke. Emotional stress, smoking, sedentary lifestyle, depression, stimulants (cocaine, amphetamines), and other lifestyle factors have similar negative effects on blood flow.

In contrast, the lifestyle medicine program described in this book improves blood flow throughout your body:

- When your brain gets more blood flow, you think more clearly and creatively, have more energy, and sleep better. You can actually grow so many new brain neurons—a process called neurogenesis—that your brain increases in size in just a few weeks! Especially those parts of your brain that you want to get measurably bigger, such as the hippocampus, which controls memory—as people age, they often start to forget someone's name or where they left their keys. Much of this dysfunction of the hippocampus now appears to be reversible, something that was thought impossible when I went to medical school. This neurogenesis helps prevent dementia later in life. More on this later.
- Your skin gets more blood flow, so you may look years younger than your biological age.
- Your heart and skeletal muscles get more blood flow, so you have more stamina and can often reverse even severe coronary heart disease. (It turns out that Roman gladiators were vegetarian because it gave them more strength and endurance that enabled them to survive in extreme battle.)
- Your eyes get more blood flow, helping to prevent blindness and sometimes even to reverse damage to blood vessels in your retina.
- Your ears get more blood flow, so the risk of hearing loss is reduced.
- Your sexual organs get more blood flow, so your potency improves. As described in Chapter 1, even a single plant-based meal caused dramatic increases in both the frequency and hardness of erections in young athletes when compared to a single meat-based meal.

When your heart doesn't receive enough blood flow to feed itself, then chest pain (angina) occurs. In our research studies, people with severe heart disease who made the diet and lifestyle changes described in this book reported a 91 percent reduction in the frequency of chest pain after only a few days to a few weeks because the blood flow to the heart increased so quickly. Within a month, there was significant improvement in blood flow to the heart and in the ability of the heart to pump blood during exercise.

In people with atrial fibrillation, two of the chambers in the heart are not pumping effectively. Because of this, blood can stagnate and increase the risk of a blood clot forming that can cause a heart attack or a stroke if it lodges in an artery. If the heart is unable to convert to a normal rhythm, doctors may prescribe blood thinners to reduce the likelihood of a blood clot forming.

Being sedentary enhances stasis and illness. One of the reasons exercise is beneficial in so many ways is that it literally and figuratively keeps everything moving. Your heart pumps blood with sufficient force to circulate your blood throughout your arteries, but the pressure in your veins is substantially lower.

When you exercise—walking, for example—the muscles in your arms and legs help to squeeze blood through your veins. It's one reason the Queen's Guards outside of Buckingham Palace in London are taught to bounce up and down on their toes when standing in one place for prolonged periods of time—otherwise, the blood would pool in their legs and they would pass out. In 2017, five guards actually did faint from standing around too long.

Spending a lot of time sitting increases your risk of a stroke due to blood clot formation. According to some studies, it increases your risk of premature death from all causes as much as smoking does!

Sitting for more than eight hours a day is associated with a *90 percent* increased risk of type 2 diabetes. Those who sit the most have a *147 percent* increased relative risk of cardiovascular events compared to those who sit the least.

Women who sit more than six hours a day are 37 percent more likely to die prematurely than those who sit less than three hours a day, even if they exercise regularly. The time spent sitting was independently associated with total mortality, regardless of physical activity level.

The combination of both sitting more than six hours a day and being less physically active was associated with a *94 percent* increase in all-cause premature death rates in women and a 48 percent increase in men compared with those who reported sitting less than three hours a day and being most active.

Why? Because even if you exercise at the gym after work, your blood has not been flowing very well earlier in the day while you've been sitting, which increases the likelihood of a blood clot forming during that time. Also, blood sugar, cholesterol levels, blood pressure, and other biomarkers are higher in people who are sedentary.

Researchers recently found that sitting for several hours at a desk significantly reduced blood flow to the brain. However, getting up and taking just a two-minute walk every half hour actually increased the brain's blood flow.

We've evolved to move and forage much of the time (e.g., walking) and also to have bursts of intense exercise. Our muscles have both fast-twitch and slow-twitch muscle fibers. So work out regularly and avoid prolonged sitting. Studies show that both are important.

One study found that the more breaks you take during the day after sitting for twenty minutes—even just getting up, walking around a minute or two, and sitting down again—the better your health. On average, each additional ten breaks per day were associated with 0.8 cm lower waist circumference, 0.3 mm lower systolic blood pressure, 3.7 percent lower triglycerides, 0.6 percent lower glucose, and 4.2 percent lower insulin.

Talk on a portable phone so you can walk around your office while having conversations—and your energy level will likely be higher as well. Take a break from sitting every twenty or thirty minutes. If you work at a desk, try a standing desk, or improvise with a high table or counter. Walk with your colleagues for meetings rather than sitting in a conference room. I invested in a treadmill desk so I can walk while doing my email or talking on the phone.

Some of the reasons not moving your body increases the risk of so many different illnesses are the effects of being sedentary on your lymphatic system—the garbage sewers of your body. It helps rid your body of toxins, waste, and other unwanted materials. Besides the lymphatic vessels, your lymphatic system includes your tonsils, appendix, thymus, and spleen. These are important parts of your immune system.

The primary function of your lymphatic system is to transport lymph, a fluid containing infection-fighting white blood cells, throughout the body. When cells in your immune system have gone to battle, the dead cells are removed via your lymphatics.

Lymph is then transported through larger lymphatic vessels to lymph nodes, where it is cleaned by white blood cells called lymphocytes. After that, lymph continues down your lymphatic system before emptying ultimately into the right or the left subclavian vein on either side of your neck.

Pressure in your lymphatic system is even lower than in your veins and relies on the contraction of your skeletal muscles—as happens in walking, for example—to squeeze the lymphatic fluid along. Also, when you take a deep breath, your diaphragm and lungs act as a bellows mechanism that changes pressure at the thoracic duct to pump the lymphatic system.

When people are sedentary, and when they breathe in a shallow way (which is common when they feel chronically stressed), their muscles aren't contracting enough to keep their lymph flowing. Because of this, the lymph can leak into their tissues and cause swelling, or edema, which predisposes them to illness. Also, when lymph is not flowing, it can leak back into the blood, causing inflammation and other problems.

The benefits of keeping things flowing in your body also helps to explain why men who have more frequent sex have less prostate cancer. One large study of almost 30,000 men in the Harvard Health Professionals Follow-Up Study found that men who said they ejaculated more than twenty-one times per month had two-thirds the risk of prostate cancer as men who ejaculated just four to seven times per month.

A follow-up study ten years later confirmed these findings, and also showed that in men who ejaculated less frequently, there was still some risk reduction. Those who reported eight to twelve ejaculations per month in their forties, for example, had a 10 percent reduction in prostate cancer risk, and those who reported thirteen to twenty ejaculations per month in their forties had a 20 percent reduction—giving a new meaning to "dose-response relationship." I'm sure the enhanced social support associated with a loving sexual relationship also plays an important role (more on this in Chapter 7).

Why would frequent ejaculation reduce the risk of prostate cancer? In modern times, most people are exposed to various carcinogens in our air, food, and water. It may be that when semen remains in your prostate gland for a longer period of time, it provides an extended exposure to any carcinogens that may be present in it, increasing the risk of prostate cancer.

By analogy, one of the reasons that dietary fiber helps to reduce the incidence of colon cancer is that it speeds up the transit of food through your intestinal tract, exposing it for a shorter period of time to carcinogens contained in it. In Chinese medicine and Ayurveda, the traditional medical system of India, blocked or stagnant energy is an underlying cause of many chronic diseases.

Better get a move on!

In summary, our lifestyle medicine program can help you reverse and prevent a wide variety of the most common chronic diseases because they share the same underlying mechanisms. And all of these mechanisms are beneficially and powerfully affected by each of these lifestyle changes.

CHAPTER 3

The Lifestyle Medicine Revolution

Science makes progress funeral by funeral: the old are never converted by
the new doctrines, they simply are replaced by a new generation.
—Max Planck

Lifestyle medicine is the most exciting movement today in health and
healing—a revolutionary tidal wave that hasn't yet even begun to crest.
You see it everywhere—after forty years of research conducted in this
area, there is now a growing awareness of the power of simple lifestyle
changes to prevent and reverse the progression of the most common
chronic diseases, often without drugs or surgery. And the only side effects are good ones!

Right Idea, Right Time, Right Now!

A convergence of forces and a growing recognition of the importance and power of lifestyle medicine finally make this the right idea at the right time.

These include an increasing body of scientific evidence documenting the limitations of high-tech medicine at the same time that there is a growing recognition of the power of lifestyle medicine to reverse and prevent a wide variety of chronic diseases. This is why Medicare and many insurance companies are now covering our lifestyle medicine program.

For example, the latest studies are showing that lifestyle changes are often actually better than drugs and surgery in treating and even reversing many of the most prevalent chronic diseases, including stable coronary heart disease and early-stage prostate cancer.

After many decades of skepticism from the old guard, lifestyle medicine is now mainstream. For example, Dr. Kim Williams was until recently the president of the American College of Cardiology (the professional society of all cardiologists nationwide). When he learned that his own cholesterol level was very high, he reviewed the medical and scientific research literature to see what alternatives might exist to going on a lifetime of cholesterol-lowering drugs, since he knew all too well what their side effects are.

He came across our research and went on our lifestyle medicine program. His LDL cholesterol fell by almost 50 percent (from 170 to 90 mg/dl), without drugs. Dr. Williams then chaired the first seminar on lifestyle medicine at the American College of Cardiology's annual scientific sessions. More than 1,000 cardiologists attended this colloquium, and others were turned away at the door.

As a few other examples that lifestyle medicine has finally arrived, Anne and I offered the first workshops on lifestyle medicine at the World Economic Forum's annual meeting in Davos, at the main TED conference in Vancouver, at the annual Summit meeting, and at the yearly Harvard Medical School symposium on lifestyle medicine, among many others. I am one of the founders of the American College of Lifestyle Medicine, a professional society of physicians and other health care professionals practicing lifestyle medicine.

In the past year, I wrote sections on lifestyle medicine for the final report of the presidential White House Advisory Group on Prevention, Health Promotion, and Integrative and Public Health as well as for the *Lancet Oncology* "Moonshot" Commission, a group of scientists worldwide who will advise on setting priorities for the billion-dollar U.S. government initiative to find a cure for cancer.

If It's Reimbursable, It's Sustainable

Most physicians I know went into medicine because they deeply want to help patients heal. But, as physicians, we're trained to use primarily drugs and surgery, and we're paid to use drugs and surgery, so that's what most doctors do. Until recently, most lifestyle medicine has not been reimbursable.

I learned a painful lesson—the importance of reimbursement—in 1993, when my colleagues and I at the nonprofit Preventive Medicine Research Institute began training hospitals and clinics in our lifestyle medicine program. We trained personnel at fifty-three sites throughout the country, including some of the most prestigious academic medical centers (such as Harvard; the University of California, San Francisco [UCSF]; and Scripps Health) as well as small community hospitals and clinics including ten sites in West Virginia, which has been number one in the United States for the highest prevalence of heart disease during the past twenty years.

Then, as now, we achieved bigger changes in lifestyle, better clinical outcomes, larger cost savings, and better adherence than had ever been documented. Unfortunately, however, because we did not have reimbursement from Medicare or most insurance companies at that time, several of these sites closed down our program even though it was highly effective.

I learned that no matter how much scientific research we published and no matter how significant our outcomes were, if it's not reimbursable, then it's not sustainable.

This is what motivated me to spend sixteen years working with leaders of the Centers for Medicare and Medicaid Services to obtain Medicare reimbursement for our reversing heart disease program as well as coverage from many private insurance companies, which my colleagues and I sincerely appreciate.

As I described in Chapter 1, when reimbursement changes, so do medical practice and medical education.

Most physicians receive almost no training in nutrition or exercise and even less in how to manage stress (even though medicine is inherently stressful) as well as how to create and nurture loving, intimate relationships in our lives. Physicians have among the highest rates of depression and suicide of any group—more than one doctor a day kills themself.

A recent survey of medical schools revealed an average of fewer than *five hours per year* are devoted to nutrition education. And even less after medical school—for example, in a thirty-five-page Accreditation Committee of Graduate Medical Education document for internal medicine residency training, from which many doctors go on to serve as primary care physicians, the word "nutrition" is completely absent.

Lifestyle Changes Are Often *Better* than Drugs and Surgery

Here are some examples in which lifestyle medicine works better than drugs or surgery in both preventing and reversing (undoing) some of the most common chronic diseases:

Lifestyle Medicine and Heart Disease

Lifestyle medicine is better than angioplasties and stents in treating most patients with stable coronary heart disease.

Although stents and angioplasties to open blocked coronary arteries have been a mainstay of treating coronary heart disease for almost forty years, many people are shocked to learn that these are largely ineffective in most patients who have stable heart disease.

A review of all eight randomized controlled trials concluded that stents don't prevent heart attacks, don't reduce the need for bypass surgery, and don't prolong life in patients with stable coronary heart disease!

Then it was thought that even if angioplasties and stents didn't prevent heart attacks, at least they reduced angina (chest pain), which justified doing these operations.

However, a recent randomized controlled trial proved that patients who underwent sham (fake) angioplasties and stent placements (where they put a tube into the heart that is usually used to place a stent but pulled the tube out without doing anything) had reductions in chest pain comparable to those who actually had the stents placed. In other words, the angioplasties and stents did not reduce angina more than doing nothing.

"All cardiology guidelines should be revised," Dr. David L. Brown of Washington University School of Medicine and Rita F. Redberg of UCSF wrote in an editorial published with this study in the *Lancet* entitled, "Last Nail in the Coffin for PCI [Stents] in Stable Angina?"

These studies clearly show that angioplasties and stents are ineffective in most stable patients. In part this is because coronary atherosclerosis (blockages) affects all coronary arteries in varying degrees, even though it is just the more severe blockages that are stented.

We even know why stents don't work in most stable patients. For many years, cardiologists believed that the more severely a coronary artery was clogged, the higher the risk of a heart attack. It turns out that arteries that are only 30–40 percent blocked are usually more likely to cause a heart attack than those that are 80–90 percent clogged. At first this seems counterintuitive.

But the reason is that by the time an artery is 80–90 percent clogged, it has usually become calcified, which makes it stable. Also, these calcifications make the artery more rigid and less likely to constrict during times of severe emotional stress.

In addition, your body has had time to grow new blood vessels, called collaterals, around these severe blockages—your body's own "bypass surgery." Even if this artery should become completely obstructed, a heart attack may not necessarily occur since there is another pathway for blood to flow around the blockage.

In contrast, when a coronary artery in your heart is only 30–40 percent blocked, it is more unstable because it's not calcified, and it has not had time to grow a protective network of collaterals. This is why these are called "vulnerable plaques"—because they are more likely to rupture and cause a sudden total obstruction, known as "catastrophic progression," which is as bad as it sounds.

What causes the vulnerable plaques to rupture and block arteries? Not surprisingly, the usual suspects—inflammation, emotional stress, diet (animal protein, sugar, saturated fat), sedentary lifestyle, smoking, stimulants such as cocaine and amphetamines, loneliness and depression, and other lifestyle factors.

Each of these can cause your arteries to constrict. When this happens, the flow of blood is reduced; the heart may not receive enough blood to maintain itself; and the reduced flow of blood (stasis) can cause it to form a clot, which can completely obstruct the flow of blood.

Also, the sudden constriction can cause rupture of vulnerable plaques, completely blocking the flow of blood. Stents are not usually placed in arteries that are only 30–40 percent blocked, yet these are the ones that are most likely to cause a heart attack or a stroke. A recent study found that even if only the most severe blockages were stented, there was still no reduction in heart attacks or premature deaths.

In contrast, the lifestyle medicine program described in this book improves all of the arteries in your heart and stabilizes arterial plaques throughout your body. Its powerful benefits are systemic.

As mentioned earlier, my colleagues and I conducted the first randomized controlled trials showing that our lifestyle medicine program can reverse the progression of even severe coronary heart disease, without drugs or surgery. Within a month, there was significant improvement in blood flow to the heart and in the ability of the heart to pump blood during exercise. There was a 91 percent reduction in the frequency of angina in the first few weeks, and most patients became free of chest pain during that time.

Within one year, even severely clogged coronary arteries often became less clogged. There was even more reversal after five years than after one year, and 2.5 times fewer cardiac events. Cardiac PET (positron emission tomography) scans revealed that blood to the heart was 400 percent higher in the group that went on this lifestyle medicine program when compared to the randomized control group—huge differences.

There is an important place for angioplasties and stents in someone who has unstable heart disease or who is in the middle of having a heart attack, in which case they can be lifesaving. But the vast majority of stents and angioplasties have been performed in stable patients who do not usually benefit.

Lifestyle Medicine and Type 2 Diabetes

Over half of the American population has type 2 diabetes or pre-diabetes, at an annual cost of over $322 billion. Yet these conditions are completely preventable in most people today by following the lifestyle medicine program described in this book. We don't need a new scientific breakthrough; we just need to put into practice what we already know.

Lifestyle medicine is better than drugs at *preventing* type 2 diabetes or pre-diabetes:

- In a study of over 23,000 European men and women, those who never smoked, were not overweight, exercised at least 3.5 hours a week, and ate primarily fruits, vegetables, and whole grains, with low meat consumption, had a *93 percent lower risk* of developing type 2 diabetes during the next eight years, as mentioned earlier.
- In the Diabetes Prevention Program, lifestyle changes worked better than drugs or placebo at preventing type 2 diabetes.
- In the Finnish Diabetes Prevention Study Group, those with pre-diabetes who reduced weight and fat intake and increased physical activity reduced the risk of developing diabetes by 58 percent. The reduction in the incidence of diabetes was directly associated with the degree of changes in lifestyle.
- A study of over 200,000 men and women for more than twenty years by the Harvard School of Public Health found that following a whole-foods plant-based diet substantially lowered the risk of developing type 2 diabetes.

Lifestyle medicine is often better than drugs alone at *treating* type 2 diabetes or pre-diabetes:

- A review article from the Mayo Clinic concluded that tight control of type 2 diabetes with drugs "burdens patients with complex treatment programs, hypoglycemia [low blood sugar], weight gain, and costs and offers uncertain benefits in return. We believe clinicians should prioritize supporting well-being and healthy lifestyles, preventive care, and cardiovascular risk reduction in these patients."

- A meta-analysis published in the *British Medical Journal* that looked at thirteen randomized controlled trials including almost 35,000 patients showed "limited benefits of intensive glucose lowering treatment [with drugs] on all cause mortality and deaths from cardiovascular causes. . . . The harm associated with severe hypoglycemia [low blood sugar] might counterbalance the potential benefit of intensive glucose lowering treatment."
- A systematic review of studies from the Therapeutics Initiative, an independent group that provides advice to physicians, said a growing body of research casts doubt on the effectiveness of type 2 diabetes drug treatment in many patients: "When intensive glucose lowering was compared with standard care, the magnitude of the harms outweighed the benefits." As such, "it is rational to emphasize lifestyle measures in these patients," including weight loss, diet, and exercise instead of medications.
- Data from two large randomized controlled trials published in the *New England Journal of Medicine* proved that tight control of blood sugar with two new drugs actually *increased* premature mortality in those with advanced type 2 diabetes and did not prevent the progression of pre-diabetes to diabetes and also failed to prevent the cardiovascular complications of diabetes, including heart attack, stroke, angina, heart failure, and need for cardiac surgery. Another study found that a different drug (empagliflozin) did show a slight but significant reduction in cardiac events in those at high cardiac risk compared to a nonintervention control group (10.5 percent versus 12.1 percent), but this was not compared to those making intensive lifestyle changes.

Lowering blood sugar with lifestyle medicine is better than with drugs alone in reversing the progression of type 2 diabetes in many patients. According to the American Diabetes Association, reducing hemoglobin A1C (a measure of average blood sugar levels during the prior two months) to below 7.0 by diet and lifestyle will help prevent these and other complications of diabetes, including amputations, impotence, kidney failure, weight gain, and blindness.

In our research, we were able to document reductions in their blood sugar (hemoglobin A1C) in almost 3,000 patients with type 2 diabetes going through our lifestyle medicine program from above 7.0 to below

7.0 after nine weeks, and they remained below 7.0 after one year, even though many patients reduced or discontinued diabetes medications during this time under their doctor's supervision.

Many patients with type 2 diabetes may initially need to be on prescribed medication if their blood sugar is very high while they are beginning to make comprehensive lifestyle changes. Ask your physician to monitor your blood sugar and to see if it comes down sufficiently due to these lifestyle changes, often enabling your doctor to reduce or, in some cases, to wean you off these medications.

In Chapter 2, I described why calorie restriction alone had no beneficial effects on life span—the *type* of food is important, not just the amount. Similarly, a large randomized controlled trial found that weight loss alone by reducing the *amount* of calories without changing the *type* of calories was not sufficient to significantly reduce the rate of cardiovascular events.

Paradoxically, statin drugs such as Lipitor, used to lower cholesterol, may significantly increase the risk of developing type 2 diabetes. One study showed that statin treatment increased the risk of type 2 diabetes by 46 percent, which is especially concerning since a major complication of diabetes is heart disease. In contrast, lowering cholesterol levels by making lifestyle changes decreases the risk of both heart disease and type 2 diabetes.

Lifestyle Medicine and Prostate Cancer

Lifestyle medicine is better than radiation or surgery in treating most patients with early-stage prostate cancer.

Prostate cancer is the most common cancer in men other than skin cancer. Most men, if they live long enough, will get prostate cancer even if it remains undiagnosed. Approximately one-third of men in their thirties or forties, one-half of men in their fifties and sixties, 70 percent of men in their seventies, and 80 percent of men in their eighties have prostate cancer even if they're not aware of it.

In other words, most men are going to die *with* prostate cancer, not *from* prostate cancer. Our immune system and other mechanisms keep it in check and it remains asymptomatic, which I discussed in Chapter 2.

What's increasingly well-documented is that the lifestyle choices you make each day have a major impact on whether or not you develop clinically significant prostate cancer. As described in Chapter 2, if your immune system is functioning effectively, then it can help keep prostate cancer from spreading—and prostate cancer is usually dangerous only when it spreads (metastasizes).

The importance of lifestyle medicine is even more relevant if you have biopsy-proven prostate cancer and want to reverse its progression. Many doctors were shocked when a major randomized controlled trial in the *New England Journal of Medicine* showed that after ten years, men diagnosed with early-stage prostate cancer who did nothing—called "watchful waiting" or "active surveillance"—lived as long as those who had surgery to remove their prostate or who underwent radiation treatments. Similar results were found in an earlier study.

Men who had surgery or radiation did have a lower rate of disease progression and metastases, but they were much more likely to become impotent, incontinent, or both—that is, maimed in the most personal ways—and they didn't live longer. Few things are more distressing and humiliating for a man than to no longer be able to have sex or to be wearing a diaper—especially when the treatments are not effective in prolonging his life.

Men who are diagnosed with early-stage prostate cancer often feel a tremendous pressure from themselves and from well-meaning friends and family to *do something* about the tumor growing in their prostate. So if the choice is between doing nothing and having radiation or surgery, most men choose the latter—even though it's unlikely to prolong their survival and very likely to reduce their quality of life.

Lifestyle medicine provides a third, better alternative. For guys who want a more macho way of putting it, let's call it "an aggressive, non-surgical, non-pharmacologic intervention."

My colleagues and I conducted the first randomized controlled trial showing that our lifestyle medicine program may slow, stop, or even reverse the progression of early-stage prostate cancer, without drugs or surgery. This was done in collaboration with Dr. Peter Carroll (chair of urology at UCSF) and the late Dr. William Fair (when he was chief of urologic surgery and chair of urologic oncology at Memorial Sloan-Kettering Cancer Center).

There is a relatively small subset of men—approximately one out of forty-nine—who have especially aggressive forms of prostate cancer and may benefit from surgery or radiation. These tend to be men who are diagnosed with prostate cancer early in life, have rapidly rising prostate-specific antigen (PSA) levels, have Gleason scores greater than 6, have tumors that are located in an area more likely to spread, or have large tumors. Dr. Carroll has developed algorithms to help identify this subset of men. Even these men needing surgery or radiation may reduce the risk of recurrence by making these lifestyle changes after this procedure.

Other studies provide insight into why these lifestyle changes have such a powerful impact on the progression of prostate cancer. For example, researchers found that men who were diagnosed with prostate cancer who ate a diet higher in red and processed meat, high-fat dairy foods, and refined grains had a significantly higher risk of both prostate-cancer-related mortality and overall mortality compared with those who ate a whole-foods plant-based diet.

They examined health and diet data from almost 1,000 men participating in the Physicians' Health Study who were diagnosed with prostate cancer and who were followed for an average of fourteen years after their diagnosis. Men who ate mostly a Western diet had a *250 percent higher risk* of prostate-cancer-related death—and a 67 percent increased risk of death from any cause. In contrast, men who ate mostly a whole-foods plant-based diet had a 36 percent lower risk of death from all causes.

Although we have not yet conducted randomized controlled trials on breast cancer, what affects prostate cancer may affect breast cancer as well. As described in Chapter 2, we found that our lifestyle medicine program downregulated oncogenes that promote breast cancer as well as prostate cancer and colon cancer in only three months.

As with prostate cancer, it is likely that some aggressive breast cancers with high potential for spreading may require chemotherapy, surgery, and/or radiation whereas others may be safely treated with lifestyle medicine alone. Even when drugs and surgery are indicated, lifestyle medicine may add additional efficacy and reduce the likelihood of recurrence. For example, women who reduced their dietary fat intake to only 20 percent (about 33 grams of fat per day) decreased their risk of breast cancer recurrence by 42 percent after five years when compared with a randomized comparison group who consumed 51 grams of fat per day.

Of course, there is a time and a place for high-tech medicine. We've all benefited from it. To be clear, drugs and surgery can be lifesaving in a crisis. And in the early stages of treating and reversing chronic diseases, drugs or surgery may be necessary in addition to intensive lifestyle changes, at least at the beginning while your body is healing. And some people may need drugs and/or surgery even when they make comprehensive lifestyle changes.

Even then, though, we need to address the underlying causes—which are usually lifestyle related, and often treatable and even reversible with lifestyle medicine.

CHAPTER 4

Eat Well

When diet is wrong, medicine is of no use.
When diet is correct, medicine is of no need.
—Ayurvedic proverb

Dean

What should you eat?

Few fields have as much controversy as nutrition—after all, everybody has to eat, and just about everyone has an opinion about it. Fortunately, the evidence is now clear.

A consensus is emerging that a whole-foods plant-based diet is the healthiest way of eating. It is low in bad carbs and bad fats; high in good carbs and with enough good fats; the right amount of plant-based protein and very low in animal protein, if any. "Whole foods" (also called "real foods") means to eat foods as close to their natural form as possible, avoiding processed foods.

In the spirit of keeping it simple, here is the way of eating that we have proven can reverse the progression of so many different chronic illnesses:

- Consume mostly plants ("good carbs" and "good protein"): vegetables, fruits, whole grains, legumes, soy products, and small amounts of nuts and seeds in forms as close as possible to their natural, unprocessed state.
- What you *include* in your diet is as important as what you *exclude*. There are many thousands of protective factors in plant-based foods that have anti-cancer, anti–heart disease, and anti-aging properties as well as being very low in disease-promoting substances.
- Minimize or, even better, eliminate animal protein and replace it with plant-based protein.
- Avoid sugar, white flour, white rice, and other "bad carbs."
- Consume 3 grams per day of "good fats" (omega-3 fatty acids).
- Reduce intake of total fat, and especially "bad fats" such as trans fats, saturated fats, and partially hydrogenated fats.
- Organic is optimal—foods taste much better, and they are much lower in pesticide residues, which can disrupt your hormones.

That's it! To undo most chronic diseases (paraphrasing Michael Pollan): Eat real foods. Just plants. Not too much sugar or fat.

The scientific evidence and mechanisms explaining why this way of eating can reverse the progression of so many chronic diseases are outlined in the first three chapters. As I mentioned in Chapter 1, the old saying about an ounce of prevention and a pound of cure is true. It usually takes a lot more changes in diet and lifestyle to reverse a disease than to prevent it.

As such, the best results come from avoiding all animal products. In our earlier studies, we included egg whites and one cup per day of either nonfat yogurt or milk—but you don't need these for good nutrition, and there is increasing evidence that it may be better to avoid dairy and eggs.

In addition to omega-3 fatty acids, I take a few supplements—vitamin C, a multivitamin without iron, vitamin D_3, turmeric (for its anti-inflammatory properties) with black pepper (*Piper nigrum*) to increase absorption, magnesium citrate, CoQ10, and a probiotic.

In this chapter, I'd like to focus on a few of the most common misconceptions about nutrition. After that, in the rest of this chapter, Anne describes how you can make the transition to this way of eating as easy and pleasurable as possible, nourishing both your body and soul.

Myth #1: It's Hard to Get Enough Protein on a Plant-Based Diet

This is the most common misconception about plant-based diets. Here's the good news—you can easily get all the protein you need on a plant-based diet. In fact, it's hard not to. If you're eating an adequate number of calories from a variety of whole foods, it's very difficult not to get enough protein.

In fact, most Americans get *too much* protein, which is as bad as not getting enough of it. Too much protein leads to increased risks of heart disease, cancer, kidney function disorders, osteoporosis, liver disease, and other chronic conditions. It also reduces autophagy, keeping your body from "cleaning house."

In 2016 the USDA dietary guidelines stated that at least half of the population is consuming too much protein.

How much protein do you need? For most people, it's only 0.36 grams of protein per pound or 0.8 grams of protein per kilogram of body weight per day. If you weigh 150 pounds, that's about 54 grams of protein per day.

Protein is essential to good health—including tissue growth and repair, digestion, metabolism, and the production of antibodies to fight infection. When you digest protein, it's broken down into its component amino acids, which are then reassembled into over 50,000 different forms your body can use for hormones, enzymes, and neurotransmitters.

Protein is formed from twenty-two different building blocks called amino acids in billions of different combinations, just as the twenty-six letters of the alphabet can combine to form a virtually endless number of words.

Your body can make thirteen of these amino acids. The other nine are called "essential amino acids," since they must be supplied in the diet. Of these, only three—lysine, tryptophan, and methionine—are worth noting, since the others are plentiful in most foods.

Plant-based foods contain these three amino acids in different proportions. By eating a variety of foods, you will obtain all of these. Legumes (beans, for example) are high in lysine but low in tryptophan and methionine. Grains (rice, for example) are low in lysine but high in tryptophan and methionine. A meal of rice and beans, therefore, provides a complete protein, no different from the protein found in eggs or meat—but without the bad stuff that can make you sick.

It used to be believed that these amino acids need to be combined in each meal. Now we know that this is not necessary—your body stores and recycles amino acids, so as long as you eat a variety of foods, including legumes, and enough calories to maintain your weight, you'll get enough protein. All plants contain protein.

Here are some examples of complete proteins:

- Rice and beans
- Tacos with beans
- Tofu with rice
- Barley and lentils
- Pasta e fagioli (pasta and beans)
- Hopping John (black-eyed peas and rice)

Here are some examples of plant-based complete proteins:

- Quinoa: 1 cup (cooked) = 8 grams of protein
- Soy (preferably organic and non-GMO):
  - 1 cup tofu = 20 grams of protein.
  - 1 cup soybeans = 30 grams
  - 1 cup soy milk = 8 grams of protein (the same amount as in 1 cup dairy milk)
- Buckwheat (also called kasha): 1 cup (cooked) = 6 grams of protein
- Unshelled pumpkin or squash seeds: 1 cup = 12 grams of protein
- Hemp seeds (shelled): 1 cup = 53 grams of protein
- Ezekiel bread (made with sprouted grains, wheat, barley, beans, lentils, millet, and spelt): 8 grams of protein in two slices (not counting what's in the rest of the sandwich)

- Hummus (chickpeas—also known as garbanzo beans—are high in lysine, and tahini is a rich source of the amino acid methionine) = 17 grams of protein per cup

A related prevailing myth is that meat makes you strong. But the word is now getting out among elite, world-class athletes that eating a whole-foods plant-based diet actually gives them a competitive advantage and even greater strength. (Remember, elephants are vegetarian.)

For example, strongman Patrik Baboumian is a vegan who broke a world record for most weight carried by a human being when he hauled over 1,200 pounds ten yards across a stage in Toronto.

Another well-known bodybuilder (and former governor), Arnold Schwarzenegger, said "Hasta la vista, baby" to meat several years ago. "I feel fantastic—if they tell you to eat more meat to be strong, don't buy it."

At age thirty-nine, Dotsie Bausch won an Olympic silver medal in cycling; she attributes her improved performance to a plant-based diet.

MMA/UFC fighters like James Wilks, Mac Danzig, and Jake Shields credit their success and tough endurance to eating plants.

Rich Roll is a vegan ultramarathon elite athlete who was named one of the "25 Fittest Guys in the World" by *Men's Fitness*. At age fifty-one! In one day, he ran forty miles and swam six miles in freezing water across twenty-six islands of the Stockholm Archipelago off Sweden as part of the grueling Ötillö Swimrun World Championship.

Myth #2: A Low-Carb, High-Protein Diet Is Good for You

I'm a veteran of so many nutritional debates and diet wars, but I thought I was done. So I wasn't planning to address this issue here. After so many studies were published showing that people on low-carb, high-fat, high-protein diets were mortgaging their health to lose weight, I was hoping that it would no longer be necessary.

But never underestimate the power of telling people what they want to hear. This diet keeps resurfacing under various names—Atkins diet, Paleo diet, ketogenic diet, and so on. What makes this diet so seductive is that it's based on a half-truth.

I debated Dr. Robert Atkins on many occasions—in front of 3,000 doctors at the American College of Cardiology's annual scientific sessions (during which he fell asleep), in the pages of the *Journal of the American Medical Association,* at the United States Department of Agriculture, in national media, and so on. He was known as the "low-carb doctor," so, unfortunately, I was often called the "low-fat doctor" (even though, as you know by now, the way of eating I recommend is so much more than just low-fat).

It's not just low-fat versus low-carb—that's a false choice. And it's not just about food. An optimal way of eating is low in fat *and* low in refined carbohydrates, as well as low as in animal protein.

The half-truth on which we all agree is that Americans *do* eat too many refined ("bad") carbohydrates, such as sugar, white flour, and white rice, as I described in Chapter 2. Because of this, if you reduce your consumption of refined carbohydrates, you'll lose weight.

What we disagree about is where you go from there. Replacing these "bad carbs" with bacon, sausage, and pork rinds is not a healthy choice. Replacing these with "good carbs" such as fruits, vegetables, whole grains, legumes, and soy products in their natural, unrefined forms is very good for you.

Here's the bottom line: the only diet that has been scientifically proven to reverse heart disease, to slow, stop, or reverse early-stage prostate cancer, and to reverse aging by lengthening telomeres (among other benefits) is a whole-foods plant-based diet low in both fat *and* refined carbohydrates.

No one has ever done a randomized trial proving that a high-fat, low-carb diet can reverse heart disease. It actually makes it worse.

For example, a Harvard study of heart attack survivors found that those eating a high-fat, low-carb diet had a 33 percent increased risk of premature death from all causes and a 51 percent increased risk of cardiovascular mortality. And the more closely they adhered to that diet, the worse were these outcomes.

Why? It's not just fats or carbs—animal protein is harmful, and plant-based proteins are protective and healing.

For example, in a study of over 130,000 men and women, animal protein intake was associated with higher premature mortality from all causes, whereas plant protein was associated with lower mortality from all causes, including heart disease, type 2 diabetes, and the most common types of cancer. Replacing animal protein with plant protein lowered the risk of premature mortality.

In almost 30,000 postmenopausal women, substituting vegetable protein for animal protein reduced premature mortality from heart disease by 30 percent.

In other studies, diets high in animal protein increased the risk of heart failure, whereas vegetable protein was protective.

It's worth repeating a study I cited in Chapter 2: in a study of over 6,000 people, those ages fifty to sixty-five who reported eating diets high in animal protein had a 75 percent increase in overall mortality, a 400 percent increase in cancer deaths, and a 500 percent increase in type 2 diabetes during the following eighteen years, whereas plant-based proteins reduced the risk of premature death in all of these categories—again, a double benefit.

It is not enough to say that people lose as much weight on a low-carb diet as on a low-fat diet. You can lose weight in lots of ways that aren't very good for you; smoking cigarettes is an effective way to lose weight, and so is chemotherapy, but no one would responsibly recommend these for weight loss.

Evidence is showing that even though people can lose weight on a high-protein, low-carb diet, they often mortgage their health in the process.

The most important question is this: what is happening in your arteries and to the other mechanisms that control your health, as described in Chapter 2?

An article in the *New England Journal of Medicine* revealed what happens in arteries on different diets:

- The top diagram (A) shows clean arteries when eating the way we recommend in this book.
- The middle graphic (B) shows arteries that are partially clogged when consuming a standard American diet (SAD—an appropriate acronym).
- The bottom graphic (C) shows arteries that are severely clogged when eating a high-protein, low-carb Atkins/paleo/ketogenic diet.

The arterial damage was caused by animal-protein-induced elevations in insulin levels and increased free fatty acids (causing inflammation) and decreased production of endothelial progenitor cells (special cells that, like Pac-Man, nibble the lining of your arteries and help keep them clean).

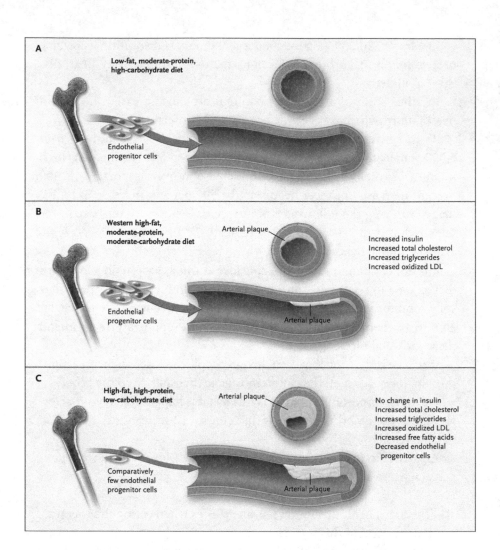

A Low-fat, moderate-protein, high-carbohydrate diet

Endothelial progenitor cells

B Western high-fat, moderate-protein, moderate-carbohydrate diet

Arterial plaque

Endothelial progenitor cells

Arterial plaque

Increased insulin
Increased total cholesterol
Increased triglycerides
Increased oxidized LDL

C High-fat, high-protein, low-carbohydrate diet

Arterial plaque

Comparatively few endothelial progenitor cells

Arterial plaque

No change in insulin
Increased total cholesterol
Increased triglycerides
Increased oxidized LDL
Increased free fatty acids
Decreased endothelial
  progenitor cells

"But wait!" you might say—"I thought the whole point of a high-fat, high-protein Atkins/ketogenic/paleo diet was that it's low in sugar and refined carbohydrates, so it keeps insulin levels lower."

In fact, meat actually *increases* insulin levels in your blood, both by raising insulin secretion and by causing insulin resistance. So does fat.

Because of this, diabetes increases as the frequency of meat consumption increases. In contrast, insulin levels are lower in those following the whole-foods plant-based diet described in this book.

A study of 37,000 men from the Harvard Health Professionals Follow-Up Study and more than 83,000 women from the Harvard Nurses' Health Study who were followed up for almost 3 million person-years found that a daily serving of red meat no larger than a deck of cards increased the risk of type 2 diabetes by 19 percent. Processed red meat proved even worse: a daily serving half that size—one hot dog or two slices of bacon, for example—was associated with a 51 percent increase in risk of diabetes.

This study also found that consumption of both processed and unprocessed red meat is associated with an increased risk of premature mortality from all causes as well as from cardiovascular disease and cancer.

Again, it's not low-fat versus low-carb—that's why it's important to eat less fat, less animal protein, *and* fewer refined carbohydrates.

Besides regulating your blood sugar level, insulin plays an important role in fat metabolism. Because insulin increases the secretion of lipoprotein lipase, an enzyme that increases the uptake of fat from your bloodstream into fat in your body's cells, when your body produces more insulin, you are more likely to convert dietary calories into body fat.

When you try to lose weight by only reducing the *amount* of food you eat instead of changing the *type* of food, your body responds not just by increasing the amount of insulin and lipoprotein lipase but also by increasing your body's sensitivity to the effects of these—a double whammy. As a result, your body increases the uptake of fat from your bloodstream and you tend to regain the lost weight. Also, when you reduce only the amount of food, your metabolism slows down so you burn calories more slowly because your body thinks you're starving.

In contrast, as mentioned earlier, patients in our Lifestyle Heart Trial lost an average of 24 pounds in the first year and kept off about half that weight five years later.

Reducing insulin levels has other benefits. Insulin also has a key role in increasing cholesterol synthesis. When your insulin levels rise, your liver makes more of an enzyme called HMG-CoA reductase, which in turn causes your body to make more cholesterol. (This enzyme is the major target of cholesterol-lowering drugs called statins.)

Besides increasing your cholesterol level, insulin enhances the growth and proliferation of arterial smooth muscle cells. These smooth muscle cells help to clog up your arteries and can lead to heart attacks. Other studies have confirmed that people with high insulin levels have higher rates of heart attacks.

Insulin also affects your stress level. When insulin levels increase, your sympathetic nervous system gets stimulated, just as it is stimulated during times of emotional stress.

Another study found higher blood flow and lower inflammation (as measured by C-reactive protein) in those following our dietary recommendations, compared with lower blood flow and higher inflammation in those on an Atkins diet. They also found that the more saturated fat consumed, the lower the blood flow.

I continue to be impressed by how dynamically food affects our well-being—for better and for worse. Just a few days of eating fatty food impairs both short-term memory and exercise performance.

In one study, scientists found that rats who were fed a low-fat diet (8 percent fat) for two months mastered a maze. All of the rats completed six or seven of the eight goals, and some did all eight on the first try. Then, half were switched to a high-fat diet (55 percent fat). After only four days, all of them performed significantly worse in the maze.

Also, their ability to exercise on a treadmill fell by 30 percent after only a few days on the high-fat diet and by 50 percent after only five days.

These researchers also found that the short-term effects of a high-fat diet on cognitive function and exercise ability were similar in humans.

Myth #3: Carb Calories Are Bad for You, and Fat Doesn't Matter—It's All About Sugar

A myth that has been repeated so often it's become a meme is that calories from carbohydrates are more likely to cause you to gain weight than an equivalent number of calories from fat.

To address this issue, Dr. Kevin Hall placed overweight people in a metabolic ward at the National Institutes of Health to determine what actually happens on different diets. They lived there for four weeks, so the researchers knew exactly what and how much they were eating.

Dr. Hall and his colleagues found that, indeed, all calories are not alike—but the *opposite* of what was predicted! The title of the journal article reporting their findings says it all: "Calorie for Calorie, Dietary Fat Restriction Results in More Body Fat Loss than Carbohydrate Restriction in People with Obesity."

Restricting dietary fat intake led to body fat loss at a rate *68 percent higher* than cutting the same number of carbohydrate calories when adults with obesity ate strictly controlled diets.

This doesn't mean that refined carbohydrates are unimportant—but it clearly shows that calories from refined carbs are *not* more likely to cause you to gain weight than the same number of calories from fat. Both are important.

Also, as stated earlier, fat has nine calories per gram whereas carbs (and protein) have only four calories per gram. So when you eat a lot of fat, you consume more calories for a given amount of food *and* you're more likely to convert that dietary fat into body fat.

For hundreds of thousands of years, the main problem for humans has been to get enough calories to survive. Precisely because fat is so much denser in calories than protein or carbohydrates, we've evolved to have a taste for fat as it gives a survival advantage if you're struggling to get enough calories to live. However, in modern times when fatty foods are so abundantly available, this same mechanism that evolved to protect us has become harmful.

The PURE study made headlines by claiming that eating more fat of all types reduced total mortality but eating more refined carbohydrates increased it. What the researchers neglected to explain was that the reason that more fat helped people live longer is that the study was done in countries where many people were barely getting enough calories to survive.

Because fat has nine calories per gram versus only four calories per gram for protein or carbohydrates, those eating more fat were able to consume more calories in a given amount of food, thus reducing premature total mortality. Those eating more fat also consumed more protein, which gave an additional survival advantage to those who were not getting enough of it in poorer countries.

There is also a lot of misinformation about saturated fat. For example, an article published in the *British Medical Journal* made headlines when it concluded in its abstract (summary): "Saturated fats are not associated with increased all-cause mortality, mortality from cardiovascular disease, or prevalence of coronary heart disease."

However, this was completely misleading. The researchers examined these data in two ways. One approach, what they called "most adjusted," analyzed the data by not including the full impact of saturated fat when it was found in association with dietary cholesterol. But foods high in dietary cholesterol are usually high in saturated fat, so removing this relationship obscures it.

The other approach, "least adjusted," included all of the data without playing with it. To me, and to most researchers, this is the more accurate way of looking at data because you're not obscuring any relationships.

The "most adjusted" analysis didn't find a relationship between saturated fats and disease, as noted in the abstract. But in the "least adjusted" analysis—the more accurate—they found that there was a significant relationship between the intake of saturated fats and increased all-cause mortality, mortality from cardiovascular disease, and prevalence of coronary heart disease.

What I find especially interesting is that *the authors didn't even report this important finding in the abstract,* which is all that most people even read. It was buried in the fine print of the manuscript.

Why would a journal do this? Unfortunately, journals are mindful of what is called their "impact factor." The more widely reported a journal article is to the general media—the more headlines it generates—the higher its impact factor. So, this article claiming that saturated fat is not harmful made headlines around the world because it told people what they wanted to hear—even though the conclusion was the exact opposite of what the more valid analysis of their data showed.

Let me reiterate yet again: it's not low-carb versus low-fat. An optimal way of eating is low in total fat and especially low in "bad fats," including trans fats and saturated fats; low in "bad carbs," such as refined carbohydrates and sugar; and low in animal protein, especially red meat.

It includes predominantly "good carbs," whole foods such as fruits, vegetables, whole grains, legumes, and soy in their natural, unrefined forms; includes 3–4 grams per day of "good fats," to provide at least 1 gram per day of omega-3 fatty acids (DHA + EPA); and is plant-based.

Another related myth that's been repeated so often that many people believe it's true is this: "Americans have been told to eat less fat; we're eating less fat but we're fatter than ever, so low-fat is dead; it's all due to sugar and refined carbohydrates."

It's true that we've been told to eat less fat—but are we?

The USDA keeps track of the entire U.S. food supply—what people are actually consuming, not what they say they're eating.

It turns out that in every decade since 1950, people have been eating more fat, sugar, meat, and calories—an average of 67 percent *more* fat, 37 percent *more* sugar, 57 pounds *more* meat, and 800 *more* calories per person. Not surprisingly, we're fatter—not because we're eating too little fat but because we're consuming too much of everything.

What happens in your arteries on different levels of fat in your diet? An important study that used very precise quantitative coronary arteriography to measure the degree of blockage in coronary arteries in the heart found:

- Those who had an overall decrease in total fat intake did *not* develop new coronary artery blockages.
- Those who had an overall increase in total fat intake *did* develop new coronary artery blockages.
- Substituting "good carbs" for fat decreased the number and severity of coronary artery blockages.

The relationship of increased fat intake to the development of new coronary artery blockages was true of *all* types of fat (total fat, polyunsaturated fat, monounsaturated fat, and saturated fat) in a dose-response relationship—the more fat people consumed, the more arterial blockages were formed.

My colleagues and I found a similar relationship in the Lifestyle Heart Trial, which proved that heart disease was reversible by making the lifestyle changes described in this book. There was a significant dose-response relationship between dietary total fat intake and changes in coronary artery blockages after one year and after five years. We found the same relationship between dietary cholesterol intake and changes in coronary artery blockages after one year and after five years.

Also, as we discussed in Chapter 3, prostate cancer only becomes clinically threatening when it spreads (metastasizes). A high-fat diet increases the likelihood of prostate cancer spreading, whereas a low-fat plant-based diet inhibits it.

Myth #4: The Mediterranean Diet Is Optimal for Reversing Heart Disease

The Mediterranean diet *is* a better diet than what most people consume, especially with its emphasis on fruits and vegetables and less red meat. But it doesn't go far enough to reverse heart disease.

In 2013, a study was published in the *New England Journal of Medicine* claiming that "the Mediterranean diet is better than a low fat diet in reducing heart attacks and strokes." It made headlines worldwide.

However, the control group did not actually follow a low-fat diet. In the "low fat" control group, total fat consumption decreased insignificantly from 39 percent to 37 percent, hardly at all —the diet we proved could reverse heart disease is closer to 10–15 percent fat—and they tended to replace fat with sugar, which is never a good idea.

Despite the claim, there was *no* significant reduction in heart attacks, death from cardiovascular causes, or death from any cause. The researchers only found a significant reduction in death from stroke.

This was likely because the Mediterranean diet group consumed more omega-3 fatty acids than the control group, which helps to keep blood clots from forming—and 90 percent of strokes are due to blood clots blocking the flow of blood to the brain. This is why for more than twenty-five years we've recommended 3 grams per day of fish oil, ground flaxseed or flaxseed oil, or plankton-based omega-3 fatty acids.

They reported the reduction in stroke rate pooled with data on heart attacks, death from cardiovascular causes, or death from any cause, which made it appear as though there were reductions in all of these.

However, when examined separately, there was no reduction in heart attacks, death from cardiovascular disease, or death from any cause— only in stroke rates. Because of methodological irregularities and errors, this study was retracted and republished in 2018.

To repeat: a Mediterranean diet is better than what most people are consuming, but it doesn't go far enough to reverse heart disease. Even better is a whole-foods plant-based diet low in fat, especially saturated/

trans fats, low in refined carbohydrates, and with sufficient omega-3 fatty acids.

What's Good for You Is Good for Our Planet

To the degree that we transition toward a whole-foods plant-based diet, it not only makes a difference in our own lives but also makes a difference in the lives of many others across the globe as well.

In 2014, NASA issued a report declaring that global warming isn't coming, it's already here. Major glaciers that are part of the West Antarctic Ice Sheet appear to have become irrevocably destabilized.

In 2018, scientists learned that Antarctica's ice sheet is melting far faster than previously thought, with more than 200 billion tons of ice flooding into oceans annually, according to new research published in the prestigious science journal *Nature*.

About 3 trillion tons of ice have disappeared since 1992. The rate of melting has accelerated threefold in the last five years, and a separate study suggests that this may lead to sea rises of ten inches by the year 2070, which would have a disastrous impact around the world.

An article in the *Journal of the American Medical Association* states, "Health is inextricably linked to climate change," including respiratory disorders, infectious diseases, water-borne diseases, and mental health disorders.

A major UN report stated that global warming could cause food shortages, mass extinctions, and flooding of major cities.

It's easy to feel overwhelmed, depressed, even nihilistic—"What can I do as one person to make a meaningful difference?" These feelings can lead to paralysis at a time when more than ever we need to take action.

So here's something to consider: *What's good for you is good for our planet. What's personally sustainable is globally sustainable.*

Many people are surprised to learn that animal agribusiness generates more greenhouse gases than all forms of transportation *combined*.

All transportation worldwide generates only about 13.5 percent of the carbon dioxide that contributes to global warming. Eating meat, on the other hand, is responsible for at least 18 percent of carbon dioxide emissions and may account for much more. Livestock also accounts for

37 percent of methane (which is twenty-three to seventy-two times more toxic to the ozone layer than carbon dioxide) and 65 percent of nitrous oxide (which is 296 times more toxic) from their manure.

The United States maintains more than 9 billion head of livestock, which consume about seven times as much grain as the entire U.S. population. Livestock now use 30 percent of all land worldwide and are causing deforestation, particularly in the Amazon, where 70 percent of the land that used to be forest is now used for grazing.

So, besides displacing land that could be used to grow food for humans, more than half of U.S. grain and nearly 40 percent of world grain is being fed to livestock rather than being consumed directly by humans. That would feed a lot of hungry people.

At a time when one in four children in the United States lacks access to enough food for a healthy life and some 800 million people in the world suffer from hunger or malnutrition, choosing to eat more plant-based foods and less red meat frees up resources for ourselves, our loved ones, and our planet.

When I was on the board of directors of the San Francisco Food Bank, I was shocked to learn that one out of five children in the affluent Bay Area goes to bed hungry each night.

That's just not acceptable—there is enough food to feed everyone on the planet if enough people move toward a plant-based diet, today. No one ever need go hungry.

It also takes significantly more energy to produce a unit of food higher on the food chain than plants. For example, it takes ten to fourteen times more resources to produce a pound of meat-based protein than a pound of plant-based protein. Producing a pound of beef requires almost 2,000 gallons of water.

Also, more than 86 percent of the $3.3 trillion in annual U.S. healthcare costs goes toward treating chronic diseases, which can often be prevented and even reversed by eating a plant-based diet, at a fraction of the cost.

Finally, eating a plant-based diet is a more compassionate way to eat. Each year, the United States grows and kills about 9 billion livestock animals. That's a lot of unnecessary suffering. I believe that what goes around comes around—for better and for worse.

When we realize that something as primal as the food we choose to put in our mouth each day makes such an important difference in addressing both global warming and personal health, as well as feeding the hungry, it empowers us and imbues these choices with meaning. As we'll discuss in Chapter 7, if it's meaningful, then it's sustainable—and a meaningful life is a longer life.

So, to the degree we choose to eat a plant-based diet, we free up tremendous amounts of resources that can benefit many others as well as ourselves. I find this very meaningful. And when we can act more compassionately, it helps our hearts as well.

- Love yourself.
- Love your family.
- Love your community.
- Love your planet.

You'll look better and feel better. Have hotter sex and a cooler planet. Feed the hungry. And reduce healthcare costs by preventing and undoing the most common chronic diseases. Sound good?

Anne

Our approach to nutrition is all about feeling good and enjoying life. When you adopt a plant-based way of eating, you'll lose excess weight and gain vibrant health. What makes eating this way sustainable is feeling deeply nourished and revitalized. May you relish this delicious and nutritious way of eating!

Eat Real Foods

One of the goals of this book is to keep it simple. Dean described the parameters of the diet we've proven can reverse—undo!—the progression of so many chronic diseases. This includes abundantly enjoying a variety of plant-based foods that are low in fat and sugar, such as fruits, vegetables, whole grains, legumes, and soy products as close as possible to the way they come in nature, with minimal processing—in other words, what are known as real foods or whole foods.

Before we get into the details of shopping, preparing, and cooking, some people find that an easy way to get started is to order prepackaged meals online or look for them in many grocery stores.

If it seems a little overwhelming to make big changes in your way of eating, we've included in Appendix A a listing of commercially available foods that fit our guidelines and which you can use to stock your pantry and freezer, as well as frozen entrées you can order online or find in many stores. (We don't have any financial relationships with these vendors; this is just presented for your convenience.)

If you eat just these foods for a week or so, because the underlying biological mechanisms we've been discussing are so dynamic, you're likely to feel so much better, so quickly, you'll be that much more motivated to learn how to shop and cook meals on your own. At that point, you can include these prepared meals on a less frequent basis, perhaps after a long day of work or a busy weekend.

They'll show you that foods can be familiar, delicious, *and* health-promoting. And you'll make the connection between what you eat and how you feel because it comes from your own experience: "When I eat this, I feel really good; when I eat that, not so good." This helps make it sustainable.

Listed in Appendix A are two weeks' worth of commercially available breakfasts, lunches, dinners, and snacks. At the time this book was written, all of these foods were available on Amazon.com, and many can be found at other online sites, including Target.com, Vitacost.com, Walmart.com, WholeFoods.com, GroceryGateway.com, FreshDirect .com, Google Express (express.google.com), Leafside Foods, Urban Remedy, and others.

A lot of these can be found in your local supermarket, and most grocery stores will special-order them for you, especially if you let them know that you'll be purchasing them on a regular basis.

Some of these foods are higher in fat or sugar than others, but think in terms of the total amount you're consuming in a given day or over several days rather than in each food item.

Also, if you follow the two-week plan in Appendix A, you'll find that some of these days have calorie totals lower than what is recommended by the USDA for an average adult. If you're trying to lose weight, this is a good thing; if not, make your portion sizes a little larger or add some items on your own that fit within our nutritional guidelines.

Now let's get into some general nutrition guidelines, building on what Dean outlined earlier in this chapter.

Just Plants ("Good Carbs")

As we've been describing, our way of eating includes a delicious abundance of foods you can enjoy. These include a wide variety of fruits, vegetables, whole grains, legumes (beans, lentils, and dried peas such as chickpeas and black-eyed peas), and soy products.

The only plant-based foods that we recommend you minimize or eliminate are those that are especially high in fat. This includes all added oils, since all oils are 100 percent fat, and avocados, which are 85 percent fat and contain about 322 calories, of which 265 calories are from fat (30 grams of fat). More on this later.

Not Too Much Sugar ("Bad Carbs")

"Bad carbs" include concentrated sweeteners such as sugar, high-fructose corn syrup, honey, maple syrup, and so on. They also include the "whites"—that is, white flour and white rice.

When you go from whole-wheat flour to white flour, or from brown rice to white rice, you turn a good carb into a bad carb because you've removed the fiber and bran that keep you healthy.

In a good carb, the fiber and bran fill you up before you get too many calories. For example, you can only eat so many apples—you'll get full before you eat too much. Also, fiber and bran slow the rate at which you absorb nutrients (including sugar) from your gut into your bloodstream.

In contrast, you can consume large amounts of sugar, white rice, and white flour without getting full because you've removed the fiber and bran. Also, the food gets absorbed very quickly—it's like injecting sugar into your veins—causing your blood sugar to spike. This, in turn, causes your pancreas to make more insulin.

As we've discussed in Chapter 2, insulin creates chronic inflammation, one of the underlying mechanisms of most chronic diseases. And the repeated surges of insulin lead to insulin resistance, metabolic syndrome, and type 2 diabetes. And these wide swings in blood sugar produced by bad carbs help to make those foods addictive—since when your blood sugar is too low, it creates a craving for more sugar.

If you're going to eat some bad carbs, eat them in the same meal with good carbs and other high-fiber foods, as the fiber in the other foods will mitigate the rapid rate of absorption into your bloodstream and keep your blood sugar in a range less likely to precipitate chronic surges of insulin.

Sugar is added to so many foods, so it's helpful to read labels. If I'm going to have some sugar, I like to save it for a treat such as a small piece of dark chocolate rather than having it disguised in so many other foods.

Alcohol causes your body to burn calories more slowly, so limit your consumption of alcohol to no more than one glass of wine, one can of beer, or one shot of hard liquor per day. Your liver's priority is to detoxify alcohol before processing anything else, so drinking slows down the burning of fat, which leads to weight gain. Drinking alcohol can also cause low blood sugar because nutrients are not transformed into energy. And it's worth noting that even one glass of wine per day increases the risk of breast cancer.

Recently, the largest study ever of the health effects of alcohol consumption in 195 countries reported:

> The widely held view of the health benefits of alcohol need revising, particularly as improved methods and analyses continue to show how much alcohol use contributes to global death and disability. Our results show that the safest level of drinking is none. This level is in conflict with most health guidelines, which espouse health benefits associated with consuming up to two drinks per day. Alcohol use contributes to health loss from many causes and exacts its toll across the lifespan. We found that the risk of all-cause mortality, and of cancers specifically, rises with increasing levels of consumption, and the level of consumption that minimizes health loss is zero.

The researchers explained that previously analyses failed, in part, to exclude people who were now nondrinkers because they had become so sick from drinking too much. This falsely elevated the risk of nondrinkers and made it seem as though having one or two drinks a day was more healthful than not drinking at all.

I'm not saying that people shouldn't drink at all—I neither prescribe it nor proscribe it. Life is not risk-free, and you have to decide if the benefits outweigh the risks. But this study shows that it would be a mistake to believe that drinking alcohol is beneficial to your health.

Some plant-based foods are higher in what's called the glycemic index—a measure of how quickly a food is absorbed from your gut into your bloodstream. In practice, since most people eat several types of foods at a meal, the fiber in low-glycemic foods tends to "cancel out" the lack of fiber in high-glycemic foods. So, in the spirit of keeping it simple, I find it's usually better not to worry about the glycemic index of a specific food if you're eating other foods that are high in fiber.

Not Too Much Fat

The way of eating that we found can reverse most chronic diseases is much lower in fat than what most people eat—closer to 10–15 percent fat than to the 40 percent in a typical American diet. This is the percentage of fat found (until recently) in the diet in countries such as China, where the prevalence of heart disease and other chronic diseases was quite low.

In practical terms, there's no need to track the amount of fat you're consuming if you only eat plant-based foods as they come in nature (other than very high-fat foods such as oils, avocados, seeds, and nuts). If you're eating commercially processed foods, try to limit your overall fat consumption to 10–15 percent of your total calories.

According to USDA dietary guidelines, recommended total calories range from 1,600 to 2,400 calories per day for adult women and from 2,000 to 3,000 calories per day for adult men. The low end of the range is for sedentary individuals; the high end of the range is for very active individuals.

In practical terms, if you're a woman eating 1,600 to 2,400 calories per day, then 10 percent fat would include about 18–27 grams of fat per day, and 15 percent fat would be about 27–40 grams of fat per day.

If you're a man eating 2,000 to 3,000 calories per day, then 10 percent fat would include about 22–33 grams of fat per day, and 15 percent fat would be about 33–50 grams of fat per day.

You only need about 4 percent of calories as fat to provide the essential fatty acids, so it's relatively hard not to get enough fat in your diet. Most people get too much.

In addition, especially try to minimize your intake of "bad fats." Trans fats are the worst, along with partially hydrogenated fats (which cause trans fats to form). Some people claim that saturated fats are not harmful, but evidence shows that they are. There is more controversy around monosaturated fats and polyunsaturated fats, but our studies and others described earlier in this chapter indicate that for reversing—undoing— chronic diseases, it's necessary to reduce the intake of *all* fats, including these.

All food labels will disclose how much fat is contained in the food. If you're eating some commercially processed foods, just keep track of how much fat you're consuming from these throughout the day.

Invest in some nonstick cookware, which makes it easier to cook without adding oil and butter. (But avoid Teflon, which may be harmful.) The recipe section of this book gives lots of examples of how to make foods taste delicious without adding extra fat and butter.

Fat is an acquired taste. Have you ever switched from drinking whole milk to low-fat or skim milk? At first, the skim milk tastes like water. After a week or two, it tastes fine—and if you go out to dinner, suddenly regular milk now tastes like cream—too rich, too greasy. The cow didn't change, but your palate adjusted. However, if you were always drinking some whole milk and some skim milk, then your palate would never have a chance to adapt.

Because of this, I find that it's paradoxically easier for people who have chronic diseases and want to reverse them to go on this reversal diet all at once rather than easing into it. In his earlier book *The Spectrum,* Dean encouraged people to make gradual changes if they're otherwise healthy—that what matters most is your *overall* way of eating and living. So, if you indulge yourself one day, eat healthier the next.

But if you're trying to reverse a life-threatening illness such as heart disease, it's actually easier to make the changes all at once, even though this may be hard to believe. Why? Because when you make big changes all at once, and because these underlying biological mechanisms we've been discussing are so dynamic, you're likely to feel so much better, so quickly, that the choices and benefits become clearer and worth making.

For example, most people who have chest pain (angina) due to heart disease find that they have much less pain—and are often pain free—within a few days to a few weeks when they closely follow our reversing heart disease program. For someone who hasn't been able to walk across the street before the light changes without getting severe chest pain, or work, or make love with their partner, or play with their kids to now find that they can do all of those things after just a short period of lifestyle change makes what they gain worth more than what they give up.

On the other hand, as described in Chapter 1, if you're only making moderate changes in what you eat, you're likely to have the worst of both worlds. You're not making changes big enough to feel that much better, but you have the hassle and deprivation of not being able to eat and do everything you want.

Therefore, if you immerse yourself in our lifestyle medicine reversal program, you're likely to feel so much better, so quickly, it makes these changes sustainable—not just to live longer (and you probably will) but also to feel better. Your palate adapts to enjoying healthier foods. After all, who wants to live longer unless you're enjoying life?

Ah, Nuts!

Although nuts and seeds are high in fat and thus in calories, we include them because numerous studies have shown that consuming these in small quantities is beneficial.

Several of the largest cohort studies, including the Adventist Study, the Iowa Women's Health Study, the Nurses' Health Study, and the Physicians' Health Study, have shown that consuming nuts and seeds correlates with a consistent 30–50 percent lower risk of cardiovascular disease, heart attacks, sudden cardiac death, and stroke.

One reason is that omega-3 fatty acids in some nuts such as walnuts help to reduce sudden cardiac death. Also, consuming nuts in small quantities reduces insulin secretion, oxidative stress, and chronic inflammation, mechanisms we've been discussing throughout this book.

In addition to these benefits, there is a germinating quality to nuts and seeds—after all, they contain concentrated energy that, when planted, can turn into a tree or plant. Although we don't have any tools in Western science to measure this "life force," other healing systems such as Ayurveda, yoga therapy, and Chinese medicine use *prana, chi, kundalini, shakti,* and other terms to describe this vital energy that is literally and figuratively packed into nuts.

One low-fat serving (around 3 grams of fat) equals any of these:

- 5 almonds
- 9 pistachios
- 1 whole walnut
- 3 pecan halves
- 2 cashews
- 6 peanuts
- 5 teaspoons of ground flaxseed
- 2 teaspoons chia seeds or shelled sunflower seeds
- 5 teaspoons pumpkin seeds

Just a Spoonful of Sugar . . .

The general consensus for sugar intake is to limit added sugars to no more than 25 grams per day (which is equivalent to 6 teaspoons) for women and less than 38 grams per day for men. Consider these as maximums; less is better.

As noted earlier, added sugars are sugars and syrups that are added to foods or beverages when they are processed or prepared. Naturally occurring sugars such as those in fruit or milk are not added sugars. Added sugars are called by many different names. An easy way to recognize sugar on a label is by recognizing the *-ose* suffix (e.g., sucrose, fructose). When you find a word that ends in *-ose* in the ingredient list, there's a good chance it is sugar. However, there are many other names for sugar that don't include *-ose:* brown sugar, corn sweetener, corn syrup and other syrups, honey, molasses, raw sugar, agave, turbinado, maltodextrin, and barley malt. To give a perspective of how much sugar this is, 1 teaspoon of sugar (or a standard sugar cube) equals 4 grams.

Eat Less Sodium

The 2015–2020 Dietary Guidelines for Americans recommends that people consume less than 2,300 milligrams (mg) of sodium per day as part of a healthy eating pattern. Less is even better, especially if you have high blood pressure, heart failure, or kidney disease. The average intake of sodium in the United States is much more than this—over 3,400 mg each day. Eating too much sodium increases the risk for high blood pressure, heart disease, and stroke.

Just 1 teaspoon of salt has 2,300 mg of sodium. Taking the salt shaker off the table is one simple strategy to minimize your sodium intake, but it is equally important to know what to look for on the label. Almost 80 percent of the salt Americans consume is hidden in processed and restaurant food. Many foods that contribute a significant amount of sodium in the diet do not taste particularly salty, such as bread and cereals. An average slice of bread can range from 80 to 230 mg of sodium, and just one serving of Kellogg's Corn Flakes contributes 200 mg.

You can also check for nutrient claims on food and beverage packages to quickly identify those that may contain less sodium. If a packaged food claims it is "low in sodium," a serving must have 140 mg or less of sodium; if it states "very low in sodium," it must have no more than 35 mg per serving. If a package notes the product is "sodium free," it can have up to 5 mg of sodium per serving.

. . . And More Fiber

The USDA's recommendation is at least 14 grams of fiber per 1,000 calories per day, which for an average intake of 2,000 calories per day is equivalent to about 25–30 grams daily. On food labels, the Daily Value (DV) shows this percentage based on 2,000 calories per day. This is a good way to use labels to check if a product is a good source of fiber. A food labeled as a "good source of fiber" provides between 10 and 19 percent of the DV of fiber per serving; a "high-fiber" food offers over 20 percent. Products low in fiber are under 10 percent of the DV.

The average intake in the United States is only 14 grams of fiber a day, which is below the USDA's recommendation. In contrast, on a typical day, the reversal diet offers closer to 40 grams.

As mentioned earlier, if all this seems a little overwhelming—so much to remember—we have curated in Appendix B a list of commercially available foods and frozen entrées that fit our guidelines and that you can order online or find in many stores. Furthermore, in Appendix A we've organized these foods into two weeks of daily shopping lists. You may even want to copy or tear out each day's list before you shop.

Raising Your Awareness About Eating: Be Mindful

For those who want to raise your awareness as to *what, why, how, where,* and *when* you eat, here are key tools, skills, and strategies to help you maintain a healthy weight while eating with greater gratification.

We've reviewed what foods are recommended for optimal health, but now it's time to consider what types of foods you enjoy the most, which foods you stock at home, and which kinds you tend to grab on the go. What kinds of snacks and meals do you make for yourself at home? Do you make food choices that nourish you and promote your health and vitality?

Mindful eating can support you in swapping out unhealthy habits and behaviors for ones that benefit your health and well-being.

Asking yourself the right questions is an effective way to be mindful about your decisions. Mindful eating can support you in swapping out unhealthy habits and behaviors for ones that benefit your health and well-being; being mindful will also deepen your awareness and make the changes needed for a healthy lifestyle. Ask yourself the five simple questions below—these will allow you to identify your eating behaviors and explore the reasons behind them.

Why Do I Eat?

Have you ever stopped to think about why you eat the way you do? When you think about it now, why do you think you eat the way you do? Is this why you've always eaten, or has it just been more recently?

The foods you eat dynamically affect how you feel, energetically and emotionally, and pretty darn quickly. Being aware of how your choices make you feel can directly inform and impact why you eat, supporting you to make healthier choices.

Being aware of how you're feeling, really feeling, allows you to determine what you really need. It's all too common to mindlessly reach for some chips when actually you're just feeling really stressed!

The key is to practice catching yourself right before succumbing to that reflex, which does come with a practice of deeper self-awareness. Tracking yourself throughout your day allows you to notice what you're really feeling, which grants you opportunities to make more satisfying choices.

You may consider taking a different kind of break, such as going for a walk or relaxing with some nice deep breathing. The chips (or whatever food may be your temptation—whatever you end up regretting) will comfort you for a minute or so, then just leave you wanting more. Unfortunately, no food will sustainably resolve your stress, sadness, anger, loneliness, or whatever feeling you're trying to escape from or numb.

Say that you usually reach for a cookie or candy in the afternoon. The next time you notice this pattern arising, pause first to mindfully check in with yourself, to see how you're really feeling. If you discover that you're actually feeling tired, instead of reaching for a quick sugar rush, which will just further fatigue you in an hour or so, experiment with going for a brisk walk or doing a yoga practice to boost your afternoon vitality.

To further explore this idea, try this practice: Close your eyes just for a moment to center yourself with a couple of full-body breaths. Ask yourself: "How am I feeling?" Give yourself the space to witness whatever arises. Take another couple of natural breaths, then ask yourself again: "How am I really feeling, right now, in this moment?" If there are mixed layers or traces of anger, sadness, fear, or guilt, perhaps along with contentment, gratitude, or calm, try to connect with the strongest, most prevailing feeling that you can sense.

Now, try to better identify your true needs as you ask yourself again, "What do I really need right now? Is it a cookie or a hug that I actually need? Is it chips or an energizing walk? Is it ice cream or some rest?"

Gently open your eyes as you exhale, relax, and reflect on another aspect of *why* you eat. Ask yourself, "Am I ready to make the necessary changes in my eating patterns to achieve my health goals?" As you reflect on your answer, find sustenance in knowing just how powerful it can be to reframe and realign *why* you eat with your determination to achieve your health goals. It imbues them with meaning while sustaining your overall way of living with a greater sense of reward and purpose.

Your self-awareness empowers you to notice your thoughts, feelings, and behaviors and discern those that are serving you from those that are not. Identifying your authentic feelings and aligning your life with a personal sense of meaning can powerfully guide you to healthier ways of nourishing yourself with what you really need.

When Do I Eat?

Eat when you're hungry. That may sound obvious, but so often people eat because of the time or the taste rather than their tummy.

Take a moment to reflect on your eating patterns to see if you can recognize what typically prompts you to eat. This also relates back to noticing why you eat. Do you sense that it is because of your body's hunger cues or familiar cravings? How often do you find that you eat because it's time—it's a lunch break, it's time for a family dinner, or you looked at the clock? Do you find yourself simply eating out of boredom or just to be with friends and family?

It's advantageous to notice the difference between your physical hunger and your emotional hunger. Emotional hunger can get triggered when your emotions get out of balance, like when you haven't eaten or you're feeling stressed or tired. At best, eating can temporarily numb your feelings and give you a quick food-high surge. Just remember that this pleasure and relief are only momentary.

Do you ever notice that when you're feeling anxious or angry, your cravings can feel like an unstoppable eruption? If so, compassionately notice under what circumstances emotional eating appears in your life. Do you eat to calm your nerves, to make yourself feel insulated and nurtured? We all have patterns; they're often created unconsciously to help us cope, to help us get through uncomfortable feelings and challenging experiences. What's productive now is that you take the time to reassess your patterns and empower yourself with greater awareness, compassion, and conscious choice.

The Hunger-Fullness Scale

The Hunger-Fullness Scale is an excellent tool for noticing when you're satisfied and help you stop short of overindulging. We recommend that you aim toward eating more in the 4–7 range, which will also help with optimizing your portions, blood sugar balance, and energy level.

1 Ravenous

2 Overly hungry

3 Hunger pangs

4 Hunger awakens

5 Neutral

6 Just satisfied

7 Completely satisfied

8 Full

9 Stuffed

10 Sick

The more aware you become of how you're feeling, the more readily you can distinguish between your physical hunger cues and your emotional triggers and begin to repattern your responses. You can develop an emotional tool bag for yourself—such as "When I feel stressed, I can use deep breathing and meditation to relax me," or "When I'm feeling sad or lonely, I can reach out to connect with a friend," or "When I am tired, I just need to get some rest." A few self-informed tools like this will go a long way toward making you feel well equipped, supported, and empowered when the urge to eat comes on.

When you practice eating mindfully, you're able to tune up your awareness to detect your hunger signals before they hijack you. Eating balanced meals and snacks on a regular basis provides the energy and fuel you need to think clearly and remain active throughout your day. This way of eating will provide you with the energy you need to move more, stress less, and love more.

Where Do I Eat?

Where do you find yourself typically eating while you're at home, at work, or out and about? Do you eat sitting at the dining table, while cooking your dinner, or simply standing up in the kitchen? Do you eat while you're working at or surfing around on your computer, or in front of the TV? Do you eat in your bed, or in your car while commuting?

Eating while sitting down and being present in a comfortable dining space is also significant in supporting you to make and maintain healthy choices. Your environment can have a compelling influence on how you feel, how you eat, and what you eat. When people eat in front of a TV, studies show, they eat 40 percent more, yet enjoy the food less.

Eating Out

Keep it simple! If you go to almost any restaurant, just ask the server to bring you a plate of whatever the chef thinks are the freshest and most delicious vegetables, legumes, and fruits on hand—you can ask for something even if it's not on the menu. Ask them to steam or stir-fry the vegetables without oil, butter, or sugar and to put any sauces on the side. Or ask for a beautiful salad with the dressing on the side. You can do this without drawing any added attention to yourself—you don't need to feel like you're Meg Ryan in *When Harry Met Sally*. ("I'll have what she's having. . . .") I often find that when my food comes, the people I'm with say, "Hey, that looks great—I didn't see that on the menu!"

With these simple tips, your new lifestyle won't keep you from dining out at your favorite restaurants and on the road.

- *Look for vegetarian restaurants.* When you're searching online, you can use certain keywords, such as "vegetarian," "vegan," or "plant-based," to further refine your selection of restaurants. You may be surprised to discover how many options you'll have. There are several handy apps that can also help you locate vegetarian restaurants, even on the road, such as Happy Cow, which searches vegetarian restaurants by location. It's often helpful to review the restaurant's menu online and plan in advance.
- *Choose favorite restaurants and try to dine at off-peak times.* Servers and chefs are often more accommodating when they are not super-

busy. Once you begin to use your new knowledge and skills in selecting restaurants and choosing food from the menu, you will begin to discover restaurants that you like and that can best accommodate your needs. If you frequent them often, it may be surprising how well they remember you and your requests (in a good way).

- *Avoid waiting to eat until you're really hungry.* Have you ever found yourself checking out at the market or going out to eat when you're ravished with hunger? Let's just say it is far more challenging to make healthy choices when you're in a famished state. Do yourself a favor and try to avoid shopping at the market or arriving at a restaurant overly hungry.

- *Bring your own.* If you know you're going to be dining out, you may find it convenient to bring travel-sized containers with your own dressing, sauce, or protein such as tofu, tempeh, or beans—but, of course, it's not necessary to do so.

- *Ask about how food is prepared.* Just because you're at a vegetarian restaurant doesn't mean that every dish on the menu is nutritionally balanced and low in fat. Always ask the key questions (in the next box) and don't be shy about requesting substitutions. For example, instead of french fries or other unhealthy sides, ask for a salad with nonfat salad dressing, or balsamic vinegar and lemon; a side of steamed or dry-roasted veggies; or fresh fruit. Review the menu, especially the specific ingredients and the sides, to see what is available so that you can ask for options and additions based on your needs and preferences.

- *Take some home.* Whenever you're served a large meal while dining out, avoid overeating by transferring a portion into a takeout container to bring home (most restaurants will provide one). It's convenient to have a healthy meal on hand the next day! In that spirit, you may find it helpful to place tempting items such as chips or buttered bread out of reach or remove them from the table.

Key Questions to Ask When Ordering from a Menu

How is the menu item prepared?

Do you use oil, butter, or other added fats?

Is it baked, fried, steamed, or roasted?

Can you please prepare this steamed, baked, or dry-roasted?

What comes with it?

Are the vegetables prepared with oil or butter?

Is oil or butter added to the sauce? (Even ask about such sauces as marinara, teriyaki, or black bean sauce.)

Is oil or butter added to the pasta?

Is the pasta made with egg?

Is whole-grain bread available?

Is brown rice available?

Is there nonfat salad dressing available, or can you provide balsamic vinegar or a fresh lemon wedge?

Are soups prepared in a meat, chicken, or seafood stock?

Is there cream or milk added?

Can you please provide healthy sides such as salad, steamed vegetables, fruit, or a plain baked potato?

Can you please give me whole-grain bread, brown rice, or whole-wheat or corn tortillas instead of their refined white counterparts?

You can also ask if menu items can be prepared differently. Politely ask if the chef could sauté the vegetables using vegetable stock. You could say, "Could I ask the chef to please sauté some mushrooms and chopped tomatoes with garlic and vegetable stock to serve over pasta?" Once your order is taken, kindly ask the server to repeat back his or her understanding of your order—everyone wants the dining experience to go well!

Tips for Ordering from Any Restaurant Menu
Here are the best things to order from just about any kind of restaurant menu while maintaining your healthy way of eating.

Mexican

- Make your own tacos, tostados, or burritos by ordering a variety of sides:
    - Black or pinto beans (ask for no oil or lard)
    - Corn tortillas
    - Dry-sautéed or steamed vegetables (ask for no oil)
    - Seasoned rice (no oil)
    - Salsa
    - Gazpacho
    - Shredded lettuce
- Taco salad: lettuce, beans

Steak House

- Baked potato stuffed with steamed broccoli and freshly diced tomatoes
- A dinner salad with nonfat salad dressing, balsamic vinegar, or lemon wedges (you can also bring your own salad dressing in a small container)
- A side of whatever beans are available there, for added protein
- Steamed or roasted vegetables without oil or butter (you can also bring your own favorite sauce from home to top them)
- An oil-free or low-fat tomato/marinara sauce for pasta

Italian

- Salad with nonfat dressing or vinegar (add white beans or chickpeas if available, for protein; ask if not on the menu)
- Minestrone (ask how the soup is prepared and what the ingredients are)
- Pasta (whole-grain if available)
    - With tomato sauce (no added oil)
    - Add tomatoes, garlic, or roasted or steamed vegetables (no added oil)

- Add dried or fresh herbs such as basil if available
- Add white beans or chickpeas if available; ask if not on the menu
- Vegan pizza (without cheese or oil)
  - Ask if they can just add pizza sauce or tomato sauce
  - Add veggies: mushrooms, tomatoes, onions, bell peppers, spinach, arugula, herbs such as fresh basil
  - For extra spice and flavor, sprinkle with red pepper flakes

Asian

- Miso soup
- Vegan sushi roll (no avocado)
- Vegan spring roll (not fried, in rice paper, no avocado)
- Steamed vegetables and tofu over rice
  - Ask for steamed, not fried or sautéed in oil
  - Ask if they have brown rice
  - Stay away from oil-based sauces such as sweet-and-sour sauce or black bean sauce
  - Ask for low-sodium soy sauce (unless you're on a sodium-restricted diet)

Indian

- Vegetable and tofu curry with steamed rice
- Lentils
- Pair chutney, a delicious condiment, with a curry or lentils
- Roti, chapatti, or naan

Traveling

Here are some highly adaptable strategies to bring your lifestyle with you wherever you go.

Be Mindful

Overall, remember to practice mindfulness and self-awareness wherever you are:

- Think about the moments and people that inspire you to be alive, healthy, and thriving—presently and in the future. These imbue your choices with meaning.
- Reaffirm your health goals and the healthy lifestyle choices that provide the greatest benefits.
- Feel proud of taking care of your health.
- Focus on what you choose to include, rather than what you choose to exclude.

Plan Ahead

Be prepared to make sure your needs are met:

- Pack lots of snacks and even instant meals. Bring dressings and sauces in travel-sized containers.
- Research the local restaurants that fit your needs and preferences.
- Research your destination's food scene.
- Request a refrigerator in your hotel room and stock it with your favorite healthy foods.
- Bring along travel-sized containers for your homemade salad dressing.

International Travel

If you're going abroad, you'll need to do a little extra work in advance.

- Research the cuisine of the culture you'll encounter.
- Know some key phrases in the destination language so that you can ask for special preparations and understand ingredients.
- Download a diet translator app that can translate the names of foods and dietary restrictions.

Pack Snacks That Travel Well

Choose snacks that aren't too perishable:

- Fresh produce, such as spiced vegetable sticks made with carrot, celery, jicama, etc.
- Hummus with carrots

- Nonfat plain yogurt with fresh fruit
- Edamame
- Roasted sweet potatoes or cauliflower
- Baked sweet potato
- Baked tofu
- Fresh fruit, such as apples, peaches, apricots, bananas, etc.

Dry snacks are also great for traveling:

- Dry roasted soy nuts/edamame
- Low-fat, low-sugar granola (less than 3 grams of fat and sugar per serving)
- Dried apricots and dried mango (no added oils, sugar, or preservatives)
- Instant soups
- Small to-go soy milks in aseptic cartons
- Energy bars: Clif Kid ZBar (honey graham), NuGgoZbar (Honey Graham), Nugo (check for the ones under 3 grams of fat)
- Instant whole grains: oatmeal, quinoa, brown rice

How Do I Eat?

You may be asking yourself, "What do you mean, 'how do I eat'? I eat through my mouth and digestive system, of course!"

However, in our high-tech, fast-paced society, exploring your eating patterns and process can be eye-opening. In fact, it's as important to be aware of *how* you eat as it is to be aware of as *what* you eat. It allows you to become more aware of your hunger so that you can sense feeling satisfied before you've become too full, which also supports better digestion.

Enhancing how you eat has a substantial influence on how much pleasure and nourishment your food can provide you. When you give your full attention to what you're eating, you enjoy it much more fully.

Digestion starts in your mouth, so chewing is essential for adequate assimilation and digestion, beginning with the saliva in your mouth. You may find that the more you chew, the less you eat. Have you ever noticed a diminishing return of pleasure after the novelty of your first few bites? Thoroughly chewing your food also plays a rich role in your sense of satiation. Slowing down your way of eating goes a long way in supporting mindful eating and allowing you to more fully enjoy your food.

To bring mindful eating to life for yourself, begin by getting centered in your chair and placing both of your feet on the ground. Close your eyes and take three slow, full-body breaths. As you slowly open your eyes, gaze down at your food as you take a moment to feel gratitude.

You'll begin by recruiting your senses into your eating experience, invoking them one by one so as to be fully present for the many pleasures waiting for you along the way. Start by simply observing what you're about to eat, noticing its shape, its color, your anticipation of its flavors. Next explore how it feels to touch it. What's the texture? Its weight? Now go ahead and simply smell it; sense the wafting of its flavors as they enter your nose.

For these next few steps, really relish each of them, as if you were doing so in sensual slow motion. First, lightly lick the food, and then let it simply rest on your tongue for a moment before chewing. Notice as saliva is secreted from the corners of your mouth, and appreciate how it enlivens a swirl of flavors in your mouth. Slowly begin to roll the food around the different areas of your mouth for a moment more before letting your teeth sink into the food.

As you slowly begin to chew, try to chew until you no longer can, until only liquid flavors are left; then swallow. Continue to slowly feed yourself small bites, savoring each one anew, noticing the confluence of sweet, sour, bitter, salty, and umami (savory) tastes on your palate. Simply slowing down to savor the entire process can heighten your senses and more deeply nourish your whole being.

Try experimenting with some form of this practice during each meal to support you in cultivating more mindful eating in your daily life. Take a moment to pause before you eat, to take a couple of deep, nurturing breaths, to center and allow yourself to be present in the moment. Appreciate the look, touch, smell, and tastes of each bite with your full array of senses. You can further stimulate your senses by simply setting your fork down between bites, to be as present as possible to experience what's already in your mouth. Try to set aside at least twenty minutes per meal to make it feel spacious.

When you pay attention to what you're eating—that is, when you eat mindfully—you get more pleasure with fewer calories. Conversely, if you eat while watching TV, you may look down at the plate and discover that it's empty because your attention was focused on the show instead of what was in your mouth. You got all the calories without much of the pleasure.

When you eat mindfully, you also become more aware of your hunger signs in such a way that your cravings tend to diminish. Ultimately, we've found that eating instincts can get recalibrated with mindfulness, so you wind up eating what you need, and even much of what you want, yet not overly so.

Just remember to ask yourself, "How much do I really need to satisfy my physical hunger and feel nourished? How much do I really need to eat in this moment?" Factor in how active you've been and are in general, as this will affect how efficiently you metabolize your food. This is easier to achieve when you're able to routinely enjoy smaller meals and snacks, instead of oversized meals once or twice per day. It also helps to keep your blood sugar more constant.

Planning ahead is key to success in so many areas of our life and essential for making healthy eating choices. Regularly preparing balanced meals and quick snacks to support you throughout your day and eating generally every three to four hours allow you to eat consistently well while providing you with the nutrition, nourishment, and energy you need.

Using smaller plates is another simple way you can support yourself in choosing optimal portions. Remember, it's quite handy to have leftovers, especially if you put them away in ready-to-eat portions. Staying well hydrated also assists in keeping cravings at bay, while cleansing your body from the inside out.

You're likely to feel and look noticeably better because your mood is more balanced when your blood sugar and brain chemistry are more balanced. Our program participants often experience that eating more mindfully leads to feeling more energy even while eating less overall, which leads to naturally losing excess weight and sustaining a healthy weight. Maintain a more consistent, vibrant energy by supersizing your mood, not your food.

You may be wondering, "How am I going to eat in this way when I'm out, or when I'm socializing or entertaining?" Don't worry! It's very common, especially in the beginning, to feel concerned or even anxious when you're eating with others. After all, this way of eating is new to you and those around you—it takes a little while for everyone to get used to it. Know that it is completely normal to have these feelings, and it's also natural to feel tempted to go along with those around you—to begin justifying why it's okay to fall off the wagon for just one meal, for just a holiday, a weekend, and so on.

It may be worth repeating, because it's so easy to get lost in complexity when you can keep it really simple: Even if it's not on the menu, just ask the waiter, "Please ask the chef to steam or stir-fry me a plate of your freshest vegetables and legumes without any added oil, butter, or sugar and to put any sauces on the side." Or ask for a "beautiful salad with the dressing on the side." Most restaurants will accommodate you—and often your friends will say, "That looks good, I didn't see it on the menu."

In such moments, remember to pause, to take a deep, nurturing breath, and reconnect with yourself in the present moment. Feel into your body and heart so that you can realign with the courage and commitment to support your health—and your life. Remind yourself that the longer you continue to live this healthy lifestyle, the better you'll feel, the easier it will become to stay the course, and the more likely it will be that you'll be around to enjoy socializing with your friends and family for a long time to come! It's powerful to practice refocusing on being with those around you by tapping into intimate social connections instead of having food be the focus. You may even inspire others to be healthier.

Here are some examples of how you could transmute common feelings that may arise as you adopt this healthy way of eating:

> "I haven't felt or looked this great in twenty years; I hope I can inspire my friends. I'm ready to start a support group so we can make living this way more fun together."
> "That steak sure looks tempting, but I know I'll feel better if I eat healthier, so I'm going to make a better choice. Besides, there are so many other delicious options."

Here are some other common feelings you may experience when socializing. See how you can practice reflecting and reframing your responses, transforming these challenges into opportunities to feel healthier and happier.

From: "I'm afraid I'm going to feel deprived at this dinner party, that there won't be anything for me to eat."

To: "I'm going to prepare my favorite dish and share it at the dinner party, so that I can enjoy eating with everyone else."

From: "My friends are not going to want to go out with me anymore when they see I'm not partaking in the same way with them."

To: "I'm just going to relax and have fun. No one is going to even notice what I order. Just be present, and enjoy being out and authentically connecting with my friends."

From: "I'm going to feel awkward, like I'm missing out during the toast at this event with my colleagues and friends."

To: "If I want to enjoy the toast, I can always enjoy one glass of whatever they're serving—then I'll just transition into enjoying sparkling water out of a wine or champagne glass to feel festive."

From: "I'm nervous about going on this trip—it's going to be so hard for me to eat along the way."

To: "I'm packing plenty of snacks for my trip, and I've identified several great local dining options and grocery stores."

If you enjoy socializing and entertaining, or even if you entertain for your business, it can be a great way to share your healthy way of living with others without proselytizing. The Ornish Kitchen recipes (see Chapter 8) give you dozens of appetizers, main courses, and even decadent desserts that you can prepare and share. A taco bar is another crowd-pleasing way to entertain. There are dozens of delicious recipes in this book for summer cookouts and for entertaining during the holidays. No one even needs to know that all the food is healthy; they will just enjoy how yummy all of the food tastes and how good they feel after eating it.

CHAPTER 5

Move More

The best things in life make you sweaty.
—Anonymous

Dean

You already know that exercise is good for you. What you may not know is just how amazingly beneficial it is, and how even a little exercise goes a very long way.

There are three basic types of exercise we recommend for just about everyone: aerobic exercise (e.g., walking), strength training (e.g., with resistance bands or lifting weights), and stretching.

In the spirit of keeping it simple, here's the bottom line about exercise: *if you like it, you'll do it.* Make it a "playout" rather than a workout. So find a type of exercise you enjoy doing in each of these three categories, and "just do it" regularly to "undo it." Everything else is a refinement of this idea.

In short: do what you enjoy, make it fun, and do it regularly. The rest is commentary.

This chapter also illustrates one of the other main themes of this book: exercise has multiple benefits because it mitigates each of the underlying mechanisms that cause chronic diseases, as described in Chapter 2.

It's not like you need to do one type of exercise to reverse heart disease, another type of exercise to reverse early-stage prostate cancer, or to lower your blood pressure, weight, cholesterol, or blood sugar levels.

You already know that exercise helps you lose weight, stay healthy, look younger, and feel better. Here are some of the many other benefits of exercise.

Exercise Helps You Live Longer

The greatest increase in longevity occurs when you go from being sedentary to doing even a little exercise every day.

For example, going from being sedentary to just walking twenty to thirty minutes per day can cut premature death rates by 20–30 percent. Another study found that walking thirty minutes five times per week reduced premature deaths by 20 percent and walking sixty minutes five times per week reduced premature deaths by 31 percent, but more intensive exercise had only incremental additional benefit in reducing mortality. Just twenty-five minutes of brisk walking a day can add as much as seven years to your life.

In the Women's Health Study involving tens of thousands of women, those who walked briskly for just sixty to ninety minutes each week— just fifteen minutes a day—cut their risk of death from heart attack and stroke in half.

But there are benefits to more intensive exercise. One of the most practical is that you can achieve most of the longevity benefits of exercise in only five minutes a day if you run instead of walk.

In one study of over 55,000 adults, eighteen to a hundred years of age, runners gained about three extra years of life compared with sedentary adults. Amazingly, these benefits were about the same whether someone ran five minutes a day or thirty minutes a day, and even at a relatively leisurely pace of ten minutes a mile or slower.

Put another way, running, whatever the pace or mileage, dropped a person's risk of premature death by almost 40 percent, a benefit that held true even when the researchers controlled for smoking, drinking, and a history of health problems such as hypertension or obesity. For every hour you spend running, you gain seven hours in your life expectancy—up to three additional years of life.

A word of caution. The risks of exercise—both musculoskeletal injury and sudden cardiac death—are directly related to the intensity. Walking gives many of the health benefits of more intensive exercise while minimizing the risks. While seven-minute high-intensity workouts appeal to busy people and may be safe for those in good shape, I'm concerned that these may create problems in some people with chronic diseases who may be vulnerable. "Slow but steady wins the race" is true both literally and figuratively. Consult with your doctor before doing high-intensity workouts, especially if you have a chronic disease.

Exercise also lengthens your telomeres. As described in Chapter 2, telomeres are the structures at the ends of your chromosomes that regulate cellular aging. As your telomeres get shorter, your life gets shorter and the risk of premature death from just about everything increases correspondingly.

People who have consistently high levels of physical activity have significantly longer telomeres than those who have sedentary lifestyles, and even longer than those who are moderately active. In one study, adults with high physical activity levels had a biologic aging advantage of nine years when compared to those who were sedentary, and seven years compared to those who were moderately active. The researchers defined "highly active" as engaging in thirty to forty minutes of jogging per day, five days a week. In other words, exercise has an anti-aging effect at a molecular level.

In another study, scientists studied men and women between the ages of fifty-five and seventy-nine who had been cycling for decades and still pedaled about four hundred miles per month. None were competitive athletes. They were biologically younger than their chronological age. Their muscles generally retained their size, fiber composition, and other markers of good health across the decades. Those riders who covered the most mileage each month displayed the healthiest muscles, whatever their age. They had an immune system, reflexes, memories, balance, and metabolic profiles that more closely resembled those of thirty-year-olds than those of the sedentary older group.

Chronic emotional stress can shorten telomeres, but exercise can also help prevent this from happening. Those who were sedentary experienced telomere shortening when feeling stressed, but those who exercised for at least fourteen minutes a day saw little to no change in telomere length even if they were stressed. In other words, cross-sectional stories showed that exercise buffered the effects of stress on their telomeres. A new study tested the effect of exercise on highly stressed elderly who were all caring for a partner with dementia. Six months of activity led to significant telomere lengthening compared to a control group.

Postmenopausal women who exercised for at least sixty minutes three or more times per week for about a year and a half had significantly longer telomeres than their sedentary peers. It showed the positive effects of both aerobic and resistance exercise.

Since identical twins have the same DNA, a study of twins and telomeres was especially interesting. Researchers found that twins who were active during leisure time were found to have longer telomeres than their inactive siblings. These findings were still significant after controlling for age, sex, nonsmoking status, weight, and physical activity at work. Again, our genes are a predisposition, but our genes are not our fate.

Exercise Makes You Happier

Even small amounts of exercise make you happier. A 2018 review of twenty-three studies with 500,000 people ranging in age from adolescents to the very old and covering a broad range of ethnic and socioeconomic groups found that exercise was strongly linked to happiness. Every one of these studies showed a beneficial relationship between being physically active and being happy.

It didn't take much—just ten minutes a week of exercise was linked with being happier! And those who worked out only once or twice a week said they felt much happier than those who never exercised. Those who worked out thirty minutes a day showed even greater benefits. Both aerobic exercise and stretching/balancing exercises were effective in improving happiness.

Even a very busy person can find ten minutes a week to exercise!

In another study, researchers pooled data from over a million men and women and found that those with the lowest fitness were 76 percent more likely to have been given diagnoses of depression than the people with the greatest fitness. The men and women in the middle third were 23 percent more likely to develop depression than those who were the most fit. In Chapter 7 we'll discuss why this is especially meaningful.

In addition to helping prevent depression, exercise can treat it—with results often equal to or even greater than a lifetime of antidepressants. A review of twenty-five randomized controlled trials concluded that "exercise had a large and significant effect on depression," in both mild and major depressive disorders. The effects were even stronger if the exercise was supervised or if the participants exercised in groups (in other words, exercise is even more beneficial in treating depression if you do it with someone else).

Even a single bout of exercise increases beneficial hormones that cause your arteries to dilate, bringing more blood flow to your brain (and everywhere else) and reducing biomarkers of inflammation.

Strength training also reduces and helps prevent depression—lifting weights lifts your mood. A 2018 meta-analysis of thirty-three clinical trials documented that men and women doing resistance exercise training consistently had fewer symptoms of depression, whether or not they were depressed at the beginning of the study. That is, if they were depressed when they began, they were less depressed after, and if they weren't depressed when they started, they had a lower chance of becoming depressed.

The frequency and amount of weight training did not seem to matter. The benefits essentially were the same whether people went to the gym twice a week or five times a week and whether they were completing lots of repetitions of each exercise or only a few. The benefits were the same for men and women, young, middle-aged, or elderly. Again, a little exercise goes a long way.

The researchers concluded that resistance exercise training is "an alternative and/or adjuvant therapy for depressive symptoms."

Exercise Makes Your Brain Bigger and Smarter!

Exercise makes you smarter. At any age.

Children who exercise in school have better grades and learn more easily. They show improvement in a broad variety of skills ranging from math to logic to reading. Similar results were obtained in young adults after twelve weeks of aerobic training.

And the benefits of exercising when you're young continue as you get older. Those who are physically active between ages fifteen and twenty-five process information faster when they become sixty-two to eighty-five years old. Although studies vary regarding the duration, intensity, and type of exercise, overall physical activity improves cognitive function in people of all ages. People who are fit are more likely to remember words and names than those who are not. Part of the reason for this is that exercise increases autophagy, which removes toxic substances from inside your cells, especially in your brain.

Fathers who exercise—even if they don't begin working out until they're adults—have smarter babies. They pass some of the brain benefits of physical activity to their children through a process called epigenetics. That is, exercise changes the brains and sperm of male animals in ways that later affect the brains and thinking skills of their offspring.

It doesn't even take very much exercise to enhance how well you think. Just standing instead of sitting makes a difference. In one study, people who were standing performed better on a test that measured selective attention than those who were seated—giving new meaning to the expression "thinking on your feet."

When I was in medical school, we were taught that you're born with a finite number of brain cells and that's all you get. If you go out and have a couple of six-packs and kill off a few thousand brain cells, you never get them back.

But here's some (literally) mind-blowing good news—your brain, like the rest of your body, has a remarkable capacity to begin healing—that is, to undo damage—if you stop doing what's causing the problem.

When you practice the lifestyle medicine program described in this book, including exercise, you can grow so many new brain cells—called neurogenesis—that your brain can get measurably bigger.

Even better news is that the part of your brain that controls memory—called the hippocampus—gets bigger. When people age, they often say,

"Where did I leave my keys?" or "What was that person's name again?" A lot of this memory loss is reversible.

For example, a randomized controlled trial of 120 older adults found that those who walked for forty minutes three times a week for a year had brain growth in the hippocampus and, as a result, improvement in their memory and cognitive function. In contrast, the brains in the comparison group who were not walking actually shrank.

Another study found that men and women with mild cognitive impairment (a precursor to Alzheimer's disease) who exercised four times a week over a six-month period (treadmill, stationary bike, or elliptical machine) experienced an increase in gray matter volume as measured by MRI and an improvement in cognitive function. In contrast, the control group showed some brain atrophy and worsening in cognitive function.

Similar findings were documented in another randomized controlled trial. After six months, those doing moderate aerobic exercise had significant increases in brain volume in both gray matter and white matter regions.

How does this happen? Exercise causes new neurons to be born, and also new connections between neurons to be made. This allows you to encode or develop new learning and memory and also provides a new vascular structure. Besides increasing the size of your hippocampus, exercise makes the connections between your neurons work more effectively and also brings more blood flow to your brain.

One of the mediators of this is a protein called brain-derived neurotrophin factor (BDNF), which stimulates neurogenesis and new connections between neurons in your brain. It fuels almost all the activities that lead to higher thought. With regular exercise, the body builds up its levels of BDNF, and the brain's nerve cells start to branch out, join together, and communicate with each other in new ways. This is the process that underlies learning: every change in the junctions between brain cells signifies a new fact or skill that's been picked up and stowed away for future use. BDNF makes that process possible. Brains with more BDNF have a greater capacity for understanding and higher cognitive function.

"It's not just a matter of slowing down the aging process," says Dr. Arthur Kramer, a research psychologist at the University of Illinois. "It's a matter of reversing it."

Lifestyle medicine, anyone?

Anne

What kinds of associations do you have with exercising? When was the last time you got a good workout? What kind of activity were you doing? Is this something you do on a regular basis? How did it make you feel in your body while you were doing it? What was your accompanying attitude throughout the experience? Were you alone or with others? Do you remember what kind of energy and mood you had afterward?

Whether you dread exercise, live to get out there and do it again, or are somewhere in between, here are some considerations to help you *move more*.

Keep it simple. Here's the essence:

1. Do activities that feel fun and energizing.
2. Do them regularly (but not more than feels comfortable on any given day).
3. Reward yourself.
4. If possible, exercise with someone else.

In that spirit, moving your body should make you feel good, not in pain. As Dean said earlier, "If it's fun, it's sustainable! If you don't enjoy it, you won't do it—at least not for long."

Can you think of activities that do feel or have felt good, even enlivening, when you're doing them—even if it was a long time ago? Note which activities come to mind. When is the last time you felt that way? How often would you like to move and feel that way? Are there other activities that you've entertained? Perhaps you have a friend who does it and has asked you to join, or perhaps you've heard of something that just sounds fun!

On the other hand, are there any ways that you move your body or activities that you do that don't feel good? Ask yourself: "What activities have made me feel uncomfortable, even in pain? What makes it worse? What helps? Are there ways to modify how I do those activities? Do I need to do them at all?"

If possible, exercise with a friend—after all, everything is better with a friend! It's like having the benefits of a trainer—you'll do it because they're with you—without having to pay for one. Even attending a class can really amp up the fun factor, and you get the benefits of social support as well.

You might find it's engaging to up the ante, so to speak, by implementing a personal reward system. Say your goal is to work out for thirty to forty minutes each day. Think of a worthwhile reward that you could grant yourself every day after you reach your goal. Honor yourself by coming up with an enticing reward, something that will act as a tantalizing "carrot" in tandem with your workout "stick"!

Dean and I have a contest going periodically where whoever exercises the most that week gets to request a special favor from the other in any aspect of our lives together and know that it will be granted. (The imagination runs wild. . . .) Works for us!

Lastly, listening to music is my go-to when it comes to making exercise (and life in general) more entertaining. I highly recommend pairing your activities with music whenever possible; it gets me out of my head and into my body, transforming any regular activity into more of a dance, with a bop here, a slide there. It becomes a fun way to relax, let loose, and liven up. What songs do this for you? You may enjoy compiling your own Move More soundtrack with some of your favorites while discovering some new ones by swapping songs with your family and friends.

What Do You Mean, *Move* More?

There are three types of exercise, and each brings its own benefits, which are synergistic with all of the others:

- Aerobic exercise
- Resistance (strength) training
- Stretching for flexibility

Here are a few guidelines for all three types of exercise:

- Always warm up before exercise, and gradually cool down when finishing.
- After eating, wait one to two hours or more before exercising.

- Discuss with your doctor how changes in your medication may affect your exercise routine, and how exercising may affect the need for medications.
- Be careful of temperature extremes.
- Avoid overexertion; you should be able to talk while exercising.
- Stay hydrated.
- Dress appropriately and invest in a good pair of shoes, which makes it more fun and safe to exercise.
- Don't exercise when you're not feeling well.
- Exercise indoors if it's cold or if there is smog or smoke.
- If you have heart disease, get a prescription from your doctor or from an exercise physiologist to let you know what a safe heart rate is for you and how and when to measure it.
- If you are diabetic, monitor your blood glucose levels before, during, and after exercising.
- Good form (e.g., keeping your back straight, bending your knees slightly) helps to prevent injuries.

Aerobic Exercise

Aerobic exercise gives you more stamina and numerous other benefits as well. It is continuous motion during a period of time that involves your large muscle groups. Examples include walking, running, biking, dancing, rowing, basketball, swimming, and so on. Great sex can be aerobic as well as intimate if it makes you sweat.

The intensity of your exercise will depend on your health and your conditioning. A good rule of thumb is to exercise hard enough so that you can talk while doing it, but not so easily that you're able to sing. As you get in shape, you'll be able to do progressively more before you reach that point.

Most studies indicate that at least three hours per week gives the best outcomes. I find it helpful to do an hour three times per week or thirty minutes six times per week. The more you move, the more you improve.

It doesn't have to be all at once. Aim for gradual progress based on where you are starting from, your medical history, and your fitness goals. Remember to always warm up and cool down.

And you can incorporate exercise into your daily life as well—for example, walk to work or to the store, take the stairs instead of the elevator, park a little farther away from wherever you're going (which has the added benefit of reducing stress because you can find a parking spot more easily). If you use the moving sidewalks at airports, *keep walking* whenever possible. If you're riding the bus or subway, get off a stop or two early and walk the rest of the way if you can spare the time. If you play golf, walk instead of riding in a golf cart. You get the idea.

Stretching

Stretching helps keep you flexible and avoid injury. Your mind affects your body: when you're stressed, the muscles in your body tense and contract to protect your inner organs during times of danger. When the stresses are chronic, the tension becomes chronic, often leading to back pain, neck pain, and more stress in a vicious cycle.

Just as your mind affects your body, your body also affects your mind. So when you stretch chronically tensed muscles slowly and gently, you allow both your body and mind to relax. Stretching should remain unforced and gentle; the focus is on moving with the control and grace of a dancer rather than a Marine drill instructor. More on this in Chapter 6.

Resistance Training

Resistance training makes you strong. Your lean muscle mass naturally decreases as you get older. So does your bone density. Resistance training helps prevent these and increases both the strength and size of your muscles. Use it or lose it!

When you lift weights or use resistance bands, you cause microscopic tears in your muscle fibers. It is during the recovery from the resistance exercise, when your muscle is repairing microscopic damage, that the muscle rebuilds and your muscles get stronger. When you increase the number of repetitions (reps), you increase glycogen storage in your muscles, which makes them bigger.

Doing resistance training no more than two or three times per week is optimal for most people, as it allows your muscles to rest, recover, heal, and grow on the days you're not exercising. So avoid back-to-back days, and vary your routine.

Muscles improve from resistance training through being overloaded— that is, working harder than they are accustomed to doing. If the overload is too much, it may be more than your body can adapt to and the chance of injury increases. But do slightly more than usual—through a heavier resistance, a different exercise, more repetitions, more sets, or a different angle of resistance—and your muscles improve.

Resistance training is based on both the amount of weight and the number of repetitions. Warm up for five to ten minutes. Choose a weight that allows you to do no fewer than eight and no more than fifteen repetitions per set. Do fewer reps with more weight to gain muscle size and strength; do more reps with less weight to gain muscle endurance. In either case, choose a weight that barely allows you to finish the last rep, as that's where the beneficial effects are the greatest.

Make your movements slow and controlled throughout the process. This will give you much better outcomes as well as decreasing the risk of injury. Breathe in as you contract, and exhale as you relax. Different areas of your body will require different weights. Stop if you have any pain or light-headedness.

You may want to invest in a set of free weights or elastic bands, but you can get the same benefit from lifting cans of food or plastic bottles of water.

In the spirit of keeping it simple, safe, and affordable, we found that elastic resistance bands (e.g., TheraBand) are worth considering for resistance training. Plus, you can take the bands with you when you travel, along with a pair of walking shoes. (Many hotels have gyms as well.) Enjoy walking and exploring new places.

Switch It Up

The exercises illustrated in the Resistance Band Programs A and B provide a comprehensive program utilizing resistance tubing. To anchor the middle of the tubing, many tubes are supplied with a figure-eight fabric loop, or loop the tubing around a sturdy, fixed structure. This program is light on leg exercise, as most aerobic exercise, which you should also be doing, utilizes the legs and involves a strength component. When you begin any movement with the band, make sure that the band has some tension in it to avoid sudden jerking, which may cause injury.

Since muscles improve through new challenges, it's best not to repeat the same exercises over and over using the same resistance. By following that repetitive pattern you would see initial improvement when the exercises are relatively new, but progress would plateau within a month or two.

So change your routine every month, switching from Program A to Program B, then back again. To add variety and change the muscle challenge, you can also change the resistance (e.g., heavier resistance with fewer repetitions, or vice versa), changing the speed of the movement, and/or holding a position for five seconds at the end of a movement for static, isometric resistance.

Breathe!

Do not hold your breath while doing resistance training, as this greatly increases the pressure within your chest cavity. Exhale when you lift, then inhale with the recovery movement.

An easy way to ensure you are exhaling is to speak. Count your repetitions, speaking as you lift, then inhale as you recover during each exercise: "one," recover, "two," recover, and so on.

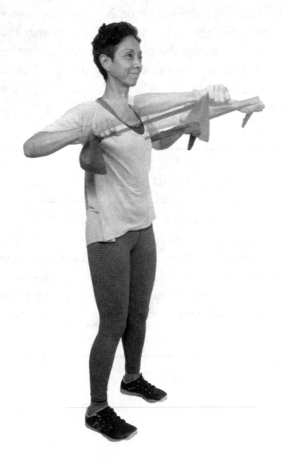

1. Chest Press

1. Fit the band around your back and under your armpits and hold the ends out in front of you.

2. Keep your knees soft (not locked) and your abdominals firm, and remain conscious of keeping an upright posture.

3. With your hands at chest level, press forward horizontally.

4. Pause the movement right before your elbows lock.

5. If you feel unsteady or just want a little more balance, stand with one foot forward.

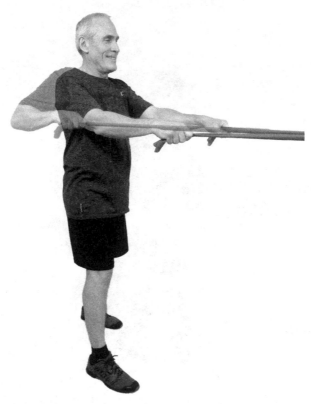

2. Standing Row

1. Loop the band around a pole or something stable while holding the ends of the band.

2. Keep your arms horizontal at chest level and lead with your elbows as you pull the ends of the band back toward your chest.

3. When your hands are close to your chest, hold that position and then pinch your shoulder blades together.

4. Keep your knees soft (not locked) and your abdominals firm, and be conscious of keeping an upright posture.

5. Stand with one foot forward if you need more balance.

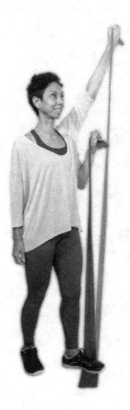

3. One-Arm Incline Press

1. Stand on one end of the band with your left foot while holding the other end in your left hand.
2. Keep a slight bend in your knees and an upright posture.
3. Begin with your elbow bent and tucked at your side.
4. Your hand should be at the level of your shoulder and palm facing forward.
5. There should be slight tension on the band in this starting position.
6. Press your hand up and toward the sky, reaching out slightly in front of your body until your arm is straight.
7. Maintain control of the movement as you lower your hand back to the starting position.
8. Repeat this exercise with the right arm.

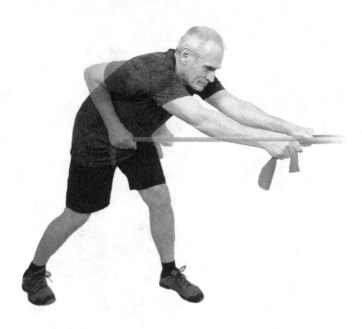

4. Lat Pull-Down

1. Secure the middle of the band around something stable so that you can grasp both ends.

2. Place one foot forward and one back, keeping your knees soft (unlocked).

3. Bend forward at your waist until your torso is at about a 45-degree angle, keeping your head in line with your spine.

4. Extend your arms toward the anchor point of the band. Arms should start fully extended and parallel with the floor.

5. While in this starting position, move backward away from the anchor point to create slight tension in the band.

6. Pull your hands back toward your waist while bending at the elbows.

7. Allow your elbows to move alongside your torso, finishing slightly beside and behind your back.

8. Maintain control of the movement as you extend your hands toward the anchor point and to the starting position.

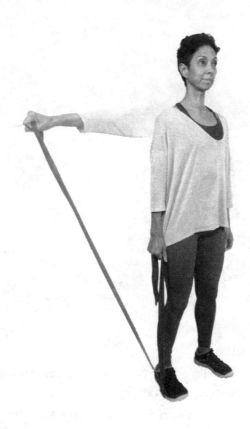

5. Side Lifts

1. Stand on the end of the band and hold the other end by your side. Be mindful of good, upright posture. Keep your knees soft.

2. Keeping your elbows soft, lift the band straight out from your body.

3. Bring your hand to shoulder height, hold the band there briefly, and then gently lower your hand back down to your side

4. If you need more balance, step forward with the foot that is not securing the end of the band.

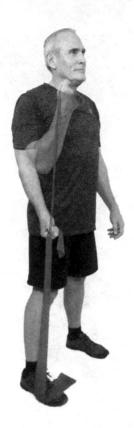

6. Hammer Curl

1. Stand on one end of the band and hold the other end by your side to start. Keep your knees soft and be mindful of good, upright posture.

2. With your palm facing inward and your thumb up, curl your hand up toward your chin.

3. Try to keep your elbow still and initiate this movement all from your hand.

4. Keep your elbows soft at the start, not locked out.

5. After two or three reps on this side, switch the band to the other foot/hand and repeat.

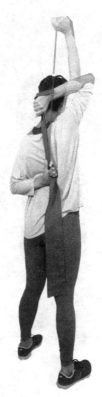

7. Overhead Triceps Pull

1. Holding one end of the band in your right hand, toss the other end gently over your right shoulder and grasp it behind your back with your left hand.

2. Your left hand will act as an anchor; keep it as still and steady as you can.

3. Now imagine you are going to throw an object upward using your right arm. Extend your right arm up over your head, straightening it all the way if you can, while keeping your elbow as still as possible throughout the movement.

4. Do a few overhead triceps pulls using your right arm, and then switch your grip and do the same on the other side.

5. Keep your knees soft and be mindful of good, upright posture throughout this exercise.

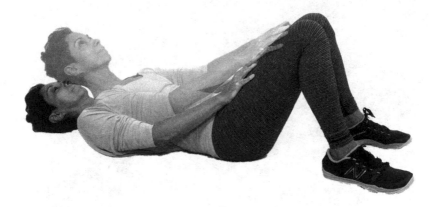

8. Abdominal Crunch

1. Lie on your back and bend both your knees, keeping your feet flat on the floor. Your arms should be extended along your sides comfortably.

2. Find a spot on the ceiling and focus on it throughout this movement.

3. On a slow exhalation, reach your arms off the ground and toward your knees, pulling your chest toward your navel and lifting your shoulder blades off the ground just a few inches.

4. Slowly lower yourself back to the floor in a controlled, gentle movement.

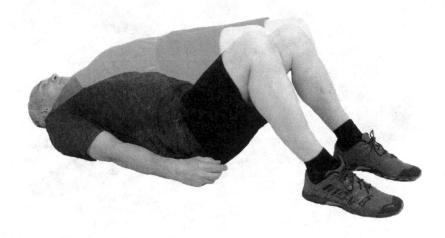

9. Hip Lifts

1. Lie on your back and bend both your knees, keeping your feet flat on the floor. Your arms should be extended along your sides comfortably.

2. Lift your hips upward, squeezing your buttocks as you go, and try to make a straight line from knees to upper body.

3. Slowly lower yourself back to the floor in a controlled, gentle movement.

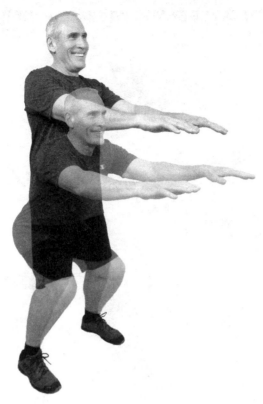

10. Leg Squats

1. Start standing with your feet shoulder width apart. Keep your eyes looking straight ahead (this will limit lower back stress).

2. With your arms out straight in front of you for balance, squat down, pushing your buttocks back as if you are sitting in a chair.

3. Try to keep your knees behind the line of your toes. If you notice that they are in front of your toes, you are putting undue stress on your knees.

4. Stand up straight again and repeat for a total of two to four times, as is comfortable.

5. If you are concerned about balance, keep an actual chair behind you and touch your buttocks lightly on the seat before standing up again.

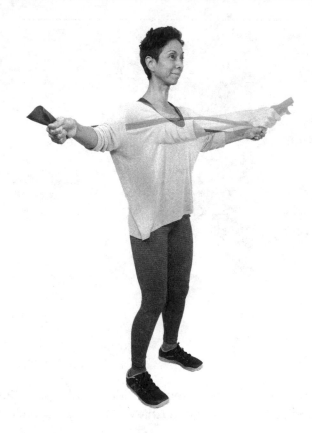

1. Chest Fly

1. Stand comfortably upright with good posture, keeping your knees soft.

2. Hold the ends of the band at shoulder height with the band under your armpits and stretched across your back. Keep your elbows slightly bent.

3. Use your chest muscles to bring your hands together in front of you. Don't stretch the band to a point where your elbows lock; keep them slightly bent.

4. Slowly release the tension on the band and bring your hands back down to where they began before starting the movement again.

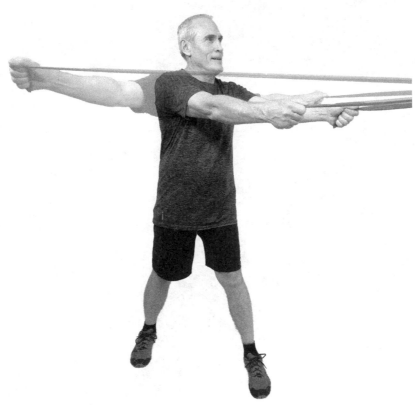

2. Rear Shoulders

1. Stand with your knees soft and with one foot forward for balance.

2. Hold both ends of the band with your arms straight and at chest level, and with some resistance (no slack) on the band.

3. Now pull your arms out as though you are spreading your wings.

4. The tension in the band will tempt you to lean forward, but maintain your upright posture and keep your abdominals tight.

5. Visualize pinching your shoulder blades together as you spread your arms wide.

6. Slowly close your arms to the starting position.

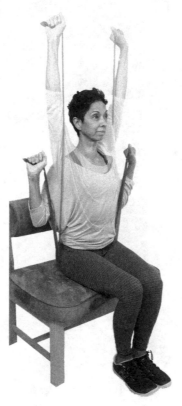

3. Seated Overhead Press

1. With good, upright posture, sit on the band on a chair, holding the ends of the band in your hands, making fists that face away from your body.
2. Reach your hands upward and over your head, stretching the band to its limit at the top of the stretch.
3. Refrain from locking your elbows or arching your back at the top of the movement.
4. Slowly release the tension on the band and bring your hands back down to chest level before starting the movement again.

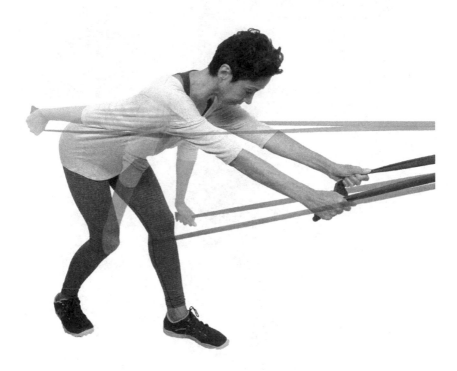

4. Standing Pull-Down

1. Secure the band to something stable and hold the band taut in front of you.
2. Keep your knees bent with one foot forward and the other back for balance.
3. Flex forward from your hips, keeping your head in line with your spine.
4. Keeping your arms extended straight—without locking your elbows—pull the band down toward your knees and then back, with your hands ending up by your hips.
5. Gently move your hands back to the start position.

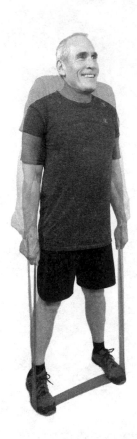

5. Shoulder Shrug

1. Stand on the middle of the band with both feet, feet shoulder width apart. Hold the ends of the band near your hips.

2. Keep your knees soft while maintaining a comfortable upright posture.

3. Keeping your arms relaxed, lift your shoulders up toward your ears, exaggerating a shrug of your shoulders.

4. Release the shrug to go back to the starting position.

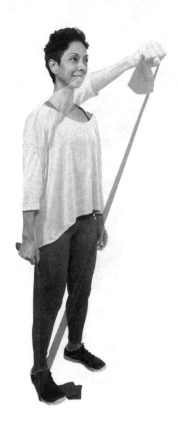

6. Front Deltoid Raise

1. Step on the end of the band with your right foot, holding the free end with your right hand.

2. Keep your knees and elbows soft and maintain a comfortable upright posture, with your palm facing backward.

3. Lift your right hand straight in front of you and in line with your body (not out to the side) so that your fisted hand is now facing the ground. Stop the movement when your fist is slightly above shoulder height.

4. Control the movement coming down. After two or three repetitions, switch sides.

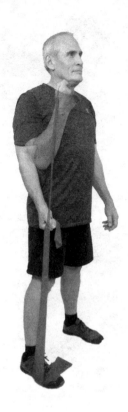

7. Biceps Curl

1. Step on the end of the band with your right foot, holding the free end with your right hand.

2. Keep your knees and elbows soft, maintaining good upright posture, with your palm facing forward.

3. Keep your elbow "glued" to your side as you lift your fisted hand up, making a 90-degree angle from your body. Try to keep your elbow very still; this movement is for your biceps, not the elbow joint.

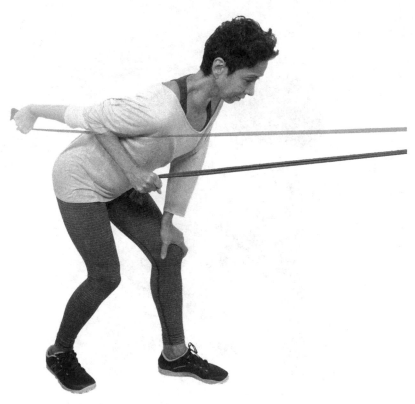

8. Triceps Kickback

1. Secure the band to something stable and step far enough back that there is tension in the band to start.

2. Stand with your feet shoulder width apart, and bend forward a little at both your knees and hips. Keep your back flat and look straight ahead.

3. Holding the band in one hand, extend it backward until your arm is straight and behind you. Keep your elbow as still as possible throughout the movement.

4. Then bring your arm back to the starting position.

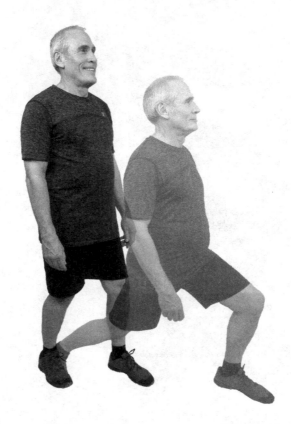

9. Lunges

1. Stand with your feet shoulder width apart, keeping your knees soft, your abdominals firm, and your posture upright.

2. Take a large step forward with one foot, bending both knees as you sink your hips straight down toward the floor.

3. To limit the stress on your knees, aim to keep your knees "behind" the line of your toes. Also look straight ahead—this will keep your spine straight.

4. When you reach the limit of your range of motion, push through your heels and return to a standing position before lunging again.

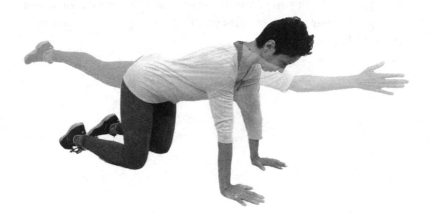

10. Alternate Arm and Leg

1. Start on your hands and knees and look down at the floor.
2. Slowly straighten out one leg, keeping it at hip level and horizontal with the floor. Extend that leg as much as is comfortably possible.
3. Slowly bring your leg down in a controlled movement.
4. Maintain engaged abdominals during each leg lift.
5. For more of a challenge, extend one leg and then bring your opposite arm up and forward, again horizontal with the floor.

In summary, there is more scientific evidence than ever documenting that exercise has powerful effects on each mechanism (described in Chapter 2) that affects our health and well-being—and how quickly these benefits can occur. Do what you enjoy; if you like it, you'll do it. The more you move, the more you improve, yet a little more movement every day goes a long way. It enables you to live longer—and, even more important, to live better.

CHAPTER 6

Stress Less

The great thing, then, in all education, is to make our nervous system our ally instead of our enemy.

—William James

Dean

Chronic stress is one of the important mechanisms underlying so many chronic diseases. It has a direct effect on our health mediated through the sympathetic nervous system, and it plays an important role via affecting each of the other mechanisms described in Chapter 2.

When it's chronic, stress can increase inflammation in your brain, which in turn can lead to or exacerbate depression. And when you're depressed, your immune system is depressed—for example, people who are HIV positive and depressed have more than double the likelihood of dying from AIDS than those who are not depressed.

Chronic stress negatively affects your health via these mechanisms in other ways as well. It shortens telomeres, adversely affects how your genes are expressed, and can have a harmful impact on the balance of the trillions of cells in your microbiome. Chronic emotional stress increases oxidative stress as well, and has negative effects on cellular metabolism and apoptosis, angiogenesis, and stasis. It causes blockages to build up faster in your arteries independent of diet.

So here's the good news: stress comes primarily not just from what happens to us but, more important, how we *react* to what happens to us. How we react, in turn, is a function of our lifestyle and our beliefs.

In short, even when we can't change what's going on in our lives, we have a lot more choice about how we react to it than we might have believed. And just as chronic stress can adversely affect our health via all of the mechanisms described above, managing stress more effectively can beneficially affect our health via all of these same mechanisms—and more quickly than had once been realized. For example, just as chronic stress can suppress your immune function, love, altruism, and compassion can enhance it.

It's the Perception of Stress

Chronic emotional stress shortens our telomeres, the ends of our chromosomes that regulate cellular aging. As our telomeres get shorter, our lives get shorter.

Taking care of a child with autism or a parent with Alzheimer's disease can be highly stressful on an ongoing, chronic basis, often for many years. It's hard to change the external stressors when your child or parent needs you for their survival on a daily basis.

In one study, my colleagues Elissa Epet and Elizabeth Blackburn studied caregivers of children with autism and found that the more stress the women reported feeling, the shorter were the length of their telomeres. Women with the highest levels of perceived stress had significantly shorter telomeres, corresponding to having telomeres thirteen average "years" shorter!

But the researchers found that it wasn't an objective measure of stress that determined its effects on their telomeres. It was how they *reacted* to the stress. Their *perceptions* of stress were more important than what was objectively occurring in their lives.

So if you *feel* stressed, you *are* stressed.

Although these women were in very similar life situations, they had dramatically different outcomes. Those who practiced the elements of the lifestyle medicine program in this book were able to buffer the stress, so it didn't affect their telomeres and health—they became more resilient. In contrast, the others showed a significant shortening of their telomeres and, as such, their lives.

This is a very empowering finding—because we can't always change what's happening to us, but we have a lot more control over how we react to it than we might realize. Again, not to blame but to empower.

The effects of stress can be debilitating or they can be enhancing. Psychologists often use analogies to talk about finding the right balance of having enough stress but not too much—like a violin string. If it's too loose, there's no music; if it's literally too high-strung, it breaks, and there's no music.

For example, a recent study showed that you can change your emotional and biological response to stress just by adjusting your mindset about it. For many people, giving a public lecture is highly stressful. But students who were trained to view stress as enhancing rather than harmful had levels of the stress hormone cortisol that were neither too high nor too low.

Interestingly, the stress-is-enhancing mindset was associated with reduced activity in high cortisol responders and increased activity in low cortisol responders to achieve an appropriate or moderate level of arousal. Just right, like Goldilocks and the Three Bears.

When you eat well, move more, and love more, then you stress less. Potentially stressful situations just don't bother you as much, giving you more degrees of freedom to react to the same situation in more productive and healing ways.

My Fuse Is Longer

When you practice these lifestyle medicine techniques on a regular basis, even a few minutes a day, your proverbial fuse gets longer as well.

We often hear patients say, "You know, I used to have a short fuse and I'd explode easily. It didn't take much to set me off. Or I'd just stuff my feelings, which made me feel even worse. But after going on your program, things just don't bother me as much. It's not like I have to hold my feelings in and make myself miserable, or explode and make everyone else around me stressed—I'm just feeling more peaceful and centered."

This allows them new degrees of freedom in how they respond. They don't have to tell themselves not to get upset; rather, things that used to be stressful don't affect them as much.

In other words, while we can't always avoid stress, we can empower ourselves with healthier, more productive ways of responding to it. You have much more control of how you react to stress than you may think! As a result, you can get more done with less stress.

Also, you become more aware of new options to change your life situation that you might not have considered before.

In all of our studies, we found that the greater the amount of time people spent practicing these stress management techniques, the more improvement we measured—at any age. Adherence to these stress management techniques was as strongly correlated with the degree of reversing heart disease as was adherence to the nutrition guidelines.

One of the recurring themes of this book is that it takes bigger changes in lifestyle to reverse (undo) disease than to prevent it—the ounce of prevention versus the pound of cure. In all of our studies on reversing chronic diseases, we asked participants to spend a total of one hour per day on these stress management techniques. Those who did more showed even greater reversal.

That's what our research shows it takes to reverse the progression of heart disease and other chronic illnesses—again, the pound of cure. We found a dose-response relationship between the frequency and duration of stress management practices and the degree of reversal.

Now, we understand that this is a significant amount of time for most people—especially when competing with so many other distractions. To put that in perspective, the average person spends over *five hours per day* on their mobile devices—plus a significant amount of time watching television.

We make time for what matters to us.

The Attention Span of a Goldfish

Although we are hyperconnected with each other via social media and other apps, studies show that we are more stressed and lonely than ever. One study revealed that people who reported spending more than two hours per day on social media were twice as likely to feel socially isolated as those who spent less than half an hour per day. And those who visited social media sites such as Facebook more than fifty-eight times per week were over three times as likely to feel socially isolated as those who visited fewer than nine times per week. More on this in Chapter 7.

Also, the time we spend on our mobile devices is shortening our attention span. A study from Microsoft found that the average attention span since the year 2000 (when smartphones were introduced) decreased by a third, from twelve seconds to only eight seconds—less than the attention span of a goldfish!

Technology is designed to be addictive. The gratification it provides is similar to that of other addictive behaviors, such as drug abuse or gambling.

So spending more time doing these stress management techniques and less time on social media will give you a double benefit. And it will help you focus better.

While at least an hour per day of stress management is optimal to reverse chronic diseases, you have a spectrum of choices for preventing them—the more you do, the more you improve. If you are otherwise healthy—the ounce of prevention—just do at least a few minutes every day. The consistency is even more important than the duration.

Of course, we have to eat every day, so with nutrition it just becomes a question of what we eat. And when we exercise, it feels like we're really doing something. But stress management is something that's easier to skip, especially when we are busiest and most need it. If you make it a habit—same time of day, same place—you're more likely to do it. Or use downtime (e.g., when you're traveling on a plane or train) to meditate instead of checking your phone.

Change Your Mind, Change Your Genes

When you're sitting with your eyes closed, it looks like you're not doing very much. In fact, though, you're doing something quite powerful.

For example, researchers at Harvard found that meditation alone can change the expression of genes that regulate inflammation, programmed cell death (apoptosis), and oxidative stress in only a few weeks.

To look at gene expression, the researchers compared non-meditators with those taught to meditate for eight weeks and also with advanced meditators. The more the participants meditated, the more it beneficially changed the expression of these genes.

In my experience, when people realize that meditation alone can actually change their genes as well as provide so many other benefits, it is usually a powerful motivator for them to do this as well as the other stress management techniques described here.

Change Your Mind, Change Your Brain

Neuroplasticity is the ability of the adult brain to change its structure and function by generating new cells and pathways. As we discussed in Chapter 2, when you eat well, move more, stress less, and love more, the part of your brain that controls memory, called the hippocampus, can get measurably bigger in only a few weeks.

New research indicates that you can actually rewire your brain to have more positive responses—seeing the proverbial glass as half full instead of half empty. We can all learn to be more positive by practicing doing so. In other words, your higher cognitive function—your thoughts—can directly influence your amygdala, the "animal" part of your brain that houses emotions like fear and anger.

I had the pleasure of speaking at a conference on happiness in Austin with Dr. Barbara Fredrickson, a leading researcher on the benefits of nurturing and reinforcing positive emotions. It was, not surprisingly, a happy experience! One way to nurture and reinforce positive emotions is to make a point of doing something, anything, every day—big or small—as an act of service, without expecting anything in return. She calls these "micro-moments of positivity"—ways to keep reinforcing positive emotions, to have a greater sense of well-being and to provide a buffer against stress and depression.

In one study, she and her colleagues trained a group of people for six weeks in what is beautifully called a "lovingkindness meditation," emphasizing kindness, love, and compassion. This resulted in an increase in positive emotions and social connectedness.

This meditation also improved function of the vagus nerve, which connects the brain to the heart and other organs. The vagus nerve is part of the parasympathetic nervous system. As described in Chapter 2, our sympathetic nervous system is stimulated during stress, but our parasympathetic nervous system relaxes the body. It counterbalances the effects of stress-induced overstimulation of the sympathetic nervous system. Among other benefits, this reduces inflammation and enables better control of blood sugar.

Dr. Fredrickson examined associations among three factors: vagal tone (the balance between sympathetic and parasympathetic nervous systems), positive emotions, and positive social connections (individual reports of positivity resonance). Her team found that an increase in one of these factors was associated with increases in the others, what she calls an upward spiral. As she puts it, "One way to think about this is that love creates health and health creates love. . . . Taking time to learn the skills to self-generate positive emotions can help us become healthier, more social, more resilient versions of ourselves."

In a related study, Dr. Richard Davidson, a pioneering neuroscientist at the University of Wisconsin, found that as little as two weeks' training in compassion and lovingkindness meditation generated changes in brain circuitry linked to an increase in positive social behaviors like generosity. He said, "Well-being can be considered a life skill. If you practice, you can actually get better at it."

Mindfulness is a form of meditation in which you observe your thoughts and feelings without judgment. According to Dr. Davidson, this form of mental training gives you "the wherewithal to pause, observe how easily the mind can exaggerate the severity of a setback, note that it is an interesting mental process, and resist getting drawn into the abyss."

Meditation causes a part of your thinking brain (the left prefrontal cortex) to send inhibitory signals to your amygdala, the emotional part of your brain that causes you to feel anger and fear. In short, we have more control over how we respond to the world than we once believed. Our thinking brain (sometimes) can overcome our emotional brain—and practice makes perfect.

In another study, those who meditated for about thirty minutes a day for only eight weeks had measurable increases in brain size in their hippocampus (leading to improved memory) and decreases in brain size in their amygdala (causing a reduction in anger and fear).

Knowing that you can beneficially change your brain and the expression of your genes (plus so many other benefits) in only two months by just meditating for a half hour daily is very inspiring!

Anne

For too many of us, "stress" has become synonymous with modern life. Historically, our ancestors learned to survive the fleeting, acute stressors they occasionally encountered outside of their caves. Today, we are faced with coping with *chronic* stress—around the clock, with no end in sight—and it is taking an epidemic toll on our health. Indeed, keeping up with the pace and demands of life often leaves us feeling tense, frazzled, and run-down.

Understand that stress in and of itself is not bad—having a positive response to it is what can help keep us alive when we are in danger.

If, for instance, you are driving home and suddenly see a child dart out into the street chasing a ball, a chain of chemical reactions happens quickly in your body, helping you brake and swerve in time before harming the child. The sight of the child causes your sympathetic nervous system to send a signal to your adrenal glands to secrete and circulate adrenaline and other stress hormones throughout your system. As described in Chapter 2, this is what's known as the fight-or-flight response.

In this state, you begin to perspire, your pupils dilate, your muscles tense up, and your breathing becomes shallow and speeds up. Your blood pressure increases, which can thicken and constrict your arteries, while your blood platelets become sticky, increasing the risk of blood clots. In acute stress, these changes can help us survive—for example, we get out of harm's way and are less likely to bleed if injured.

However, if your everyday life feels like that adrenaline-fueled swerve—you have bills to pay, deadlines to meet, and noise and advertising messages coming at you—you are likely in a state of constant hormonal arousal, and that can cause damage to the body. In the long term this stress and imbalance contribute to emotional and physical disease. And if you're not sleeping well, either, that just makes things worse, since the brain literally detoxifies when we sleep.

Stress-related diseases have been increasing for decades, including heart disease, hypertension, obesity, diabetes, addiction, anxiety, and depression. In fact, stress is linked to six leading causes of death—heart disease, cancer, lung ailments, accidents, cirrhosis of the liver, and suicide.

This is why it's so helpful to understand how you can deliberately regulate your nervous system's response to stress. Our sympathetic nervous system allows us to respond quickly to danger, but our parasympathetic nervous system relaxes the body, undoing the effects of stress while restoring good health to your mind and body. Practicing stress management techniques allows us to upregulate or turn on the parasympathetic nervous system (relaxation response) while downregulating or toning down the sympathetic nervous system (fight-or-flight response).

The takeaway for you? Practiced in combination with the nutrition, exercise, and emotional support pillars of our lifestyle medicine program, one hour a day of stress reduction has a powerful impact that has been proven to stop and undo a wide variety of chronic diseases.

When you take the time to relax and relieve your stress on a regular basis, you can experience vibrant physiological health and longevity as well as an overall sense of psychological, emotional, and spiritual well-being.

Here are five different stress reduction techniques, followed by step-by-step instructions. Do what works for you and your lifestyle.

1. *Gentle stretching.* Think of gentle stretching as healing movements that bring you back into the conscious experience of your own body, while helping you listen to signals and symptoms before they become problematic. As your body relaxes, so does your mind. The focus in this technique is on creating a relationship with your body and listening to the information it

is offering you about yourself. Benefits include increased balance and coordination, improved strength and flexibility, increased bone strength, regulated breathing rhythm, and improved body awareness.

2. *Breathing techniques.* Your breath both reflects and affects your emotions. The way we think and feel affects the way we breathe, and the way we breathe affects the way we think and feel. When we're stressed, we tend to breathe in a rapid and shallow way. Therefore, one of the easiest and quickest ways to control stress is to consciously breathe slowly and deeply. The practice of consciously guiding the direction, depth, and rhythm of your breath can restore, calm, and balance the nervous system, increase oxygen circulation in the blood, help increase awareness of internal states, and lower blood pressure and heart rate.

3. *Meditation.* Meditation is the act of steadying your concentration on one object, such as your breath, a word, or a feeling. Meditation allows us to stay centered while we observe the natural ups and downs of the mind. The benefits of meditation also include better concentration, a more consistent feeling of calm, clarity, and a sharpened mind. Those who meditate daily often comment that the things that used to bother them don't bother them as much anymore. Regular meditators report that their practice provides them with greater insight and inspiration. One study showed that meditation can change the expression of your genes in only eight weeks—turning on genes that keep you healthy and turning off ones that lead to illness—and long-term meditation caused even more improvements.

4. *Guided imagery.* Our bodies respond to mental images as though we are really experiencing what we are imagining—for better and for worse. Thus, using your imagination to invoke positive imagery can help support healing outcomes. Amazingly, developing positive imagery can induce positive mental and physical states that can repattern feelings, thoughts and behaviors that lead to healing. In contrast, when we worry and imagine an awful outcome, this can also become self-fulfilling.

5. *Deep relaxation.* Deep relaxation is one of the most healing practices of all. When you are able to deeply relax—a learned, conscious, and progressive letting go of tension and stress— you allow and support the body's natural healing process. You will find that you are able to rest and restore even more deeply than during sleep.

That's not to say that getting enough sleep isn't also crucial to our health and well-being. It is! Many studies have documented that insufficient sleep increases your risk of a wide variety of chronic conditions, including depression, heart disease, type 2 diabetes, ADHD, and Alzheimer's disease, among many others. In 2014, the Centers for Disease Control and Prevention called sleep deprivation a public health epidemic. Practicing deep relaxation and meditation before bed will help you fall asleep more easily and sleep more deeply. Getting a good night's sleep is one of the most powerful things you can do to reduce stress and gain health.

Start with the techniques you love and do more of those. Some days you may want to spend more time in, say, meditation, and the next day you might prefer to spend more time in relaxation. Give yourself permission to be flexible, but put the time in. Each one of the techniques has value, and together they are even more powerful.

We list here a wide variety of techniques within each of these categories. Choose the ones that most appeal to you—if you enjoy them, you're more likely to do them. Ask a friend to read these while you practice them, or you can make an audiotape and play it back for yourself.

Gentle Stretching

As part of the fight-or-flight response, our bodies tense up, giving us more "body armor" for battle. This helps us survive acute stresses—as long as we relax once the danger has passed. However, when the fight-or-flight response is chronically turned on, our bodies can become chronically tense and painful.

Just as our mind affects our body, our body affects our mind. So when you stretch chronically tensed muscles slowly and gently, you allow the body and mind to relax. We recommend a number of what are called yoga "poses" or "postures" for this portion of our lifestyle medicine program.

The terminology here is actually helpful—these movements are to be done very slowly and gently instead of bouncing movements that jerk you from one position to the next. Your postures should be unforced and gentle; the focus is on moving with the control and grace of a dancer rather than a Marine drill instructor.

Postures call on skills very different from those required in aerobic exercise or calisthenics. The challenge here is not to do more or to push, but to learn to move slowly enough to encourage awareness. Over time, as your body relaxes and becomes more limber, you may be able to stretch farther or hold more difficult positions, but this is not the goal. The goal is to feel peaceful and relaxed by the end of the practice.

Smooth and even breathing is particularly important while stretching. Conscious breathing promotes relaxation and health. Being aware of your breath will also help you monitor how you are reacting to different poses and will encourage you not to stretch beyond your own limits. Any dizziness, shortness of breath, flushing of the face, or pain is an important signal to stop what you are doing and rest.

Reminders for Gentle Stretching

- Move slowly and consciously, and never strain.
- Pay attention to the area being stretched.
- Stretch to a point before you feel pain, not beyond.
- Always keep your breath natural and through the nose whenever possible.
- Always remember to breathe smoothly and evenly during stretching postures.
- Full-body inhalations and exhalations help you to relax and stretch farther.
- The time you take for relaxing between the poses is as important as the postures themselves.

- Be aware of signs of stress—dizziness, shortness of breath, pain, and agitation.

- Use common sense. If it hurts, stop what you are doing.

- Hold each posture only as long as it feels comfortable.

- The goal is to feel peaceful and relaxed.

Postures require no special equipment other than a quiet room, a chair, a mat or carpet, some pillows and blankets, and loose, comfortable clothing.

It may be worth repeating that the goal is not to see how far you can stretch, but rather just to stretch as far as feels comfortable for you. Be alert for signs of strain, such as shortness of breath or pain. In this case, by doing less, you may actually be doing more. If you finish feeling peaceful and relaxed, then you have accomplished the purpose of these techniques and can carry that relaxation into your daily life.

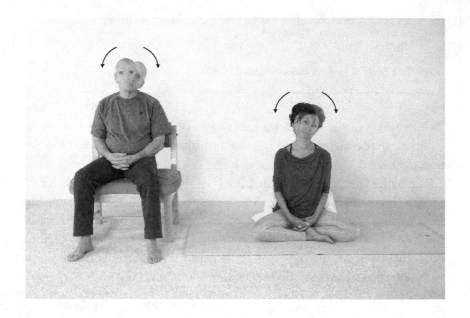

Neck Exercises

1. On your exhale, slowly lower your chin toward your chest.

2. Now inhale and slowly raise your head back to the center. Exhale and relax.

3. On your next exhale, slowly bring your right ear toward your right shoulder. (Try not to bring your shoulder up to your ear.)

4. Inhale and slowly raise your head back to the center. Exhale and relax.

5. Do the same on your left side.

Benefit: This exercise reduces tension and tightness in your neck and shoulders and it calms and quiets the nervous system. Use it anytime you need it!

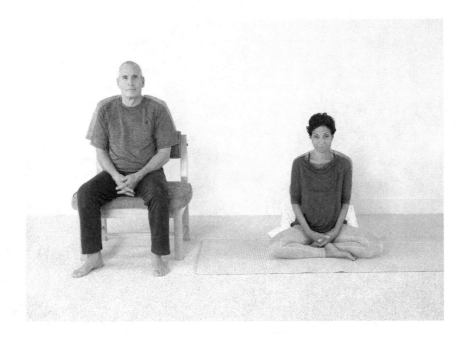

Shoulder Rolls

1. Inhale slowly as you bring both of your shoulders forward and then raise them toward your ears.
2. Exhale as you gently roll them back and down. Do this two or three times.
3. Now rotate your shoulders in the opposite direction two or three times.
4. Shake your arms out, exhale, and relax.

Benefit: This exercise relaxes tension in your shoulders while improving shoulder flexibility and range of motion. It also counteracts the effects of poor posture.

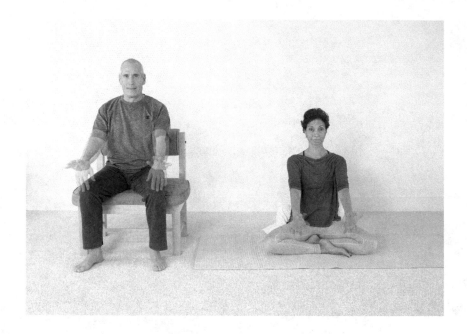

Wrist Stretch 1

1. Extend your arms out in front of you with your elbows bent. There should be no strain in your upper back or shoulders. This can also be done with your hands down alongside your body.

2. Exhale and bend your wrists so that your hands and fingers point toward the floor.

3. Inhale as you bring your hands and fingers up toward the ceiling.

4. Continue this process a few times as you continue to breathe slowly and evenly.

Wrist Stretch 2

1. Extend your arms out in front of you with your elbows bent. There should be no strain in your upper back or shoulders.

This can also be done with your hands down alongside your body.

2. Breathe slowly and evenly as you rotate your wrists in a clockwise direction, gradually increasing the size of the circle you make.

3. Now move your wrists in a counterclockwise circle.

4. Shake your hands and arms, exhale, and relax.

Benefit: These two wrist exercises articulate your joints and thereby increase wrist flexibility. Because they also help with blood circulation, they may help relieve arthritic pain.

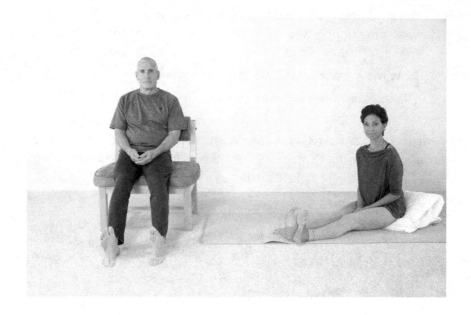

Ankle Stretch 1

1. Stretch out your legs, resting your feet on the floor.
2. As you exhale, point your toes away from your body.
3. As you inhale, bring them back toward your body.
4. Practice this movement three to five times with your own natural breath as the rhythm.

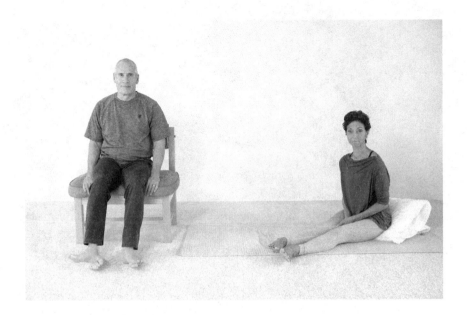

Ankle Stretch 2

1. Stretch out your legs, resting your feet on the floor.
2. Keeping your legs still, rotate your feet in a circle. Increase the size of the circle as you feel comfortable.
3. Rotate the feet in the opposite direction.

Benefit: Ankle stretches articulate the many joints in your feet. They help relieve stiffness and bring synovial fluid to the joints, which will allow for better balance and mobility when you're standing.

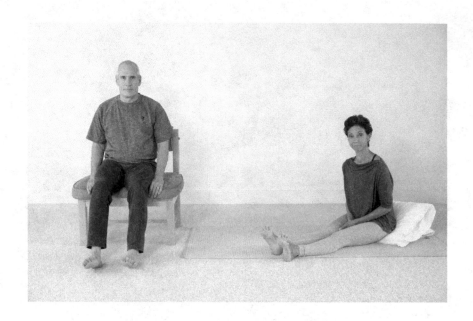

Toe Stretch

1. Alternately spread and squeeze your toes together several times.

2. Shake your legs, exhale, and relax.

Benefit: Toe stretches articulate the joints in your toes. Like ankle stretches, they help relieve stiffness and bring synovial fluid to the joints, which will allow for better balance and mobility when you're standing.

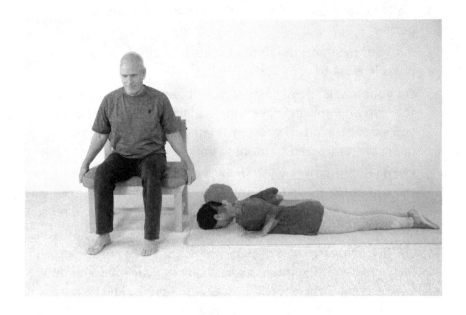

Cobra Pose

Seated in a chair:

1. Hold the sides of your chair with both hands.
2. As you exhale, gently round your spine and slowly lower your chin toward your chest.
3. On an inhale, lift your nose, chin, and chest toward the ceiling. Gently exhale, allowing your chest to expand as you roll your shoulders back and down (without straining).
4. Do this two or three times as you continue to breathe naturally and evenly.
5. Exhale and release when you are finished.

From the floor:

1. Lie facedown on the floor with your legs straight out and together.
2. Put your palms on the floor next to your chest, with your elbows in close to your body.
3. On your inhale, gently extend your head and shoulders in a forward and upward direction, feeling your chest expand as you do so. Try to feel yourself floating upward from your heart center instead of pushing yourself up with your hands.
4. Keep your breath flowing freely, fully, and evenly, pausing at the top of the movement only if you're comfortable. Exhale as you gently release yourself back down to the floor and relax.

Benefit: This pose helps tone the upper back, improves posture, expands the chest and lungs, and promotes flexibility in your spine and the cranial nerves. It may help relieve backache and shoulder and neck tension. If you're doing it on the floor, Cobra also stretches your abdominal muscles, tones abdominal organs, and circulates blood to your reproductive organs.

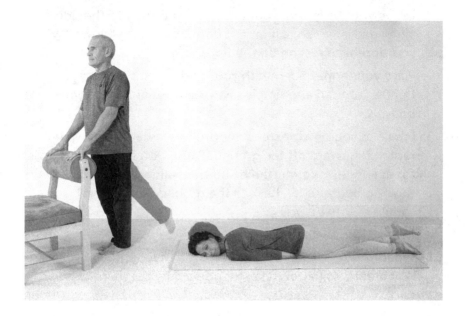

Half Locust

Using a chair:

1. Place both of your hands on the back of a chair for support.
2. Inhale as you extend your right leg behind you, tucking your toes under so that they point behind you as well. You should notice the activation of your leg and gluteal muscles.
3. If you would like a bit more of a stretch, raise your foot a couple of inches off the floor and hold the pose.
4. Pause where your leg feels comfortably extended for a couple of natural breath cycles. Release and repeat two or three times while maintaining a smooth and even breathing rhythm.
5. When you feel ready, bring your leg back into a standing position, switch legs, and repeat.
6. Exhale and relax.

From the floor:

1. Lie on your belly with your head either turned to the side, to allow one cheek to rest on the floor, or looking "down," with your forehead resting on the floor.
2. Place your arms underneath your body, palms against your thighs. (You can also simply rest your arms alongside your body.)
3. Inhale as you slowly extend your right leg backward while raising it upward off the ground. Pause at the top of this pose for as long as is comfortable and then allow your exhale to slowly guide your leg back to the ground. Rest and relax for a couple of breath cycles.
4. Repeat with the left leg.
5. When you're done with both legs, turn over and feel your natural breath while you relax for a few minutes there on your back.

Benefit: This pose helps tone the lower spine and buttocks area, and strengthens the lower back. When you do this on the floor, you also exercise your pelvis and abdomen and tone your abdominal organs. It also helps improve elimination.

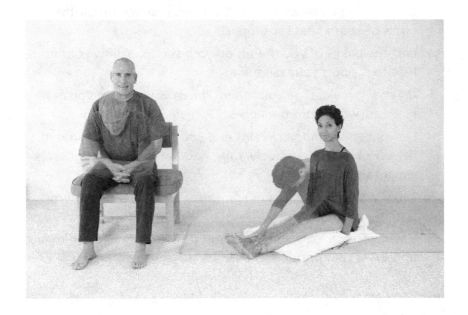

Forward Stretch

Seated in a chair:

1. On your exhale, rest your hands on your thighs as you slide your upper body forward, hinging from your pelvis. Once you find your comfortable edge, pause there for a couple of full-body breath cycles.
2. You can either fold your arms on your lap, rest your forearms on your thighs, or slide your hands down your legs.
3. Allow your spine to remain supple and your head rest forward.
4. Inhale as you slowly slide back to resume your relaxed upright seated position. Exhale and relax.

From the floor:

1. Use a small pillow under your buttocks and one under the backs of your knees for support.
2. Rest the palms of your hands on your thighs,. Allow your inhale to support your tall spine.
3. On your exhale, slide your hands down your legs as you gently hinge forward from the pelvis.
4. Let your spine and neck relax and your head incline forward. Let your breath flow freely, fully, and naturally, feeling it relax you into the stretch.
5. Pause where you find your comfortable edge; refrain from pushing or straining.
6. When you are ready, inhale as you slowly come back up to an upright seated position. Exhale and relax.

Benefit: The forward stretch improves shoulder, hamstring, and hip flexibility. It also relaxes your back and neck muscles and improves elimination.

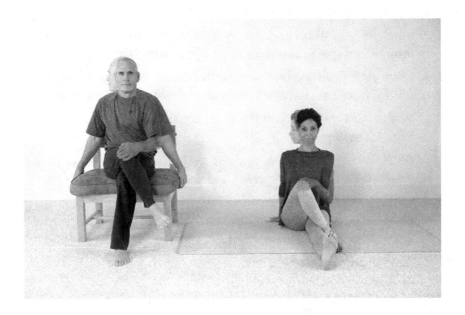

Spinal Twist

Seated in a chair:

1. Inhale as you sit up and gently extend your spine upward, creating more spaciousness between your vertebrae.
2. Cross your right leg over your left.
3. While holding the seat of the chair with your right hand, place your left hand on your right knee.
4. With your exhale, slowly begin to twist to the right while engaging your whole spine in the twist. Let your eyes gaze softly to the right as you twist, pausing at your comfortable edge.
5. On your inhale, gently unwind back to the center when you're ready. Rest your palms in your lap, exhale, and relax.
6. Repeat on the opposite side.

From the floor:

1. Extend your legs out in front of you.
2. Inhale as you sit up and gently extend your spine upward, creating more spaciousness between your vertebrae.
3. Cross your right leg over your left, placing your right foot flat on the floor somewhere between your left knee and ankle.
4. With your right hand on the floor to support you, hold your right knee with your left hand.
5. With your exhale, begin to twist to the right while engaging your whole spine in the twist. Let your eyes gaze softly to the right as you twist, pausing at your comfortable edge.
6. On your inhale, gently unwind back to your center. Rest your palms in your lap, exhale, and relax.
7. Repeat on the opposite side.

Floor variations:

- Place your foot on the inside of your extended leg instead of on the other side of it. Follow the remaining instructions for where to place your hands and when to twist.
- Sit cross-legged on the floor, instead of with your legs out in front of you. Place your right hand on your left knee and twist to the left. Repeat on the other side. This variation allows for more openness and less pressure in the abdomen.

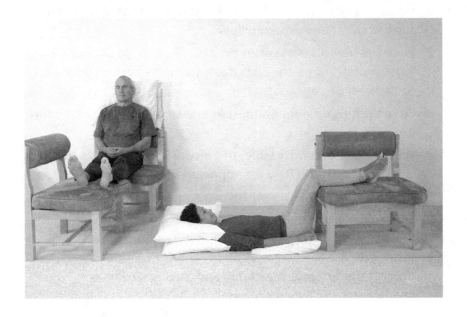

Shoulder Stand

Using two chairs:

1. Place one chair against the wall to sit on and one in front of you. Sit in the chair that is against the wall, with one or two pillows behind your upper back and shoulders for support.
2. Rest your legs upon the chair in front of you.
3. Relax your hands in your lap, close your eyes, and let your chin "soften" and relax toward your chest.
4. Relax in this pose for a couple of minutes, resting your breath awareness at your heart—gently breathe as if your heart is breathing!
5. When you're ready, open your eyes and transition slowly.

From the floor:

1. Lie on the floor with a chair in front of you with your head supported by one or two pillows.
2. Place one leg on the seat of the chair so that your entire lower leg is supported on the chair seat, from the back of your knee to the heel of your foot.
3. Lift your hips up enough to slide one small pillow under your buttocks for support.
4. When you feel comfortable, place your second leg on the chair seat so that it, too, is supported knee to heel.
5. Close your eyes and simply rest your breath awareness at your heart. Imagine that it is your heart that is breathing, nourishing you deeply from the inside and out.
6. When you are ready, slowly open your eyes and gently transition off the ground. Watch for any dizziness or light-headedness.

Benefit: This posture is considered a restorative pose for the heart. Having your legs supported on a chair gives the veins to your legs a rest and allows the blood to flow with gravity back to your heart. The position also pools blood in your carotid arteries, which sends the message to your brain that the heart has enough blood and doesn't need to pump as hard. This, in turn, lowers your heart rate and blood pressure. This practice also brings blood, energy, and balance to the thyroid gland, drains the lymphatic system (which is not a pumped system), and rests the muscles of the lower back.

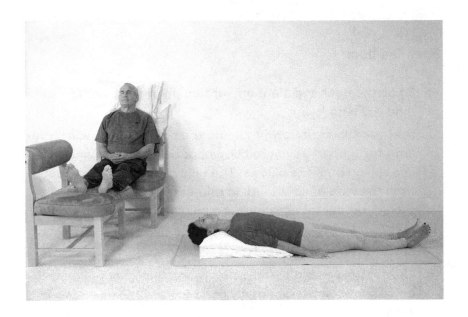

Fish Pose

Using two chairs:

1. Place one chair against the wall to sit on and one in front of you, resting your legs up on it.
2. Place a pillow lengthwise behind your back and head for support.
3. Your chest should be gently expanded and your shoulders and neck should be relaxed. Slightly lift your chin so that you are looking straight ahead.
4. Close your eyes and breathe slowly and smoothly. Imagine energy and blood flowing freely between your heart and your arms.

5. When you are ready, slowly open your eyes and transition slowly.

From the floor:

1. Sit on the floor and place one or two pillows on the floor behind you lengthwise.
2. Now ease yourself down to lie on the pillows, using your forearms for support as you roll down, or by resting on your side and rolling onto the pillows. The pillows should support you from the base of your spine to mid-ear or higher. Your head should rest back a bit; adjust the pillow(s) if you need to.
3. Let your arms relax by your sides, with palms facing up or down—whatever you find most comfortable.
4. Close your eyes and breathe slowly and smoothly. Imagine energy and blood flowing freely between your heart and your arms.
5. When you are ready, slowly open your eyes and transition slowly by putting your hands under the back of your head (to bring your head to a neutral position), and then bend your knees and roll to your side.

Variation: You can do this pose without pillows. Tuck your forearms under you to gently press and lift your chest while tilting your head back so that the back portion of the top of your head is on the floor. If you choose this variation, don't hold the pose more than several seconds at a time.

Benefit: This pose expands the chest and counteracts the effects of poor posture. It brings blood to the thyroid and parathyroid glands, stretches the muscles of the back, neck, and shoulders, and improves blood flow to the heart and lungs.

Breathing Techniques

One of the easiest and quickest ways to reduce stress is with your breath. The breath anchors us in the present moment while serving as a bridge between body and mind. After all, changes in your mind both affect and reflect your breathing.

When we are anxious, our breathing tends to be rapid and shallow. When we are relaxed, we tend to breathe more slowly and more deeply. Likewise, changes in your breathing affect your body. When we exercise quickly, our oxygen requirements go up and we breathe faster. When we exercise slowly, the oxygen requirement is less and we breathe more slowly. Lastly, changes in your breathing affect your mind. When you are a little tired, taking a few deep, full-body in-breaths creates a stimulating effect, making you feel more awake and alert. When you are feeling anxious or worried, lengthening and deepening the out-breath creates a calming effect, helping you feel more relaxed. When practiced skillfully and safely, the directed awareness of your breath can manually help to tone your mood, your nervous system, and your physiology.

Your natural breathing pattern flows much like the ocean tide, gently lapping in and out from the shore of your body, day or night, awake or asleep, unconsciously or consciously. As long as you're alive, your breath has no starting or stopping point; it's just one continuous movement. When you inhale, you are nourishing yourself with the energy from your breath. When you exhale, you are cleansing yourself by letting go of tension and toxins. Consciously attuning your attention to the rhythmic sensation of your breath is integral to receive these practice's full benefits.

In general, it's optimal to breathe through your nose for several reasons. Breathing through your mouth can lead to more rapid, shallow breathing, creating a jittery effect. However, due to the narrower nasal passageway, nostril breathing naturally slows down and deepens the breath, creating a calming effect. Your tiny nose hairs, called cilia, expand and contract to regulate your breathing while also collecting moisture and filtering foreign particles from the air entering the nasal cavity.

We recommend any of the following three types of technique: abdominal breathing, three-part breathing, or alternate-nostril breathing. With any of these breathing practices, you will learn how to use your breath as a tool to break the stress cycle, increase oxygen circulating in the blood, lower blood pressure and heart rate, and bring calm and balance to your nervous system.

A few tips before you start:

- In addition to using this technique as a part of your daily stress-reduction practice, you can do it whenever you have some free time or when you are feeling stressed.
- Since your exhale correlates with relaxation, enjoy the calming effects of gradually and gently extending the length of your exhale, so that it is longer than your inhale, for as many breath cycles as feels comfortable. When you're ready, slowly resume your natural, even breathing rhythm.
- You may be either sitting with your spine gently extended upward or lying on your back in a comfortable resting position.

Abdominal Breathing

Deep or abdominal breathing is one of the simplest yet most effective stress management techniques. You can do it anywhere, at any time. It becomes even more effective with practice. The diaphragm is a large muscle located between the chest and the abdomen. When you breathe in, this large muscle is forced downward, causing a partial vacuum that forces air into the lungs. This type of abdominal or diaphragmatic breathing increases the suction pressure in the chest, thereby improving venous return of blood to the heart.

To practice abdominal breathing, find a comfortable position, either sitting up or lying down, whichever you prefer. Begin by exhaling through your nose until empty. At the bottom of the exhalation, sense the natural gathering in at your abdomen. Begin the inhalation by slowly releasing your abdomen and allowing your lungs to refill with your next breath. Continue a few times until you feel comfortable and rhythmic with it. The objective is to sense the abdomen deflate as it gently contracts with each exhalation, then sense the abdomen slowly inflate and expand with your breath upon each inhalation.

As you breathe, feel your spine gently extend upward with your in-breath, creating length and space between your tailbone and the crown of your head. Keep your breath smooth and gentle, without strain. If at any time you feel dizzy or light-headed, discontinue the practice and allow your breathing to return to normal.

While abdominal breathing may feel stilted or unnatural at first, it will gradually become easier and quite enjoyable if you practice it on a regular basis.

Three-Part Breathing

This mode of breathing progressively tones your lungs to their fullest capacity while releasing tension and calming the mind in just a few minutes. It is an effective way to regulate shallow breathing by restoring your natural rhythm of breath, especially after exertion. It can also help prepare your body and mind for meditation, if you choose to extend your stress reduction to include meditation as well. You can do this type of deep breathing anywhere, at any time. It only becomes more effective with practice.

- *Part one:* Begin by exhaling completely through your nose. At the end of the exhalation, lightly pull your abdomen inward. Begin the next inhalation by expanding your abdomen and then filling your lungs with your breath until full.
- *Part two:* Continue to inhale, allowing your entire rib cage area to fill. Then exhale, allowing the breath to flow out of your rib cage area. At the bottom of the exhale, gently contract your abdomen in. Practice a few times until you feel comfortable with this part.
- *Part three:* Exhale through your nose until empty. At the bottom of the exhalation, gently draw your abdomen in. Begin the inhalation by slowly releasing your abdomen and allowing your next breath to refill from the bottom of your lungs, expanding into the sides and back of your lungs and up to your upper chest, so you can feel your collarbones rise slightly. On the exhalation, contract the upper chest, the rib cage, and the abdomen, one section following from the top down until you are empty of breath. Sense the abdomen deflate and naturally contract at the bottom of each exhalation. Continue a few times until you feel comfortable with it—always keeping the breathing slow, easy, deep and rhythmic, and ending with an exhalation.

Alternate-Nostril Breathing

The technique of alternate-nostril breathing is exceptionally powerful. It's been used for centuries to rebalance the equilibrium of breathing and to calm the mind and body. It equally stimulates and balances the right and left hemispheres of the brain as well as the sympathetic and parasympathetic nervous systems. It invites your awareness to turn inward while calming your body and mind. This is an ideal preparation for meditation, if you want to add meditation to your repertoire. Even a few seconds can make a meaningful difference in reducing acute stress and anxiety.

Our noses are lined with a mucous membrane that swells and shrinks during the day. Although you probably are not aware of it, the flow of air through the nose shifts from one nostril to the other during the day as the lining of each nostril expands and contracts in a biological rhythm. With this technique, we are being deliberate about the use of each nostril by simply closing off one "valve" at a time.

Traditional yoga texts instruct a person to close one nostril in a specific way, which you might want to try: make a gentle fist with the right hand's thumb and the last two fingers, allowing the index and middle finger to remain extended so those fingertips can rest between your eyebrows. The side of the thumb is used to close off the right nostril, and the side of the ring finger is used to close off the left nostril. In practice, you may find it easier to use your thumb and index finger. Some people find it easier to consciously sense and direct their breath in and out of the right or left nostril with their attention rather than physically using their fingers to do so. Do whatever is most comfortable for you.

To practice alternate-nostril breathing:

1. Sit in a tall, comfortable position with your eyes closed.
2. Exhale and inhale slowly and smoothly through both nostrils.
3. Gently close off your right nostril with your right thumb, and exhale and inhale slowly through your left nostril.
4. Now switch to gently close off your left nostril with the fourth and fifth fingers. Exhale and inhale slowly through your right nostril.
5. As another option, you may choose to apply the same three-part deep breathing method described in the previous section, expanding and contracting the abdomen, lower chest, and upper chest.
6. Continue for at least three rounds of breath, three cycles of exhaling and inhaling, changing nostrils after each inhalation.

7. If at any time you feel like you are not getting enough air, simply resume your free, natural breathing. Increase your practice time slowly, only as is comfortable for you.

8. When you are ready to stop this practice, simply allow your hand to come to your lap and breathe naturally and evenly through both nostrils.

9. Sit quietly for a moment of inner awareness. Relax with your eyes closed and your attention focused on the breath passing gently and evenly through both nostrils.

Meditation

Meditation is really just the practice of bringing your mind to one thing. It can be anything—a sound, a phrase, or an image. It can be secular or religious—whatever appeals to you the most.

The basic attitude cultivated in all forms of meditation and relaxation exercises is called "passive attention." Your attention should be on the immediate process, without any goal or outcome. Paradoxically, the more you try to relax or concentrate, the more difficult it becomes to achieve the desired state of consciousness—just as the harder you try to fall asleep, the more difficult it is to actually fall asleep. In meditation, you gently focus without forcing or trying. Stay open to all of your surroundings, and to the deepest parts of your inner experience. Your mind will rest on the object of your meditation (such as a word, a prayer, or the breath), and when it wanders away from that object, as it will—and this will happen most of the time when you're beginning—the objective is to simply observe where it goes and, without any labels or judgments, gently return to your point of focus. The idea here is that you aren't engaged in the process of thinking but rather are cultivating an attitude of "witnessing." Notice what is arising and gently let it pass.

Many studies have shown that our brain waves become more coherent when we meditate. Also, in 2011 a Harvard study showed that meditation increased gray matter in the frontal cortex of the brain. Gray matter is associated with working memory and executive decision making. A follow-up study suggests that after eight weeks of meditation there were also changes in brain volume in five different regions of the brain. Brain volume affects cognition, perspective taking, emotional regulation, compassion, and more.

In other words, meditation makes you smarter!

In addition, when you focus your mind, a number of more subtle but no less desirable things begin to occur:

- When you focus energy, you gain power. A magnifying glass can focus the sun's rays, burning through paper. A laser is a focused or coherent light and can burn through steel. Whenever you focus your attention, you perform better. World-class athletes use meditation to gain a competitive advantage. When you focus better, you think more clearly and study better.
- When you focus your attention, it can be profoundly sensual. Whether it is food, music, art, massage, or sex, when you pay attention to what you're doing, you enjoy it much more fully.
- Your mind quiets down and you begin to experience an inner sense of peace, joy, and well-being. As you feel that centeredness, you feel calm, clear, and connected.
- When you meditate deeply, you begin to experience a "double vision." That is, on one level, you can appreciate that individual human beings are separate—you're you and I'm me. But on another level, you start to see that we are part of something transcendent that connects us all. More on this in Chapter 7.

There are many schools of thought on meditation technique. We'll outline four simple/beginner techniques below. When choosing which meditation technique is best for you, consider two criteria. First, it should be the technique that feels right to you—personally resonant. Second, it should be the technique that you enjoy. If it feels right, you'll enjoy it more. And if you enjoy it, you'll get more out of it.

The four basic meditation techniques are:

- Gazing meditation
- Meditation on your breath
- Meditation on a word
- Walking meditation

It may be useful to practice each one of the four basic techniques for a short period of time to get a feel for which one suits you best. Over time it is best to choose a technique and stay with it so you can experience the depth of its benefits.

Gazing Meditation

When your eyes are still and focused, your mind will be, too. When your mind strays, your eyes will move also. Gazing meditation gives you that feedback immediately—you know your mind is wandering if you are looking around. And you know you are finding focus and stillness when you can fix your gaze steadily on something. As you become better at fixing your gaze outwardly—at a candle flame, a photograph, a beautiful flower, a sunset—you can progressively reflect more inwardly, getting more in touch with your intuition by steadying your mind.

We'll get to a short instruction soon, but here are a few tips:

- When you are just starting a gazing meditation, we recommend that you start with at least five minutes a day. You can set a timer or alarm if you feel that will help you really dedicate yourself to the effort.
- You may find that your mind starts to take over—you'll find yourself thinking about your object in other contexts. If you've chosen a candle flame, maybe you'll start to think about the candles on your last birthday cake or the small votive candles that were on the table at a restaurant you went to last night. From there, you might start to think about the people who were around the table when you blew out the birthday candles, or what you were wearing at the restaurant. The mind is funny that way; it loves to wander! If and when this starts to happen, don't beat yourself up. Just gently try to bring your focus back to the object in front of you. Bring it back to the beautiful candle flame. See if you can just focus on the candle flame itself, letting go of the surroundings, like the table and the candleholder. Keep your eyes soft—no need to open them wide or rigidly focus on the details of the flame. Another way to think of softening is to simply receive the object with your full senses instead of projecting your eyes onto the object. There is a subtle but significant difference; recruit your full senses so as to remain

awake and aware yet restive and reflective. Maintain an easy natural breath through your nose.

- When your timer goes off or when you are coming out of the meditation, bring your hands together, keeping your eyes closed, and briskly rub your palms together. This will generate some heat. Then take your warmed palms, gently cup them over your eyes, and allow the darkness and the warmth to penetrate deep into and behind your eyes. This is a soothing way to release any tension you may feel. After a few seconds, very slowly touch your fingertips to your eyelids, stroking your eyelids out toward your ears. This might sound funny to read, but when you actually do it, you'll likely feel tension or eyestrain evaporating.

Now, go ahead and try it:

1. Sit in a comfortable position.
2. Take a few deep breaths through your nose. Inhale fully, and as you exhale, let that breath out very slowly, and with it, release any tension you might feel.
3. Close your eyes briefly.
4. Now open them slowly and begin to gaze at the object you have chosen for this exercise (a candle flame, for example).
5. If your eyes become tired, allow them to close, but remain focused on the image or object you have chosen by seeing it with your memory, imagination, or "inner vision." As that image begins to fade, open your eyes again and refocus your gaze on your actual object for however long you'd like. Continue the process, gazing and sensing outward, and then closing your eyes and reflecting inward.
6. Now close your eyes if they're not already closed, and as you sit quietly, allow that image to reflect your poise and peace within. Allow a period for personal quiet time.

Meditation on Your Breath

Your breath flows in and out approximately sixteen times a minute. This meditation technique uses your breath's natural tide-like rhythm as the

"object" of your focus, connecting you to a deeper place within you—
a place where your sense of inner peace and calm flow freely.

Try it:

1. Set a timer for however long you want; try starting for at least five minutes.
2. Sit comfortably, with your spine gently upright and your body at ease.
3. Close your eyes and bring your awareness to your breathing.
4. Breathe through your nose, simply noticing the transition in the direction of your breath as it flows in and down and then comes back up and out.
5. Next, notice the depth and breadth of your breath. With each inhalation, see to what extent your breath can gently expand your lungs' capacity.
6. Notice how your chest rises and falls and how your belly moves in and out as you breathe. The whole system seems to move in rhythm with your breath's rhythm; it's amazing!
7. If your mind begins to wander from focusing on your breath, gently bring it back to the flow, in and out. The objective here is to try not to *control* your breath in any way, but instead just observe how it flows in and flows out, like the tide.
8. When your timer goes off or you are ready to come out of this meditation on your own, open your eyes slowly and look downward at your hands resting on your lap or thighs. When you feel ready, gently wiggle your fingers and toes, and make your transition back.

Meditation on the breath reduces blood pressure, decreases muscle tension, and increases alpha brain waves. It brings the heartbeat into rhythm, increases learning ability and mental clarity, and can bring feelings of peace and tranquility.

Meditation on a Word

Certain words have a great impact on us. They can evoke strong feelings and emotions. The idea in this meditation technique is to think of a word that creates a strong positive vibration in you when you hear it, see it, or say it. This can be an everyday word, a "feeling" word, a religious or spiritual word, a prayer, or a mantra.

In many cultures, people meditate on words that begin with an *A* or an *O* and end with an *M* or an *N* because these sounds have been found to be soothing—for instance, *om, shalom, amen, ameen,* and *salaam,* all of which happen to translate as the English word "peace." These words mean peace and bring peace. If you prefer a more secular word, use "one."

As you do this practice regularly, you will enjoy the benefits of peace and calmness and the ability to respond appropriately to everyday situations. At some point, you may notice that you hear this word in your mind when you are quietly going about your day and your tasks. Use it to help quiet and calm your mind when you need it. You can repeat it throughout the day even when you are not meditating to help center and focus your awareness.

Have you ever heard a song on the radio and found yourself humming it later in the day? Meditation works the same way—even a few minutes in the morning will continue subconsciously throughout the day and keep you centered in the midst of busy activity.

Try it:

1. Find a comfortable sitting position that is gently upright, relaxed, and at ease.

2. Close your eyes and notice your breath as it comes in and as it goes out.

3. Begin to slowly repeat the word you've chosen, silently or out loud. You can move your lips if you want to say the word silently. Just repeat it over and over, like a wheel turning, round and round.

4. For example, let's say you want to meditate on the word "one." Inhale fully, and then say the word "one," emphasizing the humming "nnnnnnn" sound at the end of the word until you run out of air. Inhale and repeat.

5. You may even notice the word synchronizing with your breath, but don't force it.

6. If you find it useful, imagine your word permeating and penetrating every cell in your body and every thought in your mind.

7. When your mind wanders, take notice and, without judging, analyzing, or ruminating, gently return to your word.

8. Continue the process for at least five minutes.

9. To come out of the practice, take in a deep inhalation, and as you do, feel and hear your word coming in even stronger. When you exhale, imagine breathing your word out into the world. When you feel ready, let your eyes open and look downward. Gently move your body when ready.

10. Allow for a period of personal reflection before you get up and move on to other things.

Meditation on a word lowers respiration rate, reduces blood pressure, decreases muscle tension, and increases alpha waves of the brain. It brings the heartbeat into rhythm, increases mental clarity, and can allow you to experience greater feelings of serenity and joy.

Walking Meditation

Walking meditation can be a wonderful complement to your seated meditation practice. Because your body is moving, it may be easier to be mindful of the sensations in your body and to stay anchored in the present moment. For this reason, many people find walking meditation easier than seated meditation. This technique may also be useful if you don't like sitting still or if you are uncomfortable sitting for long periods of time. Another reason many people like this technique is that it can go with you anywhere. You may want to practice outside in nature, or in the privacy of your own home. It can be done with a group or alone.

But don't misunderstand: this isn't really like taking a walk. You'll be standing up, your eyes will be open, and you'll be moving, so you'll necessarily have a bit more interaction with the outside world, even if only the room or path you've chosen. But walking meditation isn't going to give you a cardio workout! Instead, walking meditation is much slower than taking a normal walk, and involves either coordination with your breath or specific focusing practices. It looks more like meditation than like walking.

We recommend practicing walking meditation for ten to fifteen minutes. To be more effective, think about where you want to do this. If you want to be outside in nature, plot out your course in your mind, so that you can focus on your walking and breathing, and not on where to go. If you're doing this meditation in your house, set a course that won't require stairs or opening doors as you go.

Walking meditation improves balance of both the body and the mind. The rhythmic movements of body and breath begin to slow the heart rate and lower blood pressure. It calms and quiets the nervous system and the mind. It can be used both as a meditation practice in and of itself and as a transition to a sitting meditation practice.

Try it:

1. First, choose how you will hold your hands. Option one is to place your hands behind your back, holding one wrist. Option two is to rest your hands in front of your body by placing one hand in a loose fist just above your navel and the other hand gently covering your fist. Option three is to simply let your arms and hands hang gently at your sides.

2. Stand in a comfortable upright position.

3. Tune in to how your breath can support a pleasant posture. As you breathe in, feel your spine gently extend upward, as if there is an invisible string extending from your spine through the crown of your head and up to the sky. As you breathe out, feel the breath slowly wash down and out through your feet, feeling a sense of grounded contact and support.

4. Keep your head upright and your gaze slightly downward for better balance.

5. Begin to walk in a deliberate and slow way. Unlock your knees, shift your weight onto your left foot, and pick up your right foot. As your heel comes up and you feel balanced, place your right foot down in front of you, committing the weight to the foot.

6. Do the same on the other side.

7. Unless you've done this a number of times before, you'll likely start at a pace that's faster than is beneficial—it's hard to unlearn all your years of walking briskly! As you are able to slow down your pace, your mind will start to follow that slow pace.

8. Continue placing one foot in front of the other, with all of your attention on walking. You may notice that your breath finds a natural rhythm with the steps you are taking, but don't force it. You want your body and your mind to stay united and your breath to flow naturally.

9. Remember, you are not really going anywhere; there is nothing to achieve except presence in this moment.

10. When you're done, either stand for a moment and let yourself linger in stillness or follow up with a seated meditation practice.

Time-Tested Meditation Tips

- Avoid meditating immediately after a meal.

- Before early morning meditations, do a few stretches and splash some cold water on your face to help you fully wake up.

- To make sitting more comfortable, use a straight-backed chair, or place a firm cushion or pillow or a folded blanket under your buttocks.

- Make sure your clothing is comfortable and sufficiently warm (your body will cool down as you relax).

- Meditate in a well-ventilated room.

- Set up a special place in your home, even a corner, where you can have a beautiful picture, some flowers, a candle, and a nice chair, et cetera. Every time you pass that place, it will remind you of your meditation and, we hope, the peacefulness you feel when doing it. Just as walking in the kitchen encourages a feeling of hunger, even though you may not be hungry, so this place in your house will encourage you to meditate.

- Meditating regularly is very important. It is through regularity that the habit of meditation can be cultivated. Once meditation becomes a habit, you will look forward to it.

- It's best to meditate in the same place and at the same time every day. This creates a routine. Your mind will gently gravitate effortlessly toward that routine over time.

- Two sittings (or two slow walks) daily of fifteen to twenty minutes is a good start for a meditation practice. Sit in the morning when you get up and in the evening before going to bed. If you're an early bird, very early in the morning (4:00 to 7:00 a.m.), when the world is quiet and peaceful, is an especially good time to meditate.

- Postures and breathing practices help to center the mind and relax the body in preparation for meditation.

- Remember, meditation is a *process*. When your mind wanders, just bring it back to your word or sound or your breath, over and over. Everyone's mind wanders—even the minds of advanced meditators. Just the practice of bringing it back, over and over, is what makes it powerful. It's a practice that takes practice!

- Don't be anxious or disturbed by distracting thoughts coming into your mind during your practice. Don't energize them; rather, simply ignore them. Know that your intention is meditation. If these thoughts want to sit for a while in your mental "room," that's up to them. Don't try to force them out—you'll create an enemy. Learning to let go of these distracting thoughts is a valuable technique.

- Tend to the *process* of meditation rather than the goal. If you do, you will get results.

- Sometimes it may seem that your mind is more disturbed in meditation than during other times. Usually this is because you've never been still or quiet enough to notice all the "static" on your mental radio. It's always been there. Listen to the show as it goes by and enjoy the drama, romance, intrigue, and comedy, but don't get caught up in any of the scenes, no matter how dramatic. Remain a witness. Use your object of meditation as your anchor.

- Approach your practice with a sense of fun and adventure.

- If possible, be around others who meditate; you will inspire each other.

Accessing Your Inner Wisdom

One of the most powerful benefits of meditation is to be able to access our inner wisdom, which we all have. It speaks very clearly but quietly and is easily drowned out by the chatter of everyday life. Some people experience this as the "God within," the "inner teacher," or the "still small voice within."

For me, this is the voice that wakes me up in the middle of the night and says, "Hey, listen up! There's something you're not paying attention to that's important."

So at the end of a meditation or a deep relaxation, when my mind is relatively still and quiet, I ask that inner wisdom, "What am I not paying attention to that I need to hear?"

And I listen.

It's often amazing what emerges. I've learned to rely on this inner wisdom and to trust the wisdom that it provides. And because it's coming from within me, there's no one to argue with. It's quite powerful!

Because I do this regularly, I've learned to recognize that voice even in the midst of busy activities during the day. Meditation allows me to access this information more intentionally. My most creative and innovative insights often come during these times.

Guided Imagery

Your mind talks to your body by using mental images. This dialogue is going on all the time—sometimes in healing ways and sometimes in harmful ways—although much of the time you may not be consciously aware of this process. Likewise, the conscious mind and unconscious mind communicate with each other by using imagery.

Worrying is a form of negative imagery. If you have ever worried about anything, you know firsthand some of the physical effects of worrying. It can cause your palms to sweat, your mouth to dry out, and your heart to race, all from just thinking about a negative outcome. If "awfulizing" can affect the body in negative ways, consider that visualizing a positive outcome can have a positive impact on our health and well-being. Guided imagery is the practice of using focused imagination to create a positive mental and physical state.

Studies show that positive visualization can upregulate or turn on the parasympathetic response (the relaxation response), which can support health and healing. Many people find guided imagery to be one of the most valuable techniques in the healing process. It can be deeply relaxing, creative, and fun.

There are two different types of guided imagery: direct and indirect. In the practice of direct imagery, you conjure a healing image that is specific to your own health and well-being. You might imagine a clogged artery opening up, or better blood flow to and from your heart. The more personal and relevant you can make the image, the more powerful the effect.

Indirect imagery begins with bringing your body and mind to a peaceful state. This state may be induced by thinking of something that invokes a sense of calm and peace—maybe a beautiful sunset or a place in nature. From that place, you can direct healing to your whole body and mind.

To practice either type of guided imagery, first find a quiet place where you can get relaxed without interruption. You may choose to sit upright or lie on your back, whichever is most comfortable. Simply find a space where you can engage in natural, slow, full-body breathing for a minute or so.

Direct Guided Imagery

Once your muscles and your mind are relaxed, create an image in your mind's eye of what you want your body to do. This image can take several forms. For the medically sophisticated or the technically minded, it can be a precise representation of specific physiological activities. For example, you might want to visualize your coronary arteries healing and becoming less clogged. Because your brain controls the muscles surrounding the arteries, studies have shown that engaging in this kind of imagery may actually dilate your arteries and allow more blood to flow into your heart muscle.

Try it:

1. While in a relaxed state, focus your mind on your body and the particular part of your body that needs your healing attention.

2. Direct all thoughts to this area and allow yourself to experience what this part of your body feels like right now.

3. After a moment, imagine what that area actually looks like. You may be able to conjure a detailed representation of what you think that part looks like, or it could be more symbolic of how that area feels to you. Keep your attention there until you are satisfied with the picture you've brought to mind.

4. Now begin to imagine the healing process to make that area better. Whatever you sense this part of your body needs to heal, use your imagination to visualize providing that healing. Imagine with as much detail as possible that this part of your body is healing right now.

5. Spend a few minutes holding that healing picture in your mind, using it as a focusing thought. If you find your mind wandering, gently return it to the healing image. However, the picture may change, and it is important to hold a place to simply observe what happens, whatever transitions and trans-

formations may occur. Sometimes unexpected yet insightful and important information can be communicated while practicing imagery (such as unexpected compassion, spontaneous forgiveness, etc.).

6. Allow yourself to reflect on the healing image for a few minutes, several times a day. Many people discover that their images are always with them in the background. From time to time during the day, they find themselves spontaneously focusing upon their healing image, allowing it to remain there for a few moments. While your conscious imagery work will take only a few minutes each day, your unconscious and your body will continue to reap the benefits of your efforts.

Indirect Guided Imagery

Indirect guided imagery practice induces a positive mental and physical state and brings forth physiological changes within the body to promote healing and peace of mind.

1. For this imagery practice, find a quiet place to enter a relaxed state. Allow your attention to simply follow the natural rhythm of your breath, moving in and out, for a minute or so.

2. Next, imagine healing light or healing energy collecting just above the crown of your head.

3. Imagine drawing that healing energy into your body and sending it through your mind, down your spine, and through your vital organs. Imagine the healing energy filling and healing your heart.

4. Now send the healing energy through your abdomen and pelvis, down your arms to your fingers, and down your legs to your toes.

5. Allow it to touch every fiber of your being, healing at the deepest level.

6. Let that light or energy expand and glow from the inside out, wrapping your body in healing light/healing energy.

7. Sense how your breath produces energy, how it enters and expands as energy circulating throughout your body. Sense your

breath reenergizing movement in your fingers and toes, in your ankles and wrists. You might find it helpful to visualize your breath as healing light coming in and out of your body.

Deep Relaxation

If you want a pendulum to go one direction, first pull it in the other. Similarly, if you want your muscles to relax, first make them tense.

As we've discussed, one of the most common ways that the body responds to stress is with muscle tension, which can lead to pain or discomfort. Gently and progressively relaxing your muscle groups reduces muscle tension and general mental anxiety, and can often help you sleep more restfully. The difference between relaxation and sleep is consciousness. When asleep we are unconscious, but during relaxation the mind stays awake and alert yet deeply relaxed, what we call being superconscious.

Deep relaxation occurs progressively, as a learned and conscious letting go. It's meant to relax not only your physical body but also what we refer to as your "subtle" body. According to the yoga tradition, your subtle body is composed of your field of consciousness, feelings, intuition, intelligence, senses, and energy, all of which govern your physical body. Relaxing your subtle body, therefore, is a kind of reawakening and rediscovery of a place of peace, stillness, and insight deep within yourself.

One of the most important themes of this book is that our peace of mind isn't something we get from outside ourselves; rather, it is there all the time until we disturb it. In this context, these techniques don't bring you a sense of peace and relaxation. They simply help us quiet down our mind and body to enable us to experience what is already there. Think of this process as relaxing from the outside in.

Practicing deep relaxation helps the body recover from exertion, lowers blood pressure and heart rate, lowers elevated cholesterol, improves sleep, calms the mind, reduces anxiety, and promotes healing and well-being. The process will take you into the deepest parts of your being. When you practice regularly, it becomes easier to maintain regular sleep patterns and an enhanced sense of peace.

To get started, find a quiet space and a pleasant position for your body that feels both symmetrical and comfortable, either lying on the floor or sitting in a chair. If you are lying down, it can be pleasant to use the support of pillows under your knees and head for more comfort. The object is to get sufficiently comfortable so that you can allow your body to be still. During progressive relaxation, blood pressure lowers and so you may become progressively cooler. Using a blanket can help make your practice cozier and more enjoyable. You may find it helpful to set an alarm for your desired practice time; try starting with ten to fifteen minutes for the short practice and thirty to forty-five minutes for the extended version.

Deep Relaxation: Short Version
Once you've allowed your body to get settled in and still, use your imagination to travel through your body, mentally inviting each part of your body to relax.

1. First engage your intended muscle by squeezing it, and then release and relax it. Start with your feet, then legs, then hips. Now move up your body to your hands, arms, and shoulders. Next, systematically move to your buttocks, abdomen, chest, and throat. Finally, focus on your spine, all the muscles in your back and neck, and then your face and head. Remember to breathe into each part of the body and then soften and relax there on the out-breath. Aim for a "letting go" type of out-breath. It's as if you're holding a heavy ball in your hand, and then once you're able to release the grip, you can exhale in relief because it feels so good to simply let it go.

2. Scan your body and use the out-breath to consciously relax and release any remaining tension.

3. Observe your breath flowing in and out naturally, slowly, deeply, and rhythmically.

4. Observe any thoughts and feelings as they arise and dissipate.

5. Rest and allow peace and stillness to emerge from deep within you.

6. Listen to and connect with your inner voice, your intuition, and the healing happening within.

7. Take a moment for personal reflection, to acknowledge your experience.

To come out of this relaxation practice, slowly roll to one side to sit up.

Deep Relaxation: Extended Version

In this extended version of the progressive relaxation, you'll be doing a systematic survey of a more detailed version of your anatomy, tensing and relaxing each part.

As odd as it might sound, you'll add your bones and even organs to the mix. Your muscles are easier to direct: we can manually squeeze and relax each of them systematically. But you can mentally do the same for your bones and organs, gently guiding each area to relax.

1. Use your imagination to travel through your body. "Where attention goes, energy flows," so sense how you can focus your attention on breathing into each area of the body, one by one, then softening and relaxing each area on the out-breath.
2. Inhale. Gently squeeze your right leg. Exhale as you relax. Do the same with your left leg. Next, inhale and gently squeeze your right arm. Exhale as you relax. Repeat with your left arm. Next, inhale and squeeze your buttocks muscles. Exhale, relax.
3. Inhale. Expand your abdomen. Then let your abdomen completely relax as you exhale through your mouth. Repeat the same sequence with your upper chest.
4. Leaving your arms relaxed at your sides, inhale and bring your shoulders up toward your ears. Exhale, relax. Inhale, bring your shoulders together in front of your chest, exhale, relax. Inhale, push your shoulders toward your feet. Exhale, relax.
5. Slowly roll your head from side to side and allow your neck to relax. Inhale and gently squeeze together all your facial muscles, including your jaw, mouth, eyes, and forehead. Exhale and relax.
6. Relax your feet, legs, hips, hands, arms, and shoulders. Relax your buttocks, abdomen, chest, heart, and throat. Relax your spine and your back, neck, facial, and head muscles.

7. After relaxing your physical body, bring your awareness to your breathing. Without trying to change the pattern of your breathing, just observe or feel the gentle flow of air as it comes in and out and as your body and mind begin to quiet down. Feel your breath flowing in and out naturally, slowly, deeply, and rhythmically, as if you can feel your whole body breathing. Gradually allow your breaths to become progressively fuller and deeper.

8. Allow your breath to take you on a tour to discover any areas of lingering tension. When you notice an area of tightness, tension, or discomfort, steer your breath there with your attention. Feel it gently expand there on the in-breath, and then soften and relax there on the out-breath. You may even notice a sense of freedom from your physical form as physical pain and discomfort begin to ease or disappear.

9. Imagine that you are breathing in light and healing energy as well as oxygen that is revitalizing and recharging your body and mind.

10. Allow this energy to come in through your head, down your back, your spine, the front of your body, your arms to your hands, and your legs to your feet.

11. Notice whatever thoughts or feelings come up, and let them pass without trying to judge, suppress, or control them.

12. Rest and allow a place of peace and stillness to emerge from deep within yourself.

13. Listen and connect with your inner voice, your intuition, and the healing happening within.

Once you have slowed down the physical body and heightened your awareness of your subtle body, you may begin to notice your everyday thoughts and feelings more as they arise. You may begin to see or feel that you store emotional pain as well as all of the impressions from your senses in certain parts of your body. As thoughts and feelings come into your awareness, simply witness them with curiosity and compassion.

As your body, breath, and mind begin to rest in alignment, a deeper sense of stillness and peace will emerge. It is here that you can start to gain some perspective. Allow yourself to rest here in your center, listening and reconnecting with that place of stillness and peace within yourself. This practice connects you with your body of wisdom and intuition, which reflects your inner light and true self. As you rest here, listen and feel connected to your inner voice, intuition, and the healing happening within.

To experience your subtle body, step back from your streaming thoughts and feelings and simply bear witness to them. Observe without judging. Simply allow thoughts and feelings to arise, and watch as they dissipate. As you reflect on your inner observations, you may be able to gain insight into how your mind works, your thinking and feeling patterns, your triggers, your drivers, and so on. Gently allow your mind to unwind from all labeling, analyzing, ruminating, and judging. Make this a practice of self-benevolence, one of tender self-care. Try not to fall asleep, but it's fine if you do.

After resting, it is important to come out of your relaxation the same way you went in, so as not to disturb the deep sense of peace and integration that you've achieved. Begin to observe the quality of your breathing, the tone of your thoughts and feelings. Begin to take some slow, deep breaths to reenergize your organs and then your extremities. Slowly move your fingers and toes. Slowly move your hands and feet. Gently roll your arms and legs back and forth. When you are ready, slowly roll over onto your side, bend your knees, and then come to a seated position feeling refreshed and rejuvenated.

Additional Stress-Busting Techniques

Although our research has shown the five techniques we've outlined above to relieve stress and allow deep healing to occur, there are multiple effective, fun, and meaningful ways to reduce stress.

Sharing Feelings

Sharing our authentic feelings in a safe and intimate environment—among trusted friends, in a support group, with a minister or therapist—can be a powerful tool for reducing stress. When we're able to openly share our true feelings within a secure setting, it can help us to unburden ourselves and allow us to feel supported by others. Our ability to connect to ourselves and others is at the root of what makes us sick and what makes us well. More on this in Chapter 7.

Taking Care of a Pet

Owning and caring for pets is also associated with reducing stress. Studies show that people who own pets have lower blood pressure, better cholesterol numbers, lower weight, and improved stress response. A nationwide study in 2017 indicated that dog owners have a lower risk of death from cardiovascular disease and strokes. The exercise you get from walking a dog is certainly a healing factor; the unconditional love that your pet gives you at the end of your long day is also healing.

Digital Detoxing

Did you know that media overload is the sixth-leading cause of stress in the United States? Digital detox centers, where people are able to "unplug" or refrain from using electronic devices such as smartphones and computers for a period of time, are popping up around the country to help people deal with the stress and isolation from too much technology.

"Crazy busy" is a self-induced, culture-induced, technology-induced disorder that leaves us feeling frazzled, forgetful, frenzied, disorganized, and overloaded. Unplugging can have a powerful effect on the nervous system. Try it for an hour a day, even one day per week—you might not only like it but also come to crave and protect unplugged sanctuaries in your life.

Warning: May Cause Inner Peace!

When you engage in any one of these stress reduction techniques, you may notice good things starting to happen. Be on the lookout for symptoms of inner peace: a tendency to think and act spontaneously (rather than on fears based on past experience), an unmistakable ability to enjoy each moment. Peaceful traits also include a loss of interest in judging other people, a loss of interest in interpreting the actions of others, and a loss of interest in conflict in general. Marks of someone with inner peace include frequent and overwhelming episodes of appreciation, frequent attacks of smiling, and a contented feeling of connectedness with others and nature. Those with inner peace share an increasing tendency to *let* things happen rather than *make* them happen.

Overcoming Barriers to Stress Management

You can probably find endless excuses to not manage your stress; it can be all too easy to talk yourself out of doing what's good for you. However, over time those excuses turn into barriers to your health and well-being. By recognizing and naming the barriers we encounter, we can begin to overcome them. Review some of the common rationalizations below that we've heard over the years. Consider which possible solutions or reframing ideas you think you could use to overcome your barriers. These exercises are helpful to do when you find yourself struggling with practice at any time.

I'm Too Busy

- Reevaluate your priorities—your life may depend on it.
- Incorporate stress management into other activities. For example, consider using commuting time or the time right after work. If you

have a long commute via train, bus, plane, or car, this can be a time to practice breathing, relaxation, meditation, and imagery. (Of course, this is not advisable if you are the driver!)

- Do a walking meditation.
- Use stress management to wind down before bed.
- Delegate or ask for support to free up time.
- Schedule it into your day like other appointments.

I'm Too Tired

- Refresh yourself by doing physical poses.
- Figure out why you are tired.
- If you are tired because of not exercising, start moving.
- If you are tired because of insufficient sleep, plan for more hours of it and protect your plan for that rest (talk with your physician if your issue is insomnia or restless legs).
- If you're too busy, plan less and reassess your goals.

It Doesn't Work

- Research shows that it clearly does work—reevaluate your expectations.
- Look for subtle changes like less anger, more patience, and less anxiety.
- You may be very "wound up." Do stress management activities throughout the day to relieve stress.
- Use a CD or DVD to help support and guide your stress management practice, such as the DVD at the end of *The Spectrum*.
- Play music to help you relax.
- Physical exercise is great, but it offers different benefits than these stress management techniques do.

I Don't Enjoy It

- Try walking meditation, which allows you to use the movement of your body to access your awareness from the outside in.
- Play music that you *do* enjoy while you are engaged in one of these stress reduction techniques.
- Attend a class for more guidance.
- Do it with a partner.
- Create a nice atmosphere (for example, candles, dim lighting, plants, aromas).
- Determine the part you like and do more of it.

I Have an Injury

- Relaxation and guided imagery are powerful healing tools and can be used when there is an injury.
- Take care to move with awareness and do only what feels right to you. You may be surprised what you find when you start slow and small.
- Some gentle movements may actually aid in the healing process. Ask your doctor or physical therapist for recommendations.
- Ask your injury what it really needs to be healed. Then listen closely to the answer.

I Have to Calm Down Before I Start

- Sometimes our lives are very far away from our relaxation practice and we need time to transition. Take the time you need to make that transition, then practice.
- Take a short walk before you practice.
- Listen to some relaxing music prior to starting.
- Do some journaling beforehand to bring you into a more quiet state of mind.

I Fear "Feeling"

- Feelings are inescapable, so you might as well spend some time being deliberate about their release.
- Know that your feelings will come out one way or another: either directly, through stress management, or indirectly, through symptoms.
- Express feelings in other ways, like writing, talking, or journaling.
- Visualize a positive outcome.
- Question your thinking. Many feelings are pleasant and uplifting; not all feelings will be uncomfortable.

I Get Bored

- Vary your stress management activities.
- Switch among individual, partner, and group sessions.
- Explore what is underneath the boredom. Do you feel lonely? Do you feel fear? Are you feeling discomfort?
- Consider the fact that sameness and familiarity might have a silver lining: they are reassuring.
- Being still on the outside doesn't equate with boredom on the inside.
- Focus on deepening your practice, not changing it.
- Get quieter, listen to your breath, and observe more.
- See your session as a counterpoint to your busy daily life.

Setting Up Your Stress Management Practice

Whichever stress management techniques from this chapter, or combination of techniques, that you choose to do, try to practice daily to make it a habit; it will soon become a personal sanctuary within your daily routine. Our habits become our lifestyle. We notice that those individuals who organize their lives around their stress management practices are more likely to maintain their practice over time as well as staying adherent to all of the aspects of the program.

Paying attention to how much better you feel when you do these techniques makes them sustainable. In summary: if you feel stressed, you are stressed; if these techniques help you to feel less stressed, then they are beneficial to you. Remember:

- Choose a regular time—morning, evening, or anytime you won't be disturbed (preferably two to three hours after a meal or prior to a meal).
- Choose a place in your home that's quiet and free from distractions and clutter.
- Make sure your space feels comfortable and conducive to your stress management practice.
- Practice on a carpeted floor or a yoga mat, or sit in a chair.
- Have a blanket, a chair, and two pillows available to use.
- Aim for one hour minimum to make sure you are getting your full prescription.
- Set your timer or clock for however much time you're able to allot to your practice.

> Some people also find it helpful to make a written commitment of their intention to do stress management. If you think this might help you, type up and then sign a short contract with yourself, something like this:
>
> I commit to _____ total hours of daily stress management, which will include _____ minutes of poses and breathing and _____ minutes of relaxation, imagery, and meditation.
>
> Signed: _____

CHAPTER 7

Love More

> Do not feel lonely. The entire universe is inside you.
> —Rumi

Dean

So far, we've provided scientific evidence showing how your health is powerfully determined by how well you live. In this chapter, we'll review how how well you live is meaningfully influenced by how well you love and how well you are loved.

Love and Intimacy Are Healing, Loneliness and Isolation Are Deadly

The need for authentic connection and community is primal, as fundamental to our health and well-being as the need for air, water, and food.

In 1998, I wrote a book, *Love and Survival*, that reviewed what were then hundreds of research studies (and now there are tens of thousands) showing that people who feel lonely, depressed, and isolated are *three to ten times more likely to get sick and die prematurely from virtually all causes* when compared to those who have strong feelings of love, connection, and community.

It's gotten even worse since then. There is an epidemic of loneliness, isolation, and alienation in our culture. One-third of people in industrialized countries are lonely, and 40 percent of adults in the United States report feeling that way. Suicide rates have increased by 25 percent in the past twenty years.

I reviewed these data on several occasions when meeting with Dr. Vivek Murthy during his term as the U.S. surgeon general. I admire him for making alleviating loneliness and social isolation one of the primary goals of his tenure. In another sign of the times, Prime Minister Theresa May recently appointed the first "minister of loneliness" in the United Kingdom.

Here again, loneliness exerts its negative influences via the same biological mechanisms we've been describing throughout this book. Every organ system and biological mechanism is affected. No other factor has such a powerful impact on our health, well-being, and survival. This provides another dimension of scientific evidence to understand the common underlying basis of so many chronic diseases.

For example, loneliness causes chronic emotional stress and overactivation of the sympathetic nervous system. Also, inflammation is persistently increased in people who are lonely or depressed, mediated via changes in C-reactive protein, interleukins, and other mechanisms described earlier.

Researchers have documented that loneliness also turns on (upregulates) gene expression in over a thousand genes associated with chronic illnesses. These include, once again, turning on genes that promote chronic inflammation, immune activation, and cell proliferation and turning off anti-inflammatory genes.

On the other hand, love and intimacy exert their healing influences via these same mechanisms, but in positive ways. For example, social support buffers the stress response by changing gene expression in the brain, especially in the amygdala, the part of the brain that regulates stress (as described in Chapter 2).

Intimacy—anything that brings us closer together and away from isolation and loneliness—is healing. We sometimes refer to this as "horizontal intimacy." It can be the romantic love of a lover or the platonic intimacy of a friend, a child, a parent, a sibling, a teacher—even a pet.

Especially a pet, which can provide the healing experience of unconditional love. When I come home from work, my dog runs up to me, wags his tail, licks my face—he just loves me for me, no matter what kind of day I've had or what I did or didn't accomplish in the world. Studies have shown that looking a dog in the eyes can boost levels of oxytocin (a hormone involved in social bonding) in both the person and the dog, similar to what is seen when a mother looks into her baby's eyes.

Intimacy can also be transcendent, in which we realize that we are not separate from each other and from ourselves. We experience our Self in different forms, manifesting as everyone and everything. We sometimes refer to this as "vertical intimacy."

Although it is often done alone, meditation and other techniques help quiet down the mind and body, paradoxically enabling us to directly experience a greater sense of interconnectedness with each other and with ourselves. For example, a randomized controlled trial showed that just eight weeks of meditation decreases loneliness and, with it, markers of inflammation.

I *See* You!

There has been a radical shift in our culture in the past fifty years with the breakdown of social networks that used to provide a strong sense of connection and community. Back then, most people had a neighborhood with two or three generations of people living together; a job that felt secure, where they spent years with the same co-workers; an extended family they saw regularly; a church, synagogue, club, or community center where they routinely came together.

One of the healing benefits of having these real-world social networks is that people really *know* you—not just your Facebook profile or your bio sketch, but also your dark side, your demons and mistakes, where you messed up. You know that they know, and they know that you know that they know—and they're still there for you.

There's something profoundly healing about being fully seen and received, warts and all. *Sawubona,* meaning "I see you," is a South African Zulu greeting made popular in the epic film *Avatar.* It says, in essence, "I see *all* of you, your light and your darkness, and I am always here for you with respect and love." The response, *ngikhona,* means "I am here." In the Zulu village context, where everyone knows one another, it's a potent representation of understanding, recognition, and compassion.

Today, many people have none of these social networks. Since 1985, the number of people saying they have no friends with whom they discuss important matters nearly tripled. There is a deep hunger for that sense of real intimacy.

This is why Facebook has over 2 billion users, but unfortunately it doesn't really meet the need for authentic intimacy. Most people usually show only the best parts of their lives on Facebook, and if you're not careful to remind yourself of this, it can feel like everyone else has an amazingly better life than yours. The technology that was supposed to bring us together often isolates us even further.

Because of this, a recent study of over 5,000 people found that while real-world social networks were positively associated with overall well-being, the use of Facebook was actually *negatively* associated with well-being. In summary, *the more that people used Facebook, the worse they felt.* Most measures of the frequency of Facebook use in one year predicted significant decreases in self-reported physical health, depression, mental health, and life satisfaction in the following year.

We can only be intimate to the degree that we can be emotionally vulnerable—in other words, to the degree that we open our hearts to each other. And we can only do that to the degree that we feel safe.

It's not that you should make yourself emotionally vulnerable to everyone all the time—after all, there are some people out there who may try to take advantage of you. We've all experienced that at different times in our lives.

But if you have nowhere that feels safe enough to let down your emotional defenses—to open your heart—and no one whom you trust enough to do that, then those walls are always up. Today, too many people have no one with whom they feel safe enough to be open and vulnerable.

Paradoxically, if your emotional walls are always up, instead of protecting you they further isolate you—another example of how a mechanism that evolved to protect us can harm us or even cause us to die prematurely when it's chronically evoked.

Intimacy Is Healing, Joyful, Erotic, and Pleasurable

In the same spirit, whom we choose *not* to be with brings as much meaning to our lives as whom we choose to be with. For this reason, being in a committed, monogamous relationship can, paradoxically, allow more freedom and pleasure at its best:

- The more committed we are, the more we trust.
- The more we trust, the safer we feel.
- The safer we feel, the more emotionally vulnerable we are able to be with each other.
- The more vulnerable we feel, the more we can open our hearts, wider and wider.
- The more open our hearts become, the more intimacy we experience.
- The more intimate we are, the more healing, joyful, erotic, and pleasurable it becomes.
- The more healing, joyful, erotic, and pleasurable it becomes, the more meaningful and liberating it is. In this way, we make our relationships, and our lives, sacred—that is, the most special, the most ecstatic.

In this context, choosing to be monogamous is a practical strategy for having the most pleasure—it's liberating, not a repressive commandment or a moral judgment. That's what makes it sustainable—again, what we gain is so much more than what we give up.

Instead of having the same kind of relatively superficial experiences with different people, Anne and I recurrently have the most meaningful and extraordinary emotionally intimate, erotic, and transcendent spiritual experiences with each other, experiences that are way beyond anything we've even read about, much less imagined, and almost always in different ways that continue to surprise and inspire us.

When we have a date, we're not trying to control what happens in order to re-create an experience that we've already had, however wonderful that might have been. Rather, "Let's be open to all degrees of freedom, all possibilities. Let's let go of expectations and control, just surrender to our True Love, and see what emerges." And what emerges is usually so much more unique and amazing than anything we could have ever imagined.

After so many years together, we keep having new experiences, which continually keeps our relationship fresh even though we're still the same people—yet again, like never before. As far as we've come, we feel like we're only beginning.

We surrender to each other out of pleasure, choice, strength, devotion, and wisdom—not out of fear, weakness, or submission. Energy flows increasingly freely, we hold back less and less as we can each be fully met and fully received—and that capacity keeps exponentially increasing as we go deeper and deeper into intimacy, like layers of an onion being continually peeled off. This level of intimacy allows us to experience the human equivalent of quantum entanglement and mirror neurons.

In quantum physics, entangled particles remain connected so that actions performed on one affect the other, even when separated by great distances. Mirror neurons are cells in our brain that are activated not just when we perform a certain action but also when we observe someone else performing that same action. Both of these phenomena are examples of how interconnected all of nature is, including us.

Great art, great science, great music, great literature, and great sex come from the ability to approach something with a beginner's mind—that is, without preconceptions. Even our imaginations are often limited by our prior experiences.

Beginner's Mind

Shoshin (初心) is a word from Zen Buddhism meaning "beginner's mind." It refers to having an attitude of openness, eagerness, and a lack of preconceptions when studying a subject, even when studying at an advanced level, just as a beginner would. As Shunryu Suzuki wrote in his classic book Zen Mind, Beginner's Mind, "In the beginner's mind there are many possibilities, in the expert's mind there are few."

For example, you might have preconceptions about certain foods, activities, or people. However, if you can practice your ability to shake the Etch A Sketch board of your mind, to reset to be open, as if you're experiencing life anew—you can rediscover a greater sense of wonder, which can be liberating.

I studied photography for several years in college with Garry Winogrand, one of the great photographers of the twentieth century. He'd put a photograph up on the wall and say, "What do you see?" People would describe what they saw.

He'd reply, "Well, how do you know someone doesn't have a gun right outside the frame? How do you know this? How do you know that?" He was getting people to really challenge the beliefs they bring to so many aspects of their lives, which often limit them.

When Henry Ford first began building cars, he was said to have remarked, "If I had asked people what they wanted, they would have said faster horses." How would they envision something they'd never seen? It's not within their frame of reference.

To have experiences that we've never had before requires a sense of openness, curiosity, adventure, trust, surrender, and vulnerability, all of which can significantly expand the new discoveries, pleasures, and meaning available to us—allowing this way of living to be continually fresh and therefore sustainable. (More on this at the end of this chapter.)

Group Support

In the lifestyle medicine program that we offer at various sites across the country, our group support sessions are designed so you can directly experience how good it feels to authentically and deeply connect with others, which is often a transformative experience and profoundly healing. We create a place that feels safe enough for you to talk intimately about what is really going on in your life—to express your authentic feelings—without fear of being judged, abandoned, or criticized.

Once you experience this, then you're more likely to have the courage to open up in significant ways with your friends, family, and loved ones—because you now know how good it feels to experience this level of community and connection with each other.

Although this is the part of our program that many people think they may have the most difficulty with and believe is least important, they usually find it to be the most meaningful and transformative for them. It's amazing how quickly people can bond in this context.

Our group support sessions are not based on healing addictions to alcohol or drugs or even reversing chronic diseases. They are designed to enhance intimacy and to facilitate a strong community of people who are supporting each other as they go through life together. When that happens, healing often occurs.

Medicare and most insurance companies are providing seventy-two hours of our lifestyle medicine intensive cardiac rehabilitation program for reversing heart disease. We divide this into eighteen four-hour sessions, twice a week for nine weeks. During this time, people receive:

- A one-hour group support session
- A one-hour stress management session, including gentle yoga–based stretching, breathing techniques, meditation, and relaxation techniques
- A one-hour exercise session
- A group meal plus a lecture

Our twelve-day residential retreats, six hours of training per day, are also reimbursable by Medicare and many insurance companies.

In my first study forty years ago, the initial purpose of the group support session was to help people stay on the other aspects of the diet and lifestyle program. I assumed that they would be sharing recipes, shopping tips, information about different types of running shoes, and so on.

Instead, I learned that bringing people together in a supportive environment allowed them to let down their emotional defenses and to talk openly and authentically about what was really going on in their lives— about their families, their marriages, their kids, their work, their school, and so on. That's what they needed and wanted most.

In short, they taught me how creating a safe group support community is a powerful antidote to loneliness and isolation. This is the model that we use in all of our programs.

It's so meaningful that after our earlier studies ended, the participants continued to meet regularly in their support groups for decades thereafter. This is a significant reason we are achieving such high levels of adherence to our program.

There is evidence from at least fifteen randomized controlled trials with people who have cancer indicating that effective psychosocial support increases the length of life as well as improving the quality of life, whereas chronic depression predicts a poorer prognosis. The presence of chronic stress hormones such as cortisol predicts more rapid cancer progression. Inflammatory processes affect cancer growth and progression. Sympathetic nervous system activity, telomere length, telomerase activity, and oncogene expression are affected by stress and can affect cancer growth.

One classic randomized controlled trial found that women with metastatic breast cancer who attended a support group once a week for one year lived twice as long as those who did not, even though they had the same conventional treatments such as radiation and chemotherapy in both groups.

A skeptic might say, "Talking about my feelings is going to help me live longer if I have cancer? Oh, please! That sounds so touchy-feely!"

Well, it *is* empathic and compassionate—that's why it works so well! We are creatures of community. Learning to listen to our inner voice while taking care of each other has enabled us to survive as a species. We are hardwired to love and be loved.

When we work at that level, we often learn that people are much more likely to make lifestyle choices that are life-enhancing rather than ones that are self-destructive. In our research, we found that group support attendance was significantly and directly linked with blood pressure, positive health behaviors, and quality of life.

Your feelings are unique and irrefutably true for you. Your uniqueness is what makes you special, part of what provides you with a sense of value, meaning, and purpose. Your feelings are the language of connection, of community. In these group support sessions, you learn to tune in to and express your authentic feelings so that you can discover how your feelings are influencing the story of your life. Yet in sharing your feelings, you also recognize what makes us similar, what connects us all, what helps us transcend the isolation that separates us from each other and from ourselves.

Expressing your authentic feelings and deepest truths can be healing. We all have within us access to a greater wisdom, yet we may not even know that until we feel free to speak out loud.

Listening to another with empathy also can be healing. A deep trust of life often emerges when you listen to what others are truly feeling. You realize you're not alone; you're actually traveling in wonderful company. Ordinary people living their lives often become extraordinary to us once we're able to feel into their life's journey.

In our group support sessions, we create a safe environment for people to connect with the deepest parts of themselves, so that they can also connect that way with others from a place of knowing themselves. We consciously create a place that feels safe for people to be open and authentic with one another, which makes this especially meaningful for people who are not used to having that in their lives. "What goes on in the group stays in the group."

The group support sessions are laboratories for people to practice the skills of sharing feelings in a safe environment. You can replicate this process in your own life in your individual relationships. Or you can get together with a group of friends or family members and practice this together. You can all chip in and hire a moderator, or you can do it on your own. Later in this chapter, Anne will describe how to replicate this group support experience in your life.

Our feelings connect us in powerful ways. As Maya Angelou once wrote, "I've learned that people will forget what you said, people will forget what you did, but people will never forget how you made them feel."

Beginning with self-acceptance and expressing your authentic feelings is a gateway for developing compassion and respect for others to do the same. Group support increases empathy for yourself and for others.

You can make your feelings known to yourself by first intimately recognizing them, and then you can make these known to others by intimately sharing them. This process helps to decrease the emotional symptoms most commonly correlated with chronic diseases, such as isolation, anxiety, hostility, stress, depression, and anger.

We begin each group support session by asking each participant to become aware of how they're presently feeling—not how they think they *should* be feeling, but how they really are. And then we ask them to authentically give voice to those feelings with the others in the group.

For example, one man might say, "I may look like the perfect father, but my son is addicted to opioids." Instead of giving advice—"Why don't you send him to a drug rehab center?"—which tends to further isolate us, we encourage the other members of the group to share how they're feeling: "Oh, I'm so sorry and sad to hear that!" one person might say. Or "My son also is struggling with some important issues around drugs." Or "I've been taking Percocet to get to sleep at night." And so on.

In other words, group support sessions are designed not to fix problems (such as how the father can get his son off opioids, as admirable as that may be) but to help heal feelings of isolation. When the father shares his authentic feelings with the group, it helps heal his feelings of loneliness, shame, and stress.

This, in turn, enables the father to feel the support of the other group members and to better love and support himself. The more love the father feels for himself, the more love he has to share with his son, helping both to heal. Now, they're both better supported and empowered to find their own creative solutions.

In short, these are the rules of engagement, whether in a group or one-on-one:

- Identify what you're feeling.
- Express what you're feeling.
- Listen empathically to what others are feeling.

Our group support sessions allow you to witness how to use your wounds as catalysts for transforming your pain—allowing your suffering to subside, your wounds to begin healing, and your heart to begin feeling safe enough to open a little wider. In this supportive context, our wounds can be our doorways to healing.

Anne

Only close, authentic, loving relationships can support and meet your primal need to be seen, to be heard, to love, and to be loved. Dean sums it up like this: "Our supportive connections are sufficient when we can answer 'Yes' to questions such as: Do you have anyone who really cares for you? Who feels close to you? Who loves you? Who wants to help you? In whom you can confide and be vulnerable?" He adds that if you cannot answer yes to any of these questions, you may have a three to ten times higher risk of premature death and diseases from all causes. In addition to supporting our physical health, loving relationships provide our lives with meaning while promoting a deep sense of comfort, companionship, and security.

For this reason, connecting intimately in small support groups is an integral part of our clinical intervention program, which is proven to reverse chronic diseases. In our support circles, we practice skills that help us develop the ability to identify and express our feelings as a healthier way of processing our emotions. In reciprocity, we also practice listening to others with empathy and compassion as they share their feelings.

Participate in a Support Group

If you want to overcome a sense of isolation and self-paralysis, join forces with others! To make sure your best intentions become solid goals and personal commitments that don't weaken, don't go it alone.

Connecting intimately in a small support group has been an integral and an increasingly validated element of our program to reverse chronic diseases. In our support circles, we set the conditions so that each person can feel safe, known, accepted, loved, and comfortable in expressing their authentic selves. We practice connecting to our own feelings and to those of others with empathy and compassion. Sharing and connecting in this way with others who similarly yearn to improve the quality of their lives heals the isolation and dis-ease felt by so many.

This is how one of our past participants, Stefanie, described her experience:

> The aspect of the program that has had the largest impact on me is the group support. In the beginning, we developed a camaraderie by simply experiencing the program together, but ultimately the group members grew to become some of my closest friends in the world. Any of us would do anything for one another. Our bond has made us healthier and stronger. We all became so close during the program that our alumni community still functions today. Our relationship is a mixture of support and accountability. Nobody is afraid to call you if you aren't at the meetings and ask, "Why aren't you here? What's going on? What's happening with you?" We want to make sure that there isn't a serious issue, so we get on the phone to see if there's anything we can do to help. The group also motivates me; it's been very inspiring to see peo-

ple let down their shields for the sake of the group's cohesive well-being. We interact socially as well; after our meetings we usually meet at an Ornish-friendly restaurant for lunch and just stay there for an hour or two—visiting, sharing, just being together. We also meet relatively often at each other's houses. We have speakers come in and we make food for each other. We are very close.

Another past participant, Joe, shared his experience this way:

> The support group in particular helped me more than I could have imagined that it would. I live alone, so the group gave me a sense of community and of leadership that had been somewhat lacking. And it inspired me; I loved to hear the stories that other people would tell, it gave me confidence—it alerted me to new ideas about the heart. Plus, from a psychological standpoint, the group support allowed me to feel a little bit less stressed about my situation; listening to my group members gave me hope. You know, you have to be optimistic in a situation like that, and that's what the group helped with. I could have taken the viewpoint of being a victim when I had the congestive heart failure, but instead I took the viewpoint of the group. And that optimism has helped me greatly ever since.

One of the greatest benefits of participating in a support group is to be able to apply your new interpersonal skills to more meaningful relationships in your daily life. The point is that practice makes perfect—you're able to practice self-awareness and communication skills in the privacy of your group so that you can do so more readily in your life, when it matters most.

Once you become increasingly comfortable expressing your true self and are able to genuinely empathize and connect with others, the benefits you'll experience in all of your relationships will be profound. When you experience how good it feels and how meaningful it is to connect more deeply with the members of your group, you're likely to feel more motivated to do this in your other relationships as well.

Do You Love Well and Feel Loved?

This is how one participant described his experience: "As I've gotten older, I've withdrawn into a comfortable nutshell, avoiding social interaction and new friendships as much as possible. The Ornish group I participated with changed all of that. I felt accepted from the first day by the other participants with whom I was lucky to share my experience. I relaxed and opened up in a way that I haven't since high school. It seems to me that I always leave sessions feeling open, relaxed, and happy."

When you genuinely practice being more compassionate and loving on a regular basis—with everyone from strangers and acquaintances to your friends and family—it helps to boost your health and well-being while diminishing the dis-ease of isolation. Anyone who's ever felt more alone in a room full of strangers than at home in solitude knows that isolation is not just a function of the number of people you are around. Isolation is measured by the quality of the relationships in your life.

The word "intimacy" comes from the Latin *intimatus,* which means "to make known." "Health" comes from a root that means "to make whole." The word "yoga" derives from the Sanskrit word that means "to yoke," "to bring together," "union." These are old ideas whose power we are rediscovering.

The point is that you can make your feelings known to yourself by intimately recognizing them, and then you can make them known to others by intimately sharing them. This process helps to decrease the emotional symptoms most commonly correlated with chronic diseases, such as isolation, anxiety, hostility, stress, depression, and anger.

In our support groups, we create a safe environment for people to connect with themselves so that they can connect with others. Beginning with self-acceptance and expressing your authentic feelings is the gateway for developing compassion and respect for others, allowing them to do the same.

These are some of the phrases that encapsulate these shared principles:

- Group is about connection, not correction.
- We do not need to be fixed. We need to feel loved.
- We each deserve to be seen, heard, and accepted.

Another program participant, Julie, describes her experience this way:

> Each of the program's four elements (nutrition, exercise, stress management, and group support) played a role in getting me to where I am today, but the group support element stands out in my mind as being particularly impactful. Only four of the people in my cohort knew each other coming into the program, but over the course of nine weeks we became very close. During our group support sessions, we'd talk about our successes, our lives, and our struggles—and there definitely were struggles, but we overcame them together. Every one of us lost weight, every one of us felt better, every one of us made a new group of friends. That's what makes the program so sustainable; it's built on love and caring among the group.

Being social is how we've evolved, and it is still your network of close relationships that reinforces who you are today. Humans are highly social beings. The ever-rising wave of social networks and their exponential adoption rate demonstrate humans' primal need for social belonging, support, and interpersonal meaning.

Have you ever experienced a time when you felt stuck in a rough patch until someone's kindhearted listening and compassion provided a shift in your perspective? Has another's encouragement and support ever given you just the boost you needed to transmute your fear or anxiety into a deeper sense of acceptance, compassion, and fortitude?

By connecting with and loving yourself, you're able to be more intimately known by others, to more genuinely connect with others from a deeper place within yourself. This is one of the greatest benefits of cultivating more love in your life—to learn how you can overcome your fears by embracing yourself, being open and vulnerable with others, and drawing from the strength found in "loving more" together.

There's an African proverb: "If you want to go fast, go alone; but if you want to go far, go together."

Your life blooms by cultivating love for yourself and others, from the inside out. Life's sweetest, most meaningful moments are savored together, when deeply connecting with others and by loving beyond yourself. "Loving More" is about developing a deeper, true connection—to yourself, to your support circle, to your family and friends.

Loving Communication Strategies

This section reviews the strategies that provide a deeply supportive structure for intimate bonds to form and healing to occur.

- Our feelings connect us, whereas our thoughts often are perceived as judgments that isolate us. Feelings include joy, anger, peacefulness, anxiety, worry, love, and so on. Therefore, differentiate your thoughts from your feelings.
- Pay attention to your feelings.
- Express your authentic feelings.
- Listen with empathy and compassion.
- Avoid judging, criticizing, or offering advice.
- Respond with your feelings.
- Keep it confidential.

Differentiate Your Thoughts from Your Feelings

The essence of emotional well-being is being able to identify and express your true feelings in ways that foster empathy, compassion, intimacy, and support. One basic principle of good communication is that our feelings help to connect us, whereas thoughts—especially judgments— tend to isolate us. It's being able to express your feelings that connects you with others, not your thoughts.

As you read the first conversation below, notice how it makes you feel.

Emma: I don't imagine you've made the house payment yet this month?

Austin: There you go again—you always assume the worst and blame me. Just because I was late last time, it doesn't mean I will be this time. I'm not perfect, you know.

Emma: Well, we both know that you're not the best with making payments on time.

Now, as you read the second conversation below, notice how it makes you feel.

Kevin: I feel worried that we'll be late for the house payment and it will affect our credit.

Jane: I hear you and empathize with your concern. I get anxious at this time of the month myself.

Kevin: I'm sorry that you're feeling anxious too. I feel really ashamed that it was my debt that lowered our credit rating.

If you say "I think you're wrong!" then the other person is likely to feel attacked and judged—and either attack back or withdraw. Either way takes you further from intimacy and healing.

If you say "I feel angry and upset!" then the other person is actually drawn closer to you. They may respond, "Why are you feeling that way?"

The difference is that the first example is a thought, whereas the second is a feeling. Even though the second example is a "negative" feeling, anger, because it's expressed as a feeling, the other person can hear and receive it without feeling attacked or judged. Our feelings connect us.

Sometimes thoughts can masquerade as feelings. "I feel upset" is a feeling; "I feel that you're wrong" is a thought and a judgment.

Most people's experience is that these kinds of "I" messages leave a significantly different feeling than the "You" messages. "You" messages tend to be about the other person and what he or she did. A common reaction to "You" messages is feeling defensive. Often people respond with anger, by withdrawing or attacking back. People usually can't hear "You" messages without feeling threatened on some level.

Notice how the "I" statements invite you into my inner landscape, and therefore "I" messages can feel more relatable. When you use "I" statements, you're speaking about your own feelings and thoughts. While expressing your thoughts and opinions can be controversial to others and argued about, your feelings cannot be refuted, because they're true for you. Therefore, it's far more likely that other people will be able to hear you and want to listen more rather than going on the defensive.

Pay Attention to Your Feelings

Many of us learn how to bottle up our feelings. We learn certain expectations at a young age regarding how feelings should be shared or not shared.

For generations, many have been given the message to keep their feelings to themselves. Girls who expressed their emotions openly may have been called drama queens, while boys who expressed their emotions may have been called sissies.

Too often, we've learned how to please others by not expressing how we're really feeling, and gradually we can become unable to even recognize our true feelings. It's valuable to pay attention to your emotions, both the comfortable ones and the uncomfortable ones, because they hone your ability to meaningfully connect with others while navigating your life.

Try this simple check-in practice for connecting with your feelings. Start by getting grounded, comfortable, and centered in a safe place. Gently close your eyes and turn your focus inward for however long you need in order to let down your mask and your appearances and give yourself permission to get in touch with how you're truly feeling.

Bring your attention to rest at your heart, and simply notice the emotions that are present. Remaining gently at the helm of your heart, tune in and genuinely ask it, "Heart, how are you feeling?" Simply listen.

Give yourself full permission to attend to whatever you're honestly feeling in this moment. Sense a "feeling tone" word that is palpable to you, that resonates like a bell of truth within you—good, bad, or ugly. Simply hold a safe space for it inside and name it. Some feeling words include "frustrated," "depressed," "discouraged," "sad," "afraid," "worried," "anxious," "lonely," "happy," "loving," "energized," "calm," "confident," "hopeful," "grateful." Remember that all feelings are okay and intrinsically valid and valuable.

Sometimes this process may happen quickly for you, while other times it may take a little longer. Once you have come up with a word that describes how you're feeling, thank your heart for sharing its truth, and let your eyes open.

If your feeling word feels good, take a moment to celebrate and feel gratitude for however that feels for you in this moment. If your feeling word doesn't feel so good, take a moment to honor that too. Simply reflect with interest, insight, empathy, and self-care on how your feeling word feels for you in this moment.

Express Your Authentic Feelings

We practice expressing our feelings because if they're not expressed, your feelings can become trapped inside and even become debilitating to your health. It is not always easy to identify your feelings, to assign words to them. It can even be challenging to find an appropriate time when you want to talk about them.

In learning to express how you're feeling, you first learn to identify your feelings so that you can better evaluate them. With practice, you can choose how you want to relate and respond to your feelings, rather than just impulsively reacting to or feeling ruled by them.

A study conducted by UCLA professor of psychology Matthew D. Lieberman found that putting feelings into words makes sadness, anger, and pain less intense. According to Lieberman, when we feel angry we have increased activity in the part of the brain called the amygdala. The amygdala is responsible for detecting fear and setting off a series of biological alarms and responses to protect the body from danger. When the angry feeling is labeled, Lieberman and researchers noted decreased responses in the amygdala and increased activity in the right ventrolateral prefrontal cortex, a part of the brain involved with inhibiting behavior and processing emotions.

Lieberman explains it this way: "When you put feelings into words, you're activating this prefrontal region and seeing a reduced response in the amygdala. In the same way you hit the brake when you're driving when you see a yellow light—when you put feelings into words you seem to be hitting the brakes on your emotional responses. As a result, a person may feel less angry or less sad." As you learn to identify, label, and express your emotions, this area of the brain is strengthened. In turn, you're more intentionally able to respond to and express your feelings with others.

When you take time to notice and name your feelings, you create a buffer of awareness that can reduce the risk of inadvertently and unconsciously short-circuiting your system. Increasing your field of awareness with a sense of inner spaciousness expands your capacity to feel while also being able to self-regulate your experience. Ultimately, this enables you to think more clearly and creatively, making it easier to find constructive solutions.

Naming and sharing your emotions with a trusted other helps you to understand what matters most to you. Lieberman believes that this is "ancient wisdom." He says: "Putting our feelings into words helps us. If a friend is sad and we get them to talk about it, they will feel better."

Expressing your true feelings is a learned skill that you don't develop unless you practice. You can learn how to hone your emotional compass and enlarge your vocabulary by practicing communication skills in your daily interactions with others. Keep in mind that people cannot listen with empathy and compassion unless they are listening to someone who they feel is expressing genuine feelings that are important to them. Authentic communication that is connective has two qualities: you share feelings that are important to you, and you express your feelings with empathy and compassion and without judgment.

Select someone in your life with whom you can practice sharing how you're feeling, someone whom you can trust to listen with an open mind and heart.

Begin by identifying your feeling word(s), then sharing them as an "I" message—such as "I'm feeling alone and afraid." Hopefully, this will elicit the person with whom you're sharing to say something like, "Why are you feeling that way?" This is your invitation to go into more depth about what is behind your feelings.

By remaining focused on sharing your feelings, you're not just telling a story, you're telling how that story is affecting you. As you do that, it reveals more about who you really are, and it allows others to get to know you and to connect with you on a deeper level.

If you're not sure if you've expressed your authentic feelings, ask yourself, "Do I know myself better?"

Practicing expressing your true feelings also allows you to learn more about yourself by uncovering and expressing the emotions that are likely fueling your behavior choices.

As this internal muscle of awareness grows, it becomes much easier to connect within and to express your feelings more clearly and directly with others—all of your relationships will benefit.

Listen with Empathy and Compassion

Knowing how to listen is as important a communication skill as knowing how to express your feelings. Empathy is the caring and capacity necessary to understand another person's experience and feelings from their perspective—that is, the process of placing yourself in another person's skin.

When you listen to others share their feelings about something that is important to them, you may experience reactions ranging from disinterest and criticism to empathy and compassion. You are more likely to meaningfully connect with others when you unplug—literally and figuratively—so you can truly be present, meet people where they are, and listen with compassion and without judgment. This is called empathic listening.

Few of us were taught how to listen to others in order to connect deeply with them. The good news is that this is a skill that can be learned. Learning how to connect deeply with others through empathic listening increases emotional intimacy and decreases isolation and loneliness. This has been shown to have a protective effect against heart disease, cancer, depression, and other conditions.

Talking and listening can enhance emotional intimacy while decreasing detachment and loneliness. However, depending on how you communicate, talking and listening can also decrease emotional intimacy while increasing feelings of isolation and detachment.

Listening with empathy is the key to relationships because it bridges the distance between people. It is the ability to connect with the other person not just in your mind but, most importantly, in your heart. People may not feel comfortable expressing their feelings with you unless they anticipate that you will listen to them with compassion and empathy rather than criticism and judgment.

Simply put, the goal of listening with empathy is to listen nonjudgmentally. You try to see from another's perspective in order to try to understand and validate their experiences and feelings. When you are speaking, the words you use can either elicit empathy from the listener, leading to a sense of understanding and connection, or cause the listener to become defensive and resistant to what you are saying, leading to a sense of frustration and disconnection.

Empathic listening includes listening with your eyes, ears, and heart in order to understand what is being said—especially noticing the feelings behind the words. Empathic listening is not about you agreeing with somebody. It's about you having the willingness to enter into and understand the world of another person.

A famous line from the novel *To Kill a Mockingbird* explains it this way: "You never really understand another person until you consider things from his point of view—until you climb into his skin and walk around in it."

The second part of empathic listening is to communicate your understanding back to the other person. It is not enough to assume that you understand the other's experience, their situation, or how they feel about it. Even if you are accurate in your understanding, the other person will not be aware of this if you keep it to yourself. Therefore, reflecting back what you think you've just heard is an essential way of validating that the other person veritably has been heard, seen, and understood.

Reflecting back what you are hearing is a definitive way to confirm that the message sent and the message received are the same. You are affirming not only what is being said but also the feelings behind the words.

To give an example, let's say someone is telling you that her dog recently got hit by a car. An empathetic response could be, "Oh no! Your dear dog got run over—I'm so sorry to hear that! You must be feeling heartbroken . . . how can I be of support?"

A non-empathetic response would be detached and lacking in emotional connection, such as: "Your dog got run over? No way! Where? What kind of car was it?"

Take a moment now to imagine someone in your life—someone who may even be annoying or angering you, anyone who you sense deeply needs to be heard and regarded by you. Conjure a feeling inside yourself: "What might it be like to be them, with all of the circumstances that led them to be who and where they are today?"

Imagine that person is before you right now, and let them know, "I'm fully present to listen to what you have to share." Hold the space to listen to what they have to say. As you listen compassionately with your heart, track what they're sharing in your body and in your heart. Open yourself up to imagine with empathy, kindness, and compassion how it feels to be where this person is in their life.

If you feel there's still more to be shared, you could say, "I care about you and want to understand better. Would you share more?"

If you notice yourself getting distracted, making judgments, or giving advice when the other person is talking, simply notice how it creates distance between the two of you. Instead, when you notice such interferences arising—because they do for us all—simply practice returning to listening with a feeling heart.

Once this sharing feels complete, thank this person for courageously sharing their true feelings with you and wish them well.

Our human need for empathy craves to be fully seen, heard, and understood in a deeply personal way. When you are fully present in this manner, your empathic communication will promote the essence of emotional intimacy that can help heal your heart and create meaningful emotional bonds with others.

Avoid Judging, Criticizing, or Offering Advice and Reassurance

In our increasingly polarized and divided world, we need empathy more than ever before. Too often we are talking at each other, unable to listen without our judgments and opinions thwarting what would otherwise be opportunities to connect with one another.

Take a moment to reflect on a time in your life when you felt that people may have judged or criticized you. Remember how that made you feel. Did it make you feel heard, regarded, connected? More likely than not, it made you feel like shutting down emotionally and fleeing.

Now take a moment to honestly reflect on how you interact with others. Simply review the last few days and notice how you may have judged, stereotyped, or otherwise put limitations on truly understanding those around you. Replay any of those interactions in your imagination, this time changing them by taking a more open, receptive, and accepting perspective and trying to put yourself in their place.

Our judgments ultimately cloud our vision and distort what we're hearing. We've learned that when we refrain from making reflexive judgments and criticisms, we become more open to better understanding, accepting, and valuing others' feelings, issues, and needs.

Giving advice can also be a form of judgment that implies that the other person is not capable of solving their own problems. It can create more distance and isolation. And when someone offers you reassurance, such as "Everything is going to be okay" or "Just think about the positive side," what they may be really saying is, "I want you to stop talking because you're making me anxious or uncomfortable." Unfortunately, offering your point of view can create unintended disengagement, with the other person needing to take space.

Many of us don't know how to respond in a helpful way to someone who is feeling discouraged. You may feel an urge to rush in and "fix" their "problem," or to ask questions, or to tell stories of your own. While often well-intended and motivated by the desire to be supportive, giving advice and talking too much can actually create more separation and concealment. It's far more effective when you can learn to resist such urges and instead practice listening in ways that keep the other person talking, sharing, and connecting with you.

Here are strategies you can employ when listening to others, without giving advice:

- Be silent. Simply listen. Refrain from saying anything.
- Use phrases that acknowledge the other person is being heard, such as "I understand" and "I hear you."
- Rephrase back to the other person what you sense they're most trying to share with you. For example, "I can tell this is very upsetting," "It sounds like you're really frustrated," or "I can feel how much joy this brings you."
- Express your compassion, such as, "That's big," "That sounds really challenging," "That must be so difficult," "It sounds like what you are feeling is so overwhelming," or "I hear you and I feel sad that things are so hard for you right now."
- Refrain from giving unsolicited advice, like: "The way I see it, you should . . . ," or "If you continue doing this . . . ," or "You only have two choices as far as I'm concerned . . ." Remember that giving advice, even when well-intentioned, is a form of judgment implying that the other person is not capable of solving his or her own problems.
- Resist the urge to tell a long story about yourself. Keep whatever you share brief, to avoid detracting from what it is they're sharing. Be mindful that this can interrupt the flow of allowing them to express what it is they're feeling.
- Avoid asking information-seeking questions that evoke thoughts and distract from the feelings the other person is trying to share. Examples of such questions are "Who is your doctor?" or "Would you like the name of my doctor?"

Simply listen with an open heart and connect not only with what the other person is sharing but, moreover, with what they're feeling—even if they are not able to express it clearly. Opening up, listening with empathy, and giving another your full attention all help to cultivate long-lasting intimate relationships.

Respond with Your Feelings

Your role as a companion is to try to understand how it would feel to be where the other person is, and then to respond by connecting with your own feelings and experiences. When you respond to someone who is sharing their feelings by recapping what you're hearing them share and then relating it to your own feelings, the other person feels reassured, less isolated, and genuinely met because a real connection is mutually felt. Maintaining eye contact while listening and sharing is a simple yet powerful way to support and sustain the connection.

You might say, "I appreciate the bravery it takes to share that with me. I'm hearing that you're utterly exhausted and blue; after the challenges you've endured for this long, my heart really goes out to you. It reminds me of how I felt last year during my divorce. I couldn't get out of bed until I finally committed to working out, meditating in the mornings, and participating in a men's group. I went from feeling broke, burnt out, and depressed to feeling revived and supported to pursue what makes me happy again!"

Remember: once the other person has had the opportunity to feel fully heard and for their feelings to be affirmed, then it's considerate to go ahead and open up yourself. It's important to do so—if someone is open and vulnerable and you just switch the topic to something unrelated, the other person is likely to feel, "I shouldn't have made myself so vulnerable." When you open up in return, then you both feel safe.

Find a gracious moment to reiterate a poignant aspect of what someone has just shared in a way that genuinely resonates for you too. Demonstrate how you can relate to what they've just shared by sharing your own similar feelings. No one wants to feel like they're alone in feeling the way they do. Remember, it's communal listening and sharing of feelings that connect us.

In case you sense that there's a different point of view arising while someone else is sharing, simply listen. Acknowledge what you understand that you've just heard (even if you don't agree with it) before asking questions or sharing your point of view.

In his book *Nonviolent Communication*, Marshall Rosenberg wrote that the time required to reach conflict resolution is cut in half when each person agrees, before responding, to accurately repeat what the previous person had said.

Implementing this simple step of recognizing what the other person has just shared does not imply that you approve of what they said or that you agree with them. It does, however, demonstrate that you're striving to understand the other person, to make them feel regarded—in the same ways you want to feel understood and regarded in return.

It can also be a revelation to start by summarizing what you both agree on. You just may find that you disagree about less than you thought! Come back to the middle, to the heart, where you can acknowledge each other's feelings and the core values that you share. At the end of the day, we all just want to be safe, heard, seen, understood, healthy, happy, and, most of all, loved. Whatever differences we may have with one another, those differences are often minor when weighed against what's universally prevalent for us all.

You may ask yourself, "Did I make the other person feel heard and understood? Was I able to empathize with others' feelings by sharing my own similar feelings in an open and authentic way?"

Marianne Williamson eloquently says, "We are not held back by the love we didn't receive in the past, but by the love we're not extending in the present."

Your ability to connect with yourself and others is at the root of what can make you sick and what can make you well, what can cause you sadness and what can bring you happiness, what makes you suffer and what leads to healing.

Keep It Confidential

It is important that whatever someone shares with you, it remains protected, private, and confidential. If you aim to create the conditions for people to let their guard down, open up, and share their authentic feelings, you need to make them feel safe and respected. By establishing mutual confidentiality from the beginning, and reinforcing it, true feelings can emerge and intimate connections can be deepened. What goes on in the group stays in the group.

Below is a small sample of such comments from participants:

> Today, when I look at my life, I realize that I can take one of two paths; first, I could go back down the road which leads me to unhealthy eating and the emergency room, or second, I could go down what I like to call the "Ornish Highway," which leads to a longer and healthier life. My choice is easy— I'll follow this program forever. I have a wonderful daughter and a twelve-year-old granddaughter who I want to enjoy for many years to come, and I know the program will help me do that. Plus, my wife and I have been married for forty-seven years, and I'm not sure if we can make it another forty-seven, but we're certainly going to try. Overall, I want to continue my activities of biking, hiking, working out daily, Olde Tymers Softball, pickleball, and relaxing on the beach, all of which makes me feel young again. The program has changed my life.   —Sam

> Visualizing myself chasing my daughter around the house and being free of medications keeps me motivated to stay on that healthy path. With those goals in mind, I'm confident that I'll never go back to my old lifestyle.   —Jahnna

> That I'll be able to be here with my grandchildren, my children, and my wife is what really matters. You know, we all want to go to heaven—I certainly do—but not tomorrow, and not the next day either. I feel like the program will make sure that I stay right here for a while. It's given me a new lease on life, and I'm going to make the most of it. —Natalie

A support group from our 2005 prostate research study met for a long time in person, but the members eventually chose to switch to a virtual meeting. After many years of traveling, in some cases for a couple of hours each way, to meet in person, they could no longer sustain it. When asked how it felt to make the transition to meeting virtually, this is how one member described it: "Meeting online has a certain quality that I didn't expect it to have. There's something special about seeing everyone's faces on the computer screen, about being able to talk with each other once a week. These are the people I know, the people I feel comfortable with, and meeting this way gives me that human contact. That's what's important. I need that contact for my humanity. Meeting more frequently online—weekly versus monthly—has allowed us to keep meeting, to maintain this way of living." Because they first bonded while meeting in person, it makes the videoconferences that much more effective.

Get Started

Find an Ornish Lifestyle Medicine Program
Please visit ornish.com to find a program site near you. We are training hospitals, clinics, and physician groups throughout the country. As we've discussed, our lifestyle medicine program is reimbursed by Medicare and many commercial payers.

Start or Join a Free Support Group
Our site at ornish.com also has information on how to start or join a support group. Here are some considerations.

How Do I Recruit Members for a Support Group?
Consider your current social network. With whom do you share common values and goals? With whom would you like to make an effort to carve out more quality time? Who do you know who could benefit from a healthy lifestyle upgrade? Who do you think may be open and ready to take this journey with you? Jot down a list, then make old-fashioned calls or send out an invitation.

If you use social media, use it thoughtfully and judiciously, as an initial avenue to gather the right group. If you want, let it be initially word-of-mouth until you have the right size and chemistry to get started. The people you invite could be family members, friends, or new people.

What Do I Want the Goals of the Group to Be?

Decide what purpose you want the group to fulfill for you. It may be helpful for you to write down your vision for the group, so you can share its mission statement. By clarifying the group's objectives, you'll be able to recruit others who share your goals and more effectively support one another.

What Size Do I Want the Group to Be?

Consider how large you want the support group to be before you start recruiting. We've found that eight to fifteen people is just about right. Anything smaller can get too sparse, while a group that's larger can get boisterous and feel less intimate.

Do I Want the Group to Be Open or Closed?

Open support groups allow for new members—friends, family members, people you've just met—to join at any time. In closed groups, people are only allowed to join the group at certain times (e.g., from the beginning) or under certain circumstances (e.g., special events with spouses). If you'd like to cultivate deeper connections and bonds, you may want to consider having some degree of a closed group.

How Frequently Should the Group Meet?

One of the best ways to forge and maintain meaningful relationships is through built-in regularity. It's optimal when the support group becomes something you can rely on every week or two, for at least a year.

Most of our support groups meet for one to several hours each session. We recommend leaving at least one hour for the group discussion, and then the group can always decide to also integrate a meal, a walk, or another activity. We've found that regular meetings predict the healthiest outcomes, as they support you in following the lifestyle over the long term.

Will the Group Meet in Person or Virtually?

You may choose for your support group to meet in person or virtually. For the greatest convenience and largest attendance, many of our alumni communities (which began as in-person groups) choose to meet virtually. There are several friendly, often free videoconference services available today. If you're able to and you'd prefer for your group to meet in person, try to select a safe, convenient location with accessible parking, such as a group member's home, a community center, a church, a hospital, or a restaurant.

How Do I Want to Start, Run, and End the Meeting?

Be intentional and consistent with how you open, run, and close each meeting. Set the direction and feeling tone for what's shared, how people listen and behave. Our support groups emphasize practicing the simple interpersonal skills that I reviewed in greater length earlier in this chapter:

Step 1:   Identify and express what you are feeling.
Step 2:   Listen actively with empathy and compassion.
Step 3:   Acknowledge what the other person is saying.

Sharing the facilitator role with other members helps them feel more committed to and invested in the group, while also allowing you not to have to be completely responsible for those tasks. The facilitator's responsibilities include making sure that everyone has an equal opportunity to share, to be heard, and to feel heard and understood. It's also crucial to remind the group to share only feelings, rather than thoughts, judgments, or advice.

Lastly, it's critical that it is well understood by everyone that people's privacy is sacred and to be protected, and that the group's confidentiality is essential.

Do You Love and Accept Yourself?

Learning how to accept and love yourself—especially the private, "if only they really knew me" parts—is an integral practice and component of living a wholehearted life. When you are embarking on a new lifestyle, self-acceptance is vital; without it you could easily become overwhelmed and discouraged, and withdraw.

Learning to care for yourself with kindness, patience, and perseverance when things don't go as you planned or when you fall off the wagon of your healthy lifestyle practice will ensure that you don't lose your way because you lost compassion for yourself.

If you're really honest with yourself, are there ways that you've succumbed into a (dis)comfort zone, where you'd prefer not to be bothered by or take the risk of changing your lifestyle? Do you somehow feel that if you attempted, you'd fail? Or on an even deeper level, are you concerned that if you upgraded the way you live, you'd feel pressured to keep it up?

We all struggle in our own ways; we've all felt stifled and stuck at different points in our lives. It takes self-awareness and courage to look inside yourself and genuinely inquire, "Why am I struggling like this?" "How did I get here?" "What is preventing me from living the life I've always dreamed for myself?" "Why and how am I letting my lifestyle choices diminish my potential for greater health and well-being?" "What are the beliefs and values that are determining my behaviors?" "What stories or conflicts inside me are getting in the way of greater fulfillment in my life?"

If your present state of affairs is no longer working for you, have the courage now to listen to yourself, to learn why you've made the lifestyle choices you have up to now, and then to let go of those patterns. Whatever has been an obstacle in the past can be removed, and much of the damage from your prior choices can be undone with enough personal awareness and resolve to repattern whatever is no longer serving you.

Can you allow yourself to notice any residual blame or shame that you may be carrying around, like invisible weights sewn into the lining of your being? If so, see if you can trace those feelings back to the source. When, where, why, and with whom did these feelings originate? Notice how it feels to acknowledge any regrets, grudges, or setbacks that you may have encountered in the past. Now notice how it would feel to give yourself permission to liberate yourself from these burdens and prolonged suffering. How would it feel to seize this as your moment to be free of tired self-judgments, doubt, and despair? See if you can practice compassionately accepting yourself as you are, recognizing the ups and downs you've experienced as a normal and expected part of the human journey.

For the next few minutes, close your eyes and place your hands on your heart, surrounding your being with loving awareness. Allow for a tender moment to first send gratitude to your heart for all of the ways it supports and nourishes you.

Next, ask your heart, "Why do I want to live better? Longer?" Now listen for your small voice within, which speaks very quietly but very clearly. It's the voice that wakes you up at 4:00 a.m. saying, "Listen up, pay attention!" Ask it, "What am I not paying attention to that I need to?" Ask it, "How can I nourish and support my healthiest and happiest self?" Listen for as long as feels right for you to receive the honest, heartfelt message from within.

Remaining deeply connected, reflect now on a time in your life when you felt most enlivened, the most vibrantly happy, loved, and in love with life. Notice where you were, what you were doing, and with whom. Notice how you feel when you recall this experience now. Notice the feeling tone of your energy and the sentiments present in your heart. How often do you make time to feel this way? What is preventing you from feeling this way more often? What does it look like and feel like to recommit to this part of yourself, to come home to your heart? When you're ready, slowly open your eyes as you envision how this feeling could guide the choices you make today and each day forward.

With every life experience, you get to know yourself better—those experiences offer valuable mirrors. Take a moment to get reacquainted with yourself, to value what you've already experienced and accomplished, both the small things and the substantial ones. Acknowledge the qualities you've needed to recruit and cultivate during the challenging times in your life. Did what seemed to be "in your way" become "your way"? If so, how did your stumbling blocks become stepping-stones for your personal growth and evolution? It's your prerogative to determine how you're going to relate to your history, past relationships, and choices, and to how they've informed and actively link to who you are today.

Joseph Campbell, the twentieth-century scholar, referred to this as the hero's journey: "Whether small or great, and no matter what the stage or grade of life, the call rings up the curtain . . . a moment of spiritual passage, which, when complete, amounts to a dying and a birth. The familiar life horizon has been outgrown; the old concepts, ideals, and emotional patterns no longer fit; the time for the passing of a threshold is at hand."

It's your honesty and courage that will compel you to move beyond the status quo of your past, to honor what's true and real for you now, and commit to stride into a brighter future for yourself. Are you ready to take back ownership of your life by taking accountability for it? It's up to you! Is this your moment, your opportunity to make these changes that matter, that are meaningful to you? Are you determined to make new choices that integrate greater health, harmony, and love in your life?

Self-acceptance is primary to the dynamic process of your inner hero's journey—a beacon of the courage required to take the risks necessary for you to grow, to heal, to love others, and to be loved.

Practices That Connect and Heal Us

In this section we discuss five practices that can both connect us with others and heal those parts of ourselves, mind and body, that need to be healed.

- *Smile and laugh freely.* Smiling and laughing are simple yet powerful ways to lead your life with a friendly tone, to boost your mood while enhancing the mood of others.
- *Express gratitude daily.* The ability and willingness to feel and express your gratitude on a regular basis sparks joy while significantly enhancing your relationships.
- *Let forgiveness free you.* When you forgive someone else, it doesn't mean you have to forget, condone, or excuse what they've done. The far more significant opportunity is to free yourself from carrying that blame and misery any further, and from spreading your suffering out to others.
- *Support and serve others.* Lending your support and serving others boosts your mood and increases your overall well-being—because you feel like what you're doing really matters.
- *Participate in a support group.* Participating in a support group is a relatively inexpensive yet highly effective way to develop meaningful, supportive relationships while pursuing common goals.

Smile and Laugh Freely

We all know just how good it feels to laugh—especially when you're otherwise feeling stressed, fearful, or in pain. Just as stress can make our muscles tense and dampen our mood, laughter releases physical tension while boosting overall mood. Laughter can actually act as an antidepressant by causing our cells to release the neurotransmitter serotonin.

Health experts now have proof that laughter is good medicine—

especially for the heart. A good belly laugh can send 20 percent more blood flowing through your entire body. One study found that when people watched a funny movie, their blood flow increased. When you laugh, the lining of your blood vessel walls relaxes and expands.

Laughing releases endorphins in the parts of the brain responsible for reducing pain and controlling emotions, providing an overall sense of relief and well-being. Laughter can also be powerfully contagious, which can quickly forge social bonds. A shared endorphin rush from a shared laugh fosters a shared connection, a feel-good sense of social togetherness. The actress and activist Marlo Thomas noted, "When we're children, we laugh seventy-five times a day, and when we're adults, we only laugh seven times per day, so have as many good laughs as you can each day! Laughing feels good and is good medicine!"

When you smile, you're extending your warmth and goodwill. Smiling is a gesture of kindness that transcends language barriers, so it can be easily received and understood.

Have you noticed that you're drawn to people who smile a lot? People who smile are perceived as being more likable than those who don't smile, according to one 2016 study. Imparting a genial smile makes it easier to dispel social discomfort; in fact, your amiable appearance can be disarming without you needing to say a thing.

While another's kind smile can catch you off guard amid a busy day, a kindhearted nod in passing can initiate a refreshing shift and provide a mini boost. Likewise, your smile can be both magnetic and contagious, creating stronger, healthier social bonds. Growing evidence shows that our instinct for facial mimicry, such as the reflex to return another's smile, allows us to empathize with and even experience other people's positive feelings. It lifts your mood, as well as the moods of those around you. A 2010 study found that people with positive emotions have more stable marriages, better interpersonal skills, and even increased life span than people with negative emotional patterns. And in 2011, researchers at the Face Research Laboratory at the University of Aberdeen, Scotland, found that smiling can even make you appear more attractive to others. When men and women were asked to rate smiling and attractiveness, they found that they were more attracted to images of people who made eye contact and smiled than those who did not. Not very surprising, right? Check it out for yourself—make it a point to smile more today, and see what kind of reactions you get.

The free, effortless act of smiling triggers neural messages in your brain that release feel-good neurotransmitters—dopamine, endorphins, and serotonin. Endorphins act as natural painkillers, without the negative side effects that are now epidemic with opioids. Similarly, serotonin is a neurotransmitter that can act as a natural antidepressant, helping to regulate anxiety, happiness, and sexual desire and function. Now that's worth smiling about!

When practiced daily, smiling has the power to cultivate more symbiotic relationships with those around you—everyone gets a release of feel-good chemicals in their brain, reward centers get activated, mutual attractiveness is enhanced, and the chances of you all living longer, healthier lives increases. When you smile at someone, it is a gift to them.

The next time you're in a social situation and you want to connect with someone, try smiling first and see what happens. Instead of automatically becoming engrossed in your phone, look up more and gently smile at people in line, on the sidewalk, at the checkout counter. Smile at the neighbor who arrives home at the same time as you. To make smiling more of a daily practice, consider consciously choosing to surround yourself with people, places, and activities that bring cheer to your day.

Laughter also bolsters your well-being while arousing good-spirited relations with others. Therefore, consider it another part of your lifestyle prescription: allow your laughter to rise up more freely and be generously shared.

In his book *Laughter: A Scientific Investigation,* Dr. Robert Provine says that laughter can draw us together socially. His research has shown that we are thirty times more likely to laugh when we're with other people than when we are alone. He remarked, "Laughter is social glue that draws group members into the fold. Laughter is not primarily about humor but about social relationships."

And in a study published in the journal *Human Nature,* British researchers found that sharing a laugh makes people more willing to tell others something personal about themselves. This finding reinforces the synergy between laughter, the openness of sharing authentic feelings, and the formation of meaningful bonds. Laughing promotes good humor, vitality, and resilience in your relationships.

When emotions are running high, laughter can be an especially powerful tool for managing conflict and reducing tension. Sharing a good chuckle can defuse misunderstandings and disagreements. Laughter has the capacity to reunite us during difficult times.

Even if you did not grow up in a family that laughed abundantly together, you can learn to bring more laughter into your life at any stage. Reflect on the feeling tone of those around you; who makes you spontaneously smile, giggle, crack up? Who can laugh at themselves and find the humor in the everyday ups and downs? Try sharing more time with those people.

An essential ingredient for developing your sense of humor is not to dwell on the negative and not to take yourself too seriously. It feels like such a relief—for yourself and everyone around you—when you can practice laughing at yourself more. Instead of feeling defensive, share your embarrassing moments by making a humorous anecdote of them that makes others laugh.

Shared laughter is one of the most effective tools for keeping relationships fresh and exciting. Bring more humor into your conversations by asking people, "What's the funniest thing that's happened to you lately?" Equip yourself with a couple of personal anecdotes that humorously expose your humility and humanity, to get an amusing, yet substantial conversation started. Keeping your sense of humor on board will unleash more playfulness while forging more fun, open, and authentic relations with others.

The poignant words of legendary musician and producer Quincy Jones Jr. sum it up: "I've learned that a big laugh is a really loud noise from the soul saying, 'Ain't that the truth!'"

Express Gratitude Daily

The practice of expressing gratitude is another powerful antidote to the modern-day stresses of overwhelm, irritation, impatience, and plain old exhaustion. To the extent that we can take regular moments to shift our awareness to gratitude, we can effectively reframe challenging moments and persevere.

Practicing gratitude invites you to reflect on your personal priorities and values to identify what sparks joy for you, what opens your heart, what makes you feel most vibrantly alive and well. The more you practice gratitude, the more you reinforce positive behaviors and prioritize what you value most highly; it's a virtuous cycle. There are small moments waiting to be noticed all around us, and profound blessings that pervade our everyday lives, so by practicing gratitude, you invite a space for joy of all sizes to come into your heart, to be nurtured, appreciated, and paid forward.

Dr. Glen Affleck and his colleagues at the University of Connecticut found that gratitude can have a protective effect against heart attacks. Researchers also found that those patients who saw benefits and gains from their heart attack, such as becoming more appreciative of life, experienced a lower risk of having another heart attack.

As part of the pioneering work done by Robert Emmons, Ph.D., regarding the psychology of gratitude and thankfulness, he documented an inspiring list of scientifically proven benefits. Gratitude is related to 23 percent lower levels of the stress hormone cortisol. Grateful people have 16 percent lower diastolic blood pressure and 10 percent lower systolic blood pressure compared to those less grateful. Gratitude is also related to a 10 percent improvement in sleep quality in patients with chronic pain, 76 percent of whom had insomnia, and a 19 percent reduction in depression levels.

Gratitude often naturally bubbles up when you're feeling upbeat, happy, and well. Yet when you consciously practice gratitude—especially during hardship—it can actually improve your health while breeding deeper contentment and love in your life.

Researchers from Gonzaga University found that expressing gratitude strengthens relationships and increases satisfaction, which leads to partners spending more time together.

Gratitude can actually boost your mood and improve your physical health, as shown in a study by Paul J. Mills, Ph.D., and colleagues. The authors state: "We found that more gratitude in these patients was associated with better mood, better sleep, less fatigue and lower levels of inflammatory biomarkers related to cardiac health."

Letting your heart open to acknowledge the grace around you and to savor the preciousness of your life is the first step. This means shifting your awareness so that you can begin to notice the small, subtle things that spark joy and nourish your heart, such as your warm cup of morning tea, the splendor of the sunrise, or simply feeling blessed when you wake up and get to greet a new day.

Almost every person and every moment holds a blessing if you slow down enough to notice and be thankful. The more you let your heart feel waves of gratitude, both small and big, the more your mind begins to pursue opportunities to feel and express more of that gratitude.

Practicing gratitude is especially powerful when things are difficult in your life. If you're able to widen your heart's aperture to hold both the challenging situation while also counting your blessings, you can effectively reframe and resource at your heart. The practice of gratitude blooms when you appreciate, nurture, and cultivate more of what's truly meaningful and important to you.

What can you remind yourself to be grateful for when you're feeling overwhelmed, annoyed, or disappointed? As a quick practice now, take a moment to bring to mind the relationships for which you're most deeply grateful. Bring your awareness to your family, friends, co-workers, and anyone else in your life whom you truly appreciate. Allow yourself to visualize and feel their presence now. Sense what it is about them that you appreciate. How do they nourish and support you? How do they inspire you to be better? Feel into your connection with them, and find the words to express your gratitude for them in this moment, from your heart to theirs. Experience the warmth and kindness this generates between you.

Before falling asleep at night, try reflecting on your day and naming at least one new thing you're grateful for each day. Let this practice be how you check in with yourself, sum up your day, and support a more peaceful sleep. You may enjoy keeping a gratitude journal or jar—whenever you're feeling gratitude flow, write down the experiences and people that make you happy, give you strength, and provide personal meaning. Fill up your life with more gratitude!

Let Forgiveness Free You

We all make mistakes, of course—it is an unavoidable, yet forgivable, characteristic of being human. What's paramount is that we learn from our regrets and let them go.

In his book *No Regrets,* Dr. Hamilton Beazley writes: "While we cannot change a past event, we *can* change our reaction to it, our understanding of it, and what we do with it. In other words, *we can change the psychological effect of that past event on our lives.* And when we change the psychological effect of something, it is like changing the thing itself.

After all, it is the *psychological effect* that determines how the *event* influences us emotionally in the present. So for all practical purposes, we *can* change the past."

Sometimes this requires 'fessing up yourself. In this case, simply take responsibility: "I messed up," "I made a mistake," "I was wrong." Admitting that you were wrong takes character. It involves swallowing your pride and being willing to be vulnerable. The power of apologizing can be initiated with one little sentence: "I'm sorry." Just these two simple words convey that you are taking accountability and imparting your sincere desire to restore respect and harmony in the relationship.

When apologizing, do your best to keep it simple, direct, and sincere. Begin by acknowledging the harm that you've caused, without including any justifications for your words or behavior. As Benjamin Franklin is thought to have wisely advised, "Never ruin an apology with an excuse."

Is now the time to resolve your unfinished emotional business? Is there someone with whom you need to express your authentic feelings, so that you can find a way to forgive them now and let bygones be bygones, so that you can move forward in your life? Do you need to say "I'm sorry" to someone? Is that someone yourself? Are there ways that you can allow forgiveness to heal you, to regenerate the love you most want in your life? It's never too late to learn to forgive, to be forgiven, to be free.

Everything that you've experienced in your life so far is what has brought you here to this moment, where you can realize just how powerfully healing love can be, to intimately connect with, source from, and share this love inside yourself abundantly—with yourself and others. It's about laying down your burdens today, resetting a positive attitude, restoring your life force, and reclaiming a peaceful life that makes your heart sing again!

When at the end of your life you look back, what matters most isn't what you've done, what you've accomplished, but how meaningfully you're able to answer the question "Have I grown in love and wisdom?"

Support and Serve Others

Social support has well-known benefits for physical and mental health, but giving support (rather than receiving it), without expectations of reciprocity, makes you feel especially fulfilled, energized, and good inside.

You may think that you're receiving social support, but a recent study reported that the biggest health benefits may come from providing support to others. In a study published in the *American Journal of Public Health* in 2013, researchers studied 846 people over the age of sixty-five and concluded that stress did not predict mortality risk among individuals who provided support for friends or family members in the past year, such as providing transportation, running errands, preparing a meal, helping out with housework, or providing childcare. However, stress did predict mortality among those who did not provide help to others. The researchers concluded, "Help given to others is a better predictor of health and well-being than are indicators of social engagement or received social support." In fact, "social connections may be beneficial to the extent that they provide individuals with the opportunity to benefit others."

And a recent study published in the journal *Psychological Science* concluded that mortality was significantly reduced for older married adults who reported providing instrumental support to friends, relatives, and neighbors, and those who reported providing emotional support to their spouse. This pattern of findings was obtained after controlling for demographic, personality, health, mental health, and marital relationship variables. These results have implications for understanding how supporting others, especially those with whom you're the closest, influences your health and longevity.

Stanford psychologist Sonja Lyubomirsky researches the benefits of acts of kindness. She says, "There are a lot of positive social consequences to being kind—other people appreciate you, they're grateful and they might reciprocate." But it's not the altruism per se that's important; it's about cultivating meaningful relationships. Helping others can also provide you with a meaningful role that boosts your self-esteem and mood and helps you find purpose in life, which in turn can enhance your mental, emotional, and physical health.

If you have time and energy left after helping friends and family, it's also rewarding to do volunteer work in your community. Think of an organization or a cause that touches you. Who could benefit from your kind support, your helping hands? It's a wonderfully symbiotic relationship, as serving and supporting others in need can measurably enhance your own health, happiness, and longevity.

Dean

We live near Silicon Valley, where some dedicated tech leaders believe that we can live forever if we can sufficiently hack our biology. There is a common presumption that most people want to live longer.

But that's not always true. Telling someone who is isolated, lonely, and depressed that they're going to live longer isn't always that motivating when they're just trying to get through the day.

And there are a lot of depressed people—prescriptions for antidepressants have risen nearly 400 percent since 1988, according to data from the CDC.

Severe depression is a reality distortion. In other words, you think you're seeing things clearly for the first time. Things are bad. They've always been bad. They'll always be bad. And any time you thought otherwise, you were just fooling yourself. I understand how bad that can feel—I was suicidally depressed in college and wrote about this experience in two of my earlier books.

That's where the hallmark of depression, which is the helplessness and hopelessness, comes from—the mistaken belief that life will never get better. It seems that nothing can bring lasting happiness or meaning.

But I learned that just as you can take all the meaning out of life, you can also put it back. One way to do so is to consciously choose *not* to do something that you otherwise could do. For example, when you intentionally choose not to eat or not to do something that you otherwise could do, it imbues those choices with meaning and makes them sustainable instead of feeling deprived.

Most religions and spiritual paths have dietary guidelines, but they often differ from one another. In one religion you can eat this but not that, or on certain days of the week, or after midnight, or just on special holidays, or whatever. Another religion prescribes different rules.

Whatever the intrinsic health benefits of eating or not eating certain foods, just the act of choosing not to put in your mouth something that you otherwise could eat makes this choice meaningful.

And if it's meaningful, then it's sustainable and healing.

Instead of focusing on a thought such as "I can't eat everything I want," which leaves you feeling chronically stressed, you might reframe your experience as "I'm choosing not to eat certain foods because when I replace them with healthier options, I feel so much better." Many people also find it meaningful that a plant-based way of eating reduces global warming and makes more resources available to feed the hungry. This reframes these choices from feelings of deprivation to meaningful ones of transformation, joy, and pleasure. Again, what you gain is more than what you give up—and you experience those gains quickly. These are choices worth making not just for how *long* you live but also for how *well* you live.

So when we work with patients, we usually ask them, "*Why* do you want to live longer?"

"Hmm, no one's ever asked me that before. Let's see—I want to live long enough to watch my kids grow up and be there for them when they need me, to dance at their wedding, and to meet my grandchildren. I want to make love with my partner, help relieve suffering in the world, be successful in my work. I want to learn to tango." And so on.

Ask yourself what is most meaningful for you. This allows you to connect the choices that you make in your lifestyle with a profound sense of meaning and purpose. Finding meaning in suffering makes it bearable and transformative.

As you think about why you want to live longer, consider a passage from Dr. Rachel Remen's extraordinary book *Kitchen Table Wisdom,* in which she shares a parable from Roberto Assagioli of three stonecutters who were building a cathedral in the fourteenth century.

The first one says, bitterly, "Can't you see what I'm doing? I'm cutting stones into blocks and I will be doing this until the day I die!"

The second one says, warmly, "I'm earning a living so I can support my beloved family. I can provide clothing and food in our home filled with love."

The third one says, joyfully, "I have the privilege to help build a great cathedral so magnificent it will inspire people and lift their spirits for a thousand years."

Same work, but each brings very different meaning to it. We often have more choices than we realize.

Anne

This is a love-based program! What do we mean by that? In forty years of conducting scientific research, we've learned that when you feel good—I mean really good, both physically and emotionally—the upgrade to your life is so gratifying that it becomes a much more sustainable motivator than your fear of dying.

No doubt your diagnosis, pain, or fear can provide a forceful entry point, even become a catalyst for changing your lifestyle. Yet once you begin making healthier lifestyle choices, you'll feel and look much better very quickly, because the underlying biological mechanisms impacted by these choices are so dynamic. Those positive changes that you can see and feel will reframe your choice to make these changes. Instead of making them from a place of fear and suffering, they'll be coming from a place of wanting to experience more pleasure and love in your life.

These simple lifestyle changes help heal your body, yielding powerful clinical outcomes such as lowering blood pressure, triglycerides, LDL cholesterol, and stress hormones, while boosting your immune system function and arterial function.

This means that your brain will get more blood flow. You'll have more energy and need less sleep. Your skin gets more blood flow, so it doesn't age as quickly. Your sexual organs get more blood flow, so your sexual function is likely to improve—this is the same way that drugs like Viagra work, but the lifestyle changes bring about those changes without the costs and the side effects of the drugs.

You can manage stress more effectively and accomplish even more, without getting stressed or sick in the process. Your whole quality of life improves. For example, our research showed that depression scores were reduced by almost 50 percent after only twelve weeks, and most patients found that their depression lifted.

You'll feel better! And the better you feel, the more open you'll be to taking advantage of opportunities to connect with friends and loved ones. This chain of favorable feelings and events becomes self-reinforcing, empowering, and ultimately healing. You could call this virtuous cycle your feel-good feedback loop.

Over 90 percent of the participants in our lifestyle medicine program continue to follow the lifestyle for at least a year—because of the community support they receive, and because they feel so much better that they can't imagine returning to their old lifestyles.

As Dean has described, we often ask people, "Why do you want to live longer?" Here are a couple of responses that exemplify the answers we commonly hear.

> Three years ago, I would have never thought that we would be doing what we are doing now; buying a motor home, showing cars, and camping with the grandkids. We are having way too much fun in this life to check out. We are going to do whatever we can do to be around. We're looking forward to the future, and this program is going to help us live it the way that we want to. —Bob L.

> Being able to spend more meaningful time with my grandkids and my wife has been tremendous for me. I have nine grandkids, and they all want to come to the house to be here with Pap and Gram, and now I can be there for that. My relationship with my wife has also really improved. Before, I basically avoided her because she wanted to do things that I just didn't have the energy to do. But now we travel and we do things together every chance we get. Plus it really meant a lot to me that she did the program with me, and it really helped her, too—her numbers and her cholesterol went down quite a bit. We cook for each other and help each other out. Overall, the program has had a huge impact on my relationships.
>
> My wife and I used to worry about being bedridden and putting a burden on our kids, but we don't worry about that as much these days. Plus, when my wife retires in two years, we're planning on traveling throughout the United States. Honestly, I don't feel like there's anything that I can't do today, whereas just three years ago there was nothing that I felt I could do.
>
> It's been a world of difference for me. The Ornish Program is a lifesaver. —Martin

Connecting intimately with yourself and others while cultivating a sense of gratitude, meaning, and purpose in your life is what we're referring to when we say "love more"—because your emotional health is essential to your overall health.

Why do *you* want to live a better, longer life?

Take a moment now to get still, comfortable, and quiet, and reflect on what makes your life meaningful. What inspires you to live another day, another year, another decade? It may be living in the presence of certain people you love in your life. It may be things you want to learn or places you want to experience. It may be something that you want to share or to teach others. It may be a call to serve, support, and care for others.

If you had no fears, no limits, and no constraints and could live the life you most deeply desire, what would that life look like? If you let go of everything that doesn't align with your happiness and well-being, what would that feel like? Allow the insight and wisdom of your heart to guide you like a compass, to support you in living your optimal existence.

What would it look like to live life fully aligned in your heart, words, and behaviors? What makes you feel the most alive in your body and happy in your life? What does it feel like to imagine living in harmony with what's calling most deeply in your heart?

That's what our program allows you to do. It's not a diet, it's not even just a lifestyle—it's your calling to enter into your deeper self, to live full-heartedly, to experience the rewards available to you by living in accord with your highest health and well-being. For most people, these are choices worth making because they affect not just how long you live but also, and more importantly, how well you live.

This life is yours to infuse with joy and meaning. You are capable of actualizing your aspirations—and yes, you are worth it!

What Ties All of This Together

Dean

All of the mechanisms that we've been discussing throughout this book keep us healthy when they are in balance. This is known as homeostasis.

These same mechanisms can also create a wide range of chronic diseases when they are out of balance. A disturbance of this balance, this homeostasis, this dynamic equilibrium, is at the root of so many chronic illnesses.

What disturbs this balance? As we've discussed, each of these mechanisms is exquisitely sensitive to what we eat, how we respond to stress, how much exercise we get, and how much love and support we have.

But there is an even more fundamental question: what motivates us to act in ways that disturb this balance?

The belief—the misperception—that we need to get our health and happiness from outside ourselves often causes us to act in ways that disturb this balance, making us unhealthy and unhappy. In my limited understanding, this is where suffering and illness begin.

Put another way, our inherent nature when we are in balance is to be healthy and happy until we disturb what's already there. In this context, our health and well-being are not something we have to get from outside ourselves; rather, we just need to stop disturbing what we already have.

Perhaps the ultimate paradox is this: not being mindful that our true nature is to be happy, healthy, and peaceful, we run after so many things in life that we have been told will bring these to us—and in the process of striving for these, we often disturb what we could have already if we just stopped doing this.

For over thirty years I had the privilege of studying with Swami Satchidananda, a renowned ecumenical spiritual teacher. His central teaching was, "Truth is One, paths are many." In other words, all spiritual paths, properly understood, will take us to the same place.

He also liked to make puns. When asked, "What are you, a Hindu?" he replied, "No, I'm an Undo" (another reason we chose this book's title). "Peace comes not from doing, but from undoing; not from getting, but from letting go. It's there already until you disturb it. The purpose of all spiritual practices is to stop disturbing what you already have."

In other words, to stop disturbing our homeostasis.

This is a concept very different from what most of us learn growing up, which is that our health and happiness come from getting and doing rather than being. The entire advertising industry is based on the idea that if only we buy what they're selling, *then* we'll be happy and peaceful.

So much of our culture influences us to believe that "If only I had more _____, then I'd be happy and lovable, so I wouldn't feel so lonely," and we fill in the blank with the usual goals: money, power, fame, status, and so on.

Although we don't usually think about it in this context, once we buy into that view of the world, then however it turns out, we're likely to be unhappy:

- Until we get it, we're not happy, not peaceful: "I hope I get it!" The stakes are high—being happy and lovable—so the stresses go way up. We're taught that it's not just winning or losing that's on the line; it's being a winner or a loser. Winners are loved, losers are isolated. High stakes indeed.
- If someone else gets it and we don't, then it's even more stressful. It reconfirms the erroneous belief that we live in a highly competitive, dog-eat-dog world, that life is a zero-sum game—the more you get, the less there is for me.
- And even if we get what we think will bring us lasting happiness, it doesn't usually last. Initially, it's very seductive, because we are happy when we get it—"I got it! It's mine!" But that's soon followed by "Now what?"—it's not enough. Or "So what?"—it doesn't bring the lasting sense of joy and meaning that we hoped for.

Fortunately, the good news is that while it's true that nothing can bring lasting happiness, practicing our lifestyle medicine program can give you the direct experience that *you have that happiness already unless you disturb it.*

Chasing happiness is like chasing your shadow—the faster you run after it, the more it eludes you. When you stop running after your shadow, turn around, and begin walking toward the light, the shadow you were chasing is now following you.

On one level, of course, we *are* separate—you're you, and I'm me. We are *apart from* each other. But on another level we're *a part of* something larger that connects us.

We are already interconnected with each other. We can consciously choose to use these connections with each other in healing ways rather than in harmful ones—what I call "horizontal intimacy," connections that exist between each other.

For example, a Harvard study of over 12,000 people found that if one or more of your friends are obese, your risk of becoming obese is 45 percent higher. If your friend's friends are obese, your risk is 20 percent higher. And, amazingly, if your friend's friend's friends are obese, your risk is 10 percent higher—even if you've never even met them! That's how interconnected we are. This pattern is also seen with smoking, depression, happiness, altruism, and predicting epidemics, among others.

We are already connected with our transcendent, higher self, whatever name we give to that—the universal Self, by any other name, what I call "vertical intimacy." We are already whole.

As the French philosopher and Jesuit priest Pierre Teilhard de Chardin wrote, "We are not human beings having a spiritual experience. We are spiritual beings having a human experience."

The goal of all spiritual practices, whether religious or otherwise, is to quiet down our mind and body enough to directly experience this transcendent state. Beyond the moment-to-moment changes in your body and mind is the universal Self, which always remains peaceful and is unaffected by the turbulence around it.

When we experience the inner peace that comes with this transcendent state, this restores homeostasis and, with it, healing. All the biological mechanisms we've been describing throughout this book come more into balance.

In other words, our natural state is to be in a state of ease; when we disturb this, we become dis-eased. We are born fine until we de-fine ourselves as being separate and only separate from others.

It's worth emphasizing that these practices don't bring this to us; rather, they allow us to experience what's already there.

By analogy, we are the one light in a movie projector manifesting as an entire universe of people, places, and dramas on the movie screen. What we experience as different names and forms is God or the Self in varying disguises, manifesting in different ways. All divisions are man-made.

When we can maintain this double vision—seeing the different names and forms while remembering it's just a movie and experiencing the one light behind the many images—then we can more fully enjoy the movie without getting lost in it, without forgetting who we really are. We can enjoy the drama without getting caught up in it, without activating the mechanisms that cause us to develop chronic diseases, thereby allowing our bodies to begin healing. And often we can be even more successful in the world, because we have less anxiety and stress.

This vision of unity, consciousness, and oneness is found in virtually all cultures and all religions, and in secular literature as well. God or the Self is described as omniscient, omnipresent, and omnipotent. Even to give this a name is to limit what is essentially an ineffable and limitless, infinite experience of interconnectedness and oneness.

For example, when God was revealed to Moses, he asked, "When I tell the people that the God of their fathers has sent me, they will ask his name. What shall I tell them?" And God said, "*I am what I am*. Tell them *I am* has sent you."

As the Old Testament describes it, "The Lord is One." If God is everywhere, One, then we are not separate from God or from each other.

A central precept in Hinduism is "Thou art That . . . The universe is nothing but Brahman." According to Jesus, "The kingdom of God is within you." Buddha taught, "You are all Buddhas. There is nothing that you need to achieve. Just open your eyes." The prophet Muhammad, founder of Islam, wrote, "Wherever you turn is God's face . . . Whoever knows himself knows God."

These experiences occur in secular life as well as the religious or spiritual life. Albert Einstein, the greatest scientist of the twentieth century, wrote, "The true value of a human being is determined primarily by the measure and the sense in which he has attained liberation from the [separate] self."

This understanding is reflected in universal greetings found in other cultures, such as *namaste,* meaning "the light in me recognizes and honors the light in you," and *aloha,* meaning "God is in us."

This experience is sometimes described as Oneness, at other times as complete emptiness or void; or as both. This paradox—everything and nothing—is at the heart of the transcendent experience, "an immediate, nondual insight that transcends conceptualization," as the eighth-century Buddhist monk Shantideva put it. This experience is found in the mystical traditions of all religions and cultures.

Although this experience of Oneness lies beyond the intellect, it can be directly experienced. When the divisions that separate us from each other begin to fade, compassion, altruism, forgiveness, and love naturally flow from that experience of transcendence.

Aldous Huxley referred to this as the "perennial philosophy"—the essence of all religious and spiritual teachings once we get past the different rituals, names, and forms that people fight over.

This vision is at the heart of compassion. From this perspective, "Love your neighbor as yourself" is a statement of fact, of what is, rather than a commandment. As Einstein wrote:

A human being is a part of the whole, called by us the "Universe," a part limited in time and space. He experiences himself, his thoughts and feelings, as something separated from the rest—a kind of optical delusion of his consciousness.

This delusion is a kind of prison for us, restricting us to our personal desires and to affection for a few persons nearest to us. Our task must be to free ourselves from this prison by widening our circle of compassion to embrace all living creatures and the whole of nature in its beauty.

Without this double vision, it's all too easy to view other people as being The Other—that is, fundamentally separate, and only separate. And once they are seen as different, and only different, then our societies may devolve into tribalism, Us versus Them, or worse: racism, anti-Semitism, sexism, and all of the other destructive "isms." It becomes much easier to do bad things to other people, or to feel that we're better than they are—because they're not us, they're Other. Sadly, and ominously, we're experiencing the rise of these trends in our current political arena.

Our language reflects how we view the world. Expressing chronic anger and hostility has been consistently shown to significantly increase the risk of premature illness and mortality.

For example, in a study of 148 million Twitter messages (tweets) across 1,347 counties in the United States, language patterns reflecting negative social relationships, disengagement, and negative emotions—especially anger—emerged as risk factors for premature death; positive emotions and psychological engagement emerged as protective factors. These predicted heart disease mortality significantly better than did a model that combined ten common demographic, socioeconomic, and health risk factors, including smoking, diabetes, hypertension, and obesity.

This way of viewing the world—that we are separate and only separate—is the antithesis of love, compassion, and healing. George Lucas described the progressive isolation that results from this way of being in the world using his *Star Wars* metaphor in an interview with Bill Moyers:

One of the themes throughout the films is that the Sith lords, when they started out thousands of years ago, embraced the dark side. They were greedy and self-centered and they all wanted to take over, so they killed each other. Eventually, there was only one left, and that one took on an apprentice. And for thousands of years, the master would teach the apprentice, the master would die, the apprentice would then teach another apprentice, become the master, and so on.

But there could never be any more than two of them, because if there were, they would try to get rid of the leader, which is exactly what Vader was trying to do, and that's exactly what the Emperor was trying to do. The Emperor was trying to get rid of Vader, and Vader was trying to get rid of the Emperor. And that is the antithesis of a symbiotic relationship, in which if you do that, you become cancer, and you eventually kill the host, and everything dies.

When we hurt others, we hurt ourselves, for we are not fundamentally separate from them.

For the same reason, when we help others, we help ourselves. It even makes us beautiful. Take a moment and remember the beautiful faces of those you know who have touched you with their love and kindness or who lead lives of service.

In summary, compassion naturally flows when the divisions that separate us from one another begin to fade. It helps to free us from anger and chronic stress, which are often manifestations of the misperception that we are separate and only separate.

The connection with one another and with our soul and spirit is already there. Behind the dramas of our lives is always the light of the projector. We are That.

At the times when we feel most vulnerable, that which is invulnerable within us becomes uncovered and easier to recognize. When our hearts begin to open, we are able to feel it, like opening a window shade and letting in the sunshine that's been there all along, waiting patiently to be allowed inside.

CHAPTER 8

The Ornish Kitchen/True Love Recipes

The globally inspired recipes offered here are for every palate! Each recipe has been professionally tested to ensure only the highest standards of taste, simplicity, nutrient density, and balance. All recipes meet the nutrition guidelines of our lifestyle medicine program, are simple to make at home, and, most important, are savor-worthy!

We've made it easy for you to search the recipe collection by main dishes, breakfasts, salads, sides, snacks, soups, desserts, condiments, and beverages. Our Ornish-certified chef's notes share insights regarding each recipe's ingredients and cooking techniques, such as optional substitutions and additions.

Each recipe provides you with a standard (FDA) nutritional label along with an enhanced profile of the nutrients that the recipe is a good or excellent source of, so that you can make informed choices to promote health and balanced eating.

Note: Percent Daily Values are based on a 2,000-calorie diet. Your daily values may be higher or lower depending on your calorie needs.

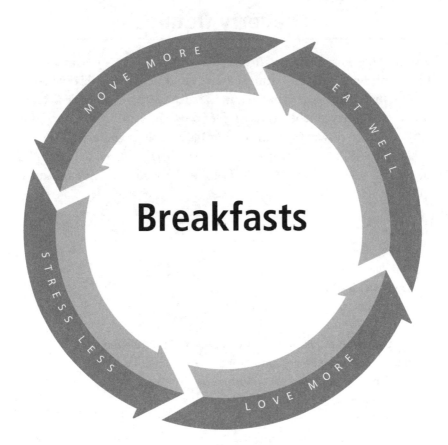

MOVE MORE

EAT WELL

Breakfasts

STRESS LESS

LOVE MORE

Blueberry Oatmeal

Feeling blue this morning? If you're spooning up this creamy, berry-filled, and fiber-rich hot oatmeal, that's good news. This flexible recipe can be made with any nondairy milk, such as soy, rice, or low-fat almond milk. Juicy blueberries are full of powerful antioxidants including anthocyanins, resveratrol, and flavonoids as well as vitamin C, but you can also try using other fruits, such as blackberries, diced apples, or bananas. For best texture, use old-fashioned rolled oats, not instant or quick-cooking oats.

Serves: 4
    Serving Size: ½ cup
    Prep Time: N/A
    Cook Time: 10–15 minutes
    Ready Time: 10–15 minutes

1 cup unsweetened nondairy milk, plus more as needed
½ teaspoon ground cinnamon, plus more as needed
¼ teaspoon powdered stevia (optional)
⅛ teaspoon fine sea salt
1 cup old-fashioned rolled oats
1 cup fresh or frozen blueberries
4 teaspoons flaxseed meal (optional)

1. In a small saucepan over medium heat, bring 1 cup water, milk, cinnamon, stevia if using, and salt to a boil.
2. Add oats. Reduce heat to medium-low and simmer, stirring frequently, until oats are cooked through and mixture has thickened to desired consistency, 10–15 minutes.
3. Stir in blueberries. Cook until blueberries have warmed through. If desired, add additional milk and/or stevia, as needed. Garnish each serving with a teaspoon of flaxseed meal and/or a sprinkle of cinnamon, as desired.

Nutrition Facts

Serving Size: ½ cup
Servings: 4

AMOUNT PER SERVING
Calories: 119
Calories from Fat: 27

	AMOUNT PER SERVING	% DAILY VALUE
Total Fat:	3 g	5%
Saturated Fat:	0 g	0%
Trans Fat:	0 g	
Cholesterol:	0 mg	0%
Sodium:	83 mg	3%
Total Carbohydrate:	20 g	7%
Dietary Fiber:	4 g	16%
Sugars:	4 g	
Protein:	4 g	8%

GOOD SOURCE OF: fiber

Country Sweet Potatoes

Planning a hearty breakfast or brunch? Try serving Tofu Vegetable Scramble (page 254) alongside these satisfying home fries, made with orange sweet potatoes for extra vitamin A, potassium, and fiber. This recipe can also be made with Yukon Gold potatoes.

Serves: 8
 Serving Size: ½ cup
 Prep Time: 10 minutes
 Cook Time: 15 minutes
 Ready Time: 25 minutes

1¼ pounds sweet potatoes
1 cup thinly sliced red onion
1 cup low-sodium vegetable broth, plus more if needed
2 teaspoons chopped fresh thyme or 1 teaspoon dried, divided
1¼ teaspoons chili powder, divided
½ teaspoon dried oregano
½ teaspoon garlic powder
¼ teaspoon fine sea salt
⅛ teaspoon freshly ground pepper
8 lime wedges, for garnish (optional)

1. Peel sweet potatoes and chop into ½-inch chunks. You should have about 4½ cups.
2. In a 12-inch heavy-bottomed skillet over high heat, combine the sweet potatoes, onions, vegetable broth, 1 teaspoon fresh thyme (or ½ teaspoon dried), ¾ teaspoon chili powder, oregano, garlic powder, salt, and pepper. Bring to a boil.
3. Reduce heat to medium-high. Cook, stirring frequently, until potatoes are tender and liquid is mostly evaporated, about 10 minutes. If liquid evaporates before potatoes are tender, add additional vegetable broth as needed.
4. Stir in remaining 1 teaspoon fresh thyme (or ½ teaspoon dried) and ½ teaspoon chili powder. Taste for seasoning, adding more

salt and/or pepper as needed. Serve warm, with lime wedges if desired.

```
┌─────────────────────────────────────────────────────┐
│                                                       │
│  Nutrition Facts                                      │
│  ───────────────────────────────────────────────     │
│                                                       │
│  Serving Size: ½ cup                                  │
│  Servings: 8                                          │
│                                                       │
│  AMOUNT PER SERVING                                   │
│  Calories: 72                                         │
│  Calories from Fat: 0                                 │
│                                                       │
│                    AMOUNT PER SERVING  % DAILY VALUE  │
│  Total Fat:                  0 g            0%        │
│  Saturated Fat:              0 g            0%        │
│  Trans Fat:                  0 g                      │
│  Cholesterol:                0 mg           0%        │
│  Sodium:                   142 mg           6%        │
│  Total Carbohydrate:        17 g            6%        │
│  Dietary Fiber:              3 g           12%        │
│  Sugars:                     4 g                      │
│  Protein:                    2 g            4%        │
│  EXCELLENT SOURCE OF: vitamin A                       │
│  GOOD SOURCE OF: fiber, manganese                     │
│                                                       │
└─────────────────────────────────────────────────────┘
```

Tofu Vegetable Scramble

Get a healthy, satisfying start on the day with this flavorful tofu scramble, rich in vitamins, nutrients, and plant protein. We've suggested using extra-firm sprouted tofu made from soybeans that have been sprouted before being processed, as some people find it easier to digest. However, you can also use regular tofu, either firm or extra-firm.

Serves: 4
    Serving Size: 1 cup
    Prep Time: 10 minutes
    Cook Time: 15 minutes
    Ready Time: 25 minutes

2 cups extra-firm tofu, preferably sprouted (8 ounces)
2 teaspoons curry powder, divided (see Chef's Notes)
1 teaspoon garlic powder, divided
¼ teaspoon fine sea salt, divided
⅛ teaspoon freshly ground black pepper, divided
1 cup roughly chopped red bell pepper
1 cup roughly chopped onion
1 cup roughly chopped zucchini
1 cup small cherry tomatoes, quartered
¼ cup chopped fresh basil
4 basil sprigs, for garnish (optional)
Sriracha or other hot sauce for garnish (optional)

1. Using paper towels, pat tofu dry, pressing firmly on all sides to remove any excess liquid. Crumble the tofu into a bowl and press again with a fresh paper towel to release any remaining liquid.
2. Add 1 teaspoon curry powder, ½ teaspoon garlic powder, ⅛ teaspoon salt, and a pinch of black pepper to the tofu. Stir to combine flavors. Set aside.
3. In a 12-inch sauté pan over high heat, combine the red peppers, onions, zucchini, ¼ cup water, and remaining 1 teaspoon curry powder, ½ teaspoon garlic powder, ⅛ teaspoon salt, and black pepper. Bring mixture to a boil. Reduce heat to medium and cook,

stirring frequently, until vegetables are tender and liquid has evaporated, about 10 minutes.

4. Stir in the cherry tomatoes. Cook until tomatoes have released some of their moisture, 2–3 minutes. Add the tofu and chopped basil and cook, stirring, until mixture is warmed through. Taste for seasoning, adding additional salt, black pepper, and/or curry powder as needed. Top with basil sprigs, if using, and serve warm, accompanied by hot sauce, if desired.

Chef's Notes

Curry powders, like any spice blend, can vary greatly in flavor—some are well-rounded and aromatic, others unpleasantly bitter. They can also lose their aroma and taste over time. Taste your curry powder before using to make sure you like it. It's also wise to buy a fresh jar every 6 to 8 months, and store it in a cool, dry place. Never store your spices directly over the stove.

Nutrition Facts

Serving Size: 1 cup
Servings: 4 servings

AMOUNT PER SERVING
Calories: 107
Calories from Fat: 36

	AMOUNT PER SERVING	% DAILY VALUE
Total Fat:	4 g	6%
Saturated Fat:	0 g	0%
Trans Fat:	0 g	
Cholesterol:	0 mg	0%
Sodium:	165 mg	7%
Total Carbohydrate:	10 g	3%
Dietary Fiber:	4 g	16%
Sugars:	4 g	
Protein:	8 g	16%

EXCELLENT SOURCE OF: vitamin A, vitamin C, vitamin K
GOOD SOURCE OF: fiber, vitamin B_6, iron, manganese, molybdenum

Apple Spice Muffins

Full of warm spices and sweet apple, these wholesome muffins make a healthy start to the day. They can also serve as a delightful afternoon snack or dessert. Look for fruit spreads that are sweetened only with fruit juice or fruit juice concentrate, not sugar or corn syrup.

Serves: 12

Serving Size: 1 muffin
Prep Time: 15 minutes
Cook Time: 35 minutes
Ready Time: 50 minutes

2 tablespoons flaxseed meal
1½ cups whole-wheat flour or gluten-free flour
½ cup old-fashioned rolled oats
2 teaspoons cinnamon or pumpkin pie spice (see Chef's Notes)
¾ teaspoon baking powder
¾ teaspoon baking soda
¾ teaspoon fine sea salt
½ teaspoon powdered stevia
1¼ cups unsweetened applesauce
½ cup apricot fruit spread, fruit-juice-sweetened only
1 cup grated apple (about 1 apple)
2 teaspoons vanilla extract
½ cup raisins

1. In a small bowl, mix flaxseed meal with ¼ cup water. Set aside for 10 to 15 minutes. The flax will absorb the water and create a thick gel.
2. Preheat oven to 350°F. Line a nonstick muffin pan with paper liners or spray the pan lightly with cooking spray. If using spray, gently wipe with a paper towel to remove excess oil.
3. In a medium bowl, whisk together flour, rolled oats, cinnamon, baking powder, baking soda, salt, and stevia until well mixed.
4. In a large bowl, stir together the applesauce, apricot fruit spread, grated apple, flax mixture, and vanilla. Stir in half the dry ingredi-

ents, then add the remaining half and stir gently until combined. Add raisins and stir lightly to mix.

5. Spoon ⅓ cup batter into each muffin cup. Bake muffins until a toothpick inserted into the center of a muffin comes out clean, about 25 minutes. Be careful not to overbake.

6. Remove muffins from the oven and let cool in the muffin pan for a few minutes. Remove muffins from the pan and let them cool on a cooling rack. These muffins are best served shortly after baking but will keep in a sealed container for several days.

Chef's Notes

We love the convenience of pumpkin pie spice, a warm, autumn-y blend of cinnamon, ginger, and cloves (and sometimes allspice, nutmeg, and/or mace, too) that's sold in the spice section of most supermarkets. It's great for adding a dash of sweet spice to apple, pear, and pumpkin desserts and baked goods. If you don't have it on hand, you can make your own using 1 teaspoon ground cinnamon, ½ teaspoon ground ginger, ¼ teaspoon ground nutmeg, and ⅛ teaspoon ground allspice.

Nutrition Facts

Serving Size: 1 muffin
Servings: 12

AMOUNT PER SERVING
Calories: 132
Calories from Fat: 9

	AMOUNT PER SERVING	% DAILY VALUE
Total Fat:	1 g	2%
Saturated Fat:	0 g	0%
Trans Fat:	0 g	
Cholesterol:	0 mg	0%
Sodium:	248 mg	10%
Total Carbohydrate:	29 g	10%
Dietary Fiber:	3 g	12%
Sugars:	12 g	
Protein:	5 g	10%

EXCELLENT SOURCE OF: manganese
GOOD SOURCE OF: fiber, selenium

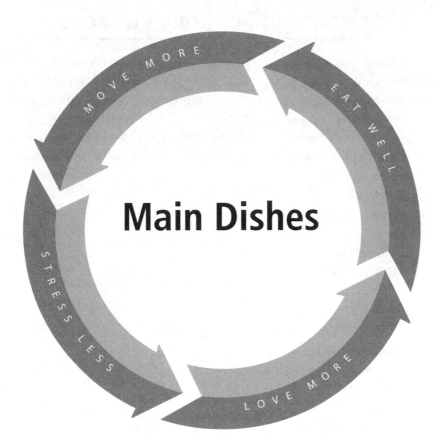

Main Dishes

MOVE MORE

EAT WELL

LOVE MORE

STRESS LESS

Spinach and Mushroom Lasagna

Love lasagna? This favorite Italian dish has been transformed into a heart-healthy Ornish classic, with whole-grain noodles layered with a vitamin-rich filling of spinach, mushrooms, and roasted garlic. This recipe makes enough to feed a crowd, so it's perfect for a big get-together or potluck—or just plenty of delicious leftovers! Every delicious bite is packed with phytochemicals and antioxidants that promote heart health.

Serves: 12

Serving Size: one 3 × 3-inch square
Prep Time: 1 hour
Cook Time: 1 hour
Ready Time: 2 hours

32 ounces frozen chopped spinach, thawed
16 ounces cremini or white button mushrooms
¼ teaspoon fine sea salt, divided
¼ teaspoon freshly ground black pepper
⅔ cup Roasted Garlic puree (page 410)
24 ounces firm tofu, blotted dry and finely crumbled
¼ cup nutritional yeast
½ cup firmly packed fresh basil leaves, finely chopped
1 tablespoon chopped fresh oregano or 1 teaspoon dried
⅛ teaspoon cayenne (optional)
1 package (13.25 ounces) whole-wheat or brown rice lasagna noodles
     (14 to 16 noodles)
2 jars (26 ounces) low-fat marinara sauce
⅓ cup chopped flat-leaf parsley, for garnish (optional)

1. Preheat oven to 375°F. To make the filling, place thawed spinach in a colander in the sink or over a deep bowl. Using your hands, squeeze or press spinach vigorously to remove excess liquid. Continue to squeeze and press spinach until it is almost dry; excess liquid left in the spinach will make a soggy lasagna. Once drained, you should have about 3 cups spinach. Set aside.

2. Working in batches as necessary, place mushrooms in a food pro-

cessor fitted with a metal blade. Pulse 6–8 times, until mushrooms are finely diced but not pureed. Place diced mushrooms in a bowl. Repeat with remaining mushrooms.

3. In a large sauté pan over medium heat, sauté diced mushrooms with ⅛ teaspoon salt and black pepper, stirring occasionally, until the mushrooms release their liquid and liquid evaporates, 15–20 minutes.

4. In a medium bowl, combine mushrooms, spinach, roasted garlic puree, tofu, nutritional yeast, basil, oregano, remaining ⅛ teaspoon salt, and cayenne, if using. Season to taste with more basil, oregano, and/or cayenne as needed.

5. In a large pot over high heat, bring 4 quarts of water to a boil. When water is boiling, add lasagna noodles one at a time, criss-crossing the layers of noodles so they don't stick.

6. Turn off heat and let noodles soften in hot water for 6 minutes. (They will seem undercooked.) Drain. If you need to hold the noodles before assembly, return noodles to pot and cover with cold water; drain and pat dry thoroughly before using.

7. To assemble the lasagna, spread 1 cup marinara sauce over the bottom of a 9½ × 13 × 2-inch baking pan. Cover sauce with 3 to 4 noodles. Spread one-quarter (about 2 cups) of the spinach-tofu filling over the noodles.

8. Repeat 3 times, using the same amounts of sauce, noodles, and filling each time. Top finished lasagna with 1 cup marinara sauce. (Any remaining marinara sauce can be spooned over the lasagna at serving time or reserved for another use.)

9. Place lasagna on middle rack of the oven and bake, uncovered, for 40 minutes. Cover lasagna with foil and bake for an additional 20 minutes.

10. Remove from oven and discard foil. Let lasagna rest for 10 minutes before serving. While lasagna is resting, heat remaining marinara sauce, if desired. Cut lasagna into squares with a serrated knife. Serve with extra warmed marinara sauce and garnish each serving with chopped parsley if desired.

Chef's Notes

Make sure to follow instructions for drying the tofu, spinach, and cooked noodles before adding them to the lasagna. Use clean tea towels or several layers of paper towels to blot dry the tofu before crumbling. Make sure to blot dry the drained, soaked noodles before assembling the lasagna. And most importantly, squeeze out as much liquid as possible from the thawed frozen spinach before adding it to the filling. Taking care of each of these steps will prevent a soggy final result.

Nutrition Facts

Serving Size: one 3 × 3-in square
Servings: 12

AMOUNT PER SERVING
Calories: 275
Calories from Fat: 45

	AMOUNT PER SERVING	% DAILY VALUE
Total Fat:	5 g	8%
Saturated Fat:	0 g	0%
Trans Fat:	0 g	
Cholesterol:	0 mg	0%
Sodium:	475 mg	20%
Total Carbohydrate:	41 g	14%
Dietary Fiber:	11 g	44%
Sugars:	7 g	
Protein:	19 g	38%

EXCELLENT SOURCE OF: fiber, vitamin A, vitamins B_1, B_2, B_3, B_6, B_{12}, iron, folate, calcium
GOOD SOURCE OF: potassium, vitamin C, magnesium

Indian Vegetable Curry

Tantalizing Indian spices bathe an abundance of health-promoting vegetables in this delicious one-pot dish. To get the most vibrant flavors in this dish, be sure to check your spices before starting. If they don't smell fragrant and bright, replace with fresh ones. Store spices in a closed drawer or pantry cupboard away from direct heat.

Serves: 6
Serving Size: 1⅓ cups
Prep Time: 10 minutes
Cook Time: 20–30 minutes
Ready Time: 40–50 minutes

2 teaspoons curry powder
1½ teaspoons ground cumin
1½ teaspoons ground coriander
1 teaspoon ground turmeric
¼ teaspoon ground cardamom
Pinch cayenne
1 can (28 ounces) crushed tomatoes
1½ cups unsweetened soy or almond milk
1 cup diced onion
1 tablespoon finely chopped ginger
2 teaspoons finely minced garlic
½ teaspoon fine sea salt
3 cups (1 pound) cubed sweet potato
16 ounces (3 cups) cauliflower florets
12 ounces green beans, cut into 1-inch lengths
1½ cups cooked or 1 can (15 ounces) chickpeas
Paprika, for garnish (optional)

1. In a large heavy-bottomed pot over medium heat, lightly toast the curry powder, cumin, coriander, turmeric, cardamom, and cayenne, stirring constantly, until they turn slightly darker in color and become aromatic, 1–2 minutes.
2. Add the tomatoes, almond or soy milk, ¾ cup water, onion, gin-

ger, garlic, and salt. Bring to a simmer and let cook, stirring occasionally, for 10 minutes.

3. While the curry sauce is simmering, place steamer basket in a saucepan and add water to just below bottom of steamer basket. Over high heat, bring water to a boil. Add sweet potato chunks to steamer. Cover and steam until sweet potatoes are just tender, 6–7 minutes.

4. Working in batches in a blender or food processor, puree half the sweet potatoes (about 1½ cups) with tomato mixture until creamy. Return pureed sweet potato and tomato mixture to the pot as well as the remaining sweet potatoes.

5. Return vegetable steamer to the saucepan, adding more water if necessary. Over high heat, bring water to a boil. Add cauliflower and green beans to the steamer. Cover and steam until both cauliflower and green beans are tender, about 5 minutes.

6. Add cauliflower and green beans to tomato mixture, followed by chickpeas. Stir to coat with tomato mixture. Bring back to a gentle simmer, cooking just until chickpeas are heated through. Taste for seasoning, adding more salt as necessary. Garnish with a sprinkle of paprika, if desired.

Nutrition Facts		
Serving Size: 1⅓ cups		
Servings: 6		
AMOUNT PER SERVING		
Calories: 260		
Calories from Fat: 25		
	AMOUNT PER SERVING	**% DAILY VALUE**
Total Fat:	3 g	4%
Saturated Fat:	0 g	0%
Trans Fat:	0 g	
Cholesterol:	0 mg	0%
Sodium:	520 mg	23%
Total Carbohydrate:	48 g	17%
Dietary Fiber:	12 g	43%
Sugars:	14 g	
Protein:	13 g	25%

EXCELLENT SOURCE OF: fiber, vitamin A, vitamin B_6, vitamin C, potassium, iron, calcium, copper

GOOD SOURCE OF: vitamin E, vitamins B_1, B_2, B_3, folate, magnesium, phosphorus

Tuscan Marinara with White Beans and Spinach

This meatless Mediterranean-inspired pasta dish is hearty and soul-satisfying. The marinara sauce is enhanced by meaty mushrooms, heady garlic, protein-rich cannellini beans, and chlorophyll-laden spinach. It's a perfect marriage of flavorful ingredients, and it's as easy as one-two-three.

Serves: 4

Serving Size: 1 cup pasta, ¾ cup sauce with beans
Prep Time: 15 minutes
Cook Time: 30 minutes
Ready Time: 45 minutes

3 cups sliced cremini mushrooms (8 ounces)
1 tablespoon minced garlic
1 jar (24 ounces) low-sodium marinara sauce (3 cups)
1⅓ cans (22.5 ounces) no-salt-added cannellini beans, rinsed and
   drained (2 cups)
16 ounces uncooked whole-grain penne
4 cups fresh spinach (4 ounces)
2 tablespoons chopped fresh basil

1. In a large skillet, add mushrooms and garlic over high heat. Cook, stirring frequently, until mushrooms are tender and all liquid has been absorbed, about 15 minutes.
2. Put a large pot filled with water over medium-high heat.
3. Add marinara sauce and beans to the mushrooms. Reduce heat to low and let simmer for 10–15 minutes, allowing flavors to meld.
4. Cook the pasta until al dente, still a little firm to the bite. Drain pasta.
5. Fold spinach and fresh basil into marinara sauce and serve alongside the cooked penne. Garnish with extra basil if desired.

Chef's Notes

Prep ahead: The marinara sauce can be made a day in advance. If making in advance, stir in the spinach and basil just before serving.

Nutrition Facts

Serving Size: 1 cup pasta, ¾ cup sauce with beans
Servings: 4

AMOUNT PER SERVING
Calories: 250
Calories from Fat: 18

	AMOUNT PER SERVING	% DAILY VALUE
Total Fat:	2 g	3%
Saturated Fat:	0 g	0%
Trans Fat:	0 g	
Cholesterol:	0 mg	0%
Sodium:	350 mg	15%
Total Carbohydrate:	71 g	24%
Dietary Fiber:	12 g	48%
Sugars:	0 g	
Protein:	18 g	36%

EXCELLENT SOURCE OF: fiber, vitamin A, vitamin C, vitamin K, thiamine, riboflavin, niacin, folate, iron, magnesium, phosphorus, zinc
GOOD SOURCE OF: pantothenic acid, calcium, potassium, selenium

Asian Stir-fry

This gorgeous dish features a rainbow of vegetable colors: green beans and zucchini, red bell peppers, and purple eggplant. As we learn more about antioxidants and phytochemicals—the disease-fighting compounds found in plants—we're discovering that many of them also happen to be the very pigments that give fruits and vegetables their vibrant colors. To maximize health benefits, we need to eat as many different colors of veggies as we can every day, in order to absorb all these different compounds. This stir-fry makes eating a rainbow of vegetables both simple and delicious.

Serves: 6
Serving Size: 1 cup stir-fry over generous ⅔ cup rice
Prep Time: 30 minutes
Cook Time: 25 minutes
Ready Time: 55 minutes

1½ cups uncooked long-grain brown rice
18 ounces extra-firm tofu (preferably sprouted), drained, patted dry, and diced
⅓ cup hoisin sauce
1 tablespoon unseasoned rice vinegar
1 tablespoon chili garlic sauce
1½ teaspoons lime juice
1½ cups chopped onion
1 tablespoon minced garlic
1 tablespoon finely chopped ginger
4 ounces long beans or green beans, cut into 2-inch lengths
1½ cups diced zucchini
1½ cups diced eggplant, preferably Asian (see Chef's Notes)
1½ cups diced red bell pepper
¼ cup chopped basil or Thai basil

1. Prepare rice according to package instructions. (One and a half cups uncooked rice will yield about 5 cups cooked.) Keep warm.
2. Line a baking sheet with paper towels and spread out diced tofu.

Press down on tofu periodically with more paper towels to help release any extra moisture.

3. To make stir-fry sauce, in a medium bowl, whisk together hoisin, ⅓ cup plus 2 tablespoons water, rice vinegar, chili garlic sauce, and lime juice. Set aside.

4. In a wok or large sauté pan, combine onions, garlic, and ginger with ½ cup water. Bring to a boil over high heat. Reduce heat to a simmer and cook until onions are tender and liquid has evaporated, 8–10 minutes. Add ½ cup water and long beans. Raise heat to high and cook for 3 minutes. Add zucchini, eggplant, and bell pepper. Cook for 5 minutes, stirring frequently, until vegetables are tender and liquid has evaporated. Add a little more water if necessary.

5. While veggies are cooking, add tofu to stir-fry sauce and gently stir to coat. Add tofu and sauce to vegetables. Stir until incorporated and cook until tofu is warmed through, about 3 minutes. Remove from heat. Fold in basil. Season to taste with more chili garlic sauce, if desired. Serve hot over cooked brown rice.

Chef's Notes

We love sprouted tofu! For some recipes, its more dense and firm texture is a benefit. Sprouting, a common procedure with legumes and grains, gives foods more bang for their nutritional buck by making the nutrients more available to us. Sprouted tofu offers a higher protein content and nutritional value, plus it's easier to digest. We recommend it for this dish because it releases less water, so it works very well in a stir-fry. If not available, use an extra-firm tofu. If packaged in water, first drain out all the water, then press the excess water from the tofu. There are several ways to press the excess water from tofu. A quick and simple way is to place tofu on a plate lined with paper or a kitchen towel, then place another towel on top of the tofu. Place a plate or cutting board on top of the tofu and weigh it down with the heavy weight of a few cans or a book or carefully press on it. Be careful not to press too hard and crumble the tofu.

Asian eggplant (sometimes called Chinese or Japanese eggplant) has thinner skin and fewer seeds (and therefore less bitterness) than a traditional globe eggplant. Overall, the Asian eggplant has a more delicate flavor than the globe eggplant. We prefer the Asian variety for this dish, but globe eggplant makes a fine substitute and lends more of an eggplant flavor. A slender Italian eggplant is another good choice.

Nutrition Facts

Serving Size: 1 cup stir-fry over generous ⅔ cup rice
Servings: 6

AMOUNT PER SERVING
Calories: 320
Calories from Fat: 63

	AMOUNT PER SERVING	% DAILY VALUE
Total Fat:	7 g	11%
Saturated Fat:	0 g	0%
Trans Fat:	0 g	
Cholesterol:	0 mg	0%
Sodium:	290 mg	12%
Total Carbohydrate:	55 g	18%
Dietary Fiber:	6 g	24%
Sugars:	9 g	
Protein:	13 g	26%

EXCELLENT SOURCE OF: fiber, vitamin A, vitamin C, vitamin K, calcium

GOOD SOURCE OF: vitamin B_6, folate, iron, manganese, molybdenum

Smoky Bean Tacos

Black beans, pinto beans, and corn come together in this taco filling with a sauce of tomatoes, poblano peppers, and smoky chipotle peppers simmered with oregano and cumin. This dish offers lots of fiber, plant-based protein, and heart-healthy vitamins.

Serves: 6

Serving Size: 2 tacos
Prep Time: 10 minutes
Cook Time: 20 minutes
Ready Time: 30 minutes

1 can (28 ounces) no-salt-added, diced fire-roasted tomatoes
1 cup diced onion
1 cup diced seeded poblano pepper (2 medium, about 8 ounces)
1 tablespoon minced garlic
1 tablespoon fresh oregano or 1 teaspoon dried
1 teaspoon ground cumin
1½ teaspoons chopped canned chipotles in adobo sauce
½ teaspoon fine sea salt
1 can (15 ounces) no-salt-added black beans, rinsed and drained
    (1½ cups)
1 can (15 ounces) no-salt-added pinto beans, rinsed and drained
    (1½ cups)
2 cups corn kernels, fresh or frozen
12 corn tortillas, 6½-inch diameter
⅓ cup chopped cilantro
3 cups chopped romaine lettuce
6 cilantro sprigs, for garnish (optional)

1. In a medium skillet over medium heat, combine tomatoes, onions, poblano pepper, garlic, oregano, cumin, chopped chipotle, and salt. Cook, stirring occasionally, until onions are softened and flavors have begun to meld, about 10 minutes.
2. Stir in beans and corn. Bring to a simmer and let cook, stirring occasionally, for 10 minutes.

3. While beans are cooking, warm tortillas, either in the oven or on the stovetop. To warm in the oven, preheat oven to 375°F. Wrap corn tortillas in aluminum foil and place in the oven. Heat until tortillas are warmed through, about 10 minutes. Alternatively, turn a stovetop gas burner to high. Using tongs, place one tortilla directly over the flame. Let tortilla cook for 2–3 seconds, then turn with tongs. Repeat, turning the tortilla every 2–3 seconds, until warmed through and browned along the edges. Repeat with remaining tortillas.

4. Just before serving, stir chopped cilantro into corn and bean mixture. Taste for seasoning and add additional salt and chopped chipotle as needed.

5. To serve, spread ½ cup romaine lettuce on each warm tortilla, followed by ½ cup bean filling. Garnish with cilantro sprigs.

Chef's Notes

You can add (or swap out the beans for) veggie crumbles (suggested brand: Yves Garden Veggie Crumbles) to create a meaty-style taco. This is a great vegan option for those who crave a classic ground beef taco, but without the fat, cholesterol, and animal protein. All the flavor and rich texture, yet packed with heart-healthy benefits.

Nutrition Facts

Serving Size: 2 tacos
Servings: 6

AMOUNT PER SERVING
Calories: 329
Calories from Fat: 18

	AMOUNT PER SERVING	% DAILY VALUE
Total Fat:	2.5 g	3%
Saturated Fat:	0 g	0%
Trans Fat:	0 g	
Cholesterol:	0 mg	0%
Sodium:	535 mg	22%
Total Carbohydrate:	65 g	22%
Dietary Fiber:	14 g	56%
Sugars:	9 g	
Protein:	13 g	26%

EXCELLENT SOURCE OF: fiber, vitamin A, vitamin C, iron
GOOD SOURCE OF: potassium, calcium, magnesium, phosphorus, zinc

Fast and Sloppy Joes

Could a soy-based meat alternative do justice to this hot and messy American classic? We discovered that even the pickiest kids could enjoy this heart-healthy version. It captures the taste and texture of the original, minus the fat and cholesterol. These sandwiches can be served closed or open-faced on whole-grain buns, whole-grain English muffins, even sliced whole-grain sandwich bread. Just don't forget the forks—and be sure to pass around plenty of napkins. A sturdy gluten-free bun or bread will work, too.

Serves: 6

Serving Size: 1 sandwich
Prep Time: 5 minutes
Cook Time: 10 minutes
Ready Time: 15 minutes

1 package (12 ounces) vegetarian ground-meat alternative (suggested brands: Yves Veggie Ground or Lightlife Smart Ground)
1 can (15 ounces) pinto beans, rinsed and drained (1½ cups)
½ cup prepared barbecue sauce (see Chef's Notes)
⅓ cup tomato paste
½ cup chopped scallions, divided
2 teaspoons apple cider vinegar
½ teaspoon smoked paprika
¼ teaspoon freshly ground black pepper
6 whole-grain buns

1. In a medium saucepan over medium heat, combine ground meat alternative, pinto beans, and barbecue sauce. In a small bowl, whisk together tomato paste and water until smooth. Add tomato paste to bean mixture along with ¼ cup scallions, vinegar, smoked paprika, and pepper.
2. Reduce heat to low and cook, stirring occasionally, until mixture is warm and flavors have melded, 5–7 minutes. While filling is cooking, toast buns.
3. To serve as a closed sandwich, spoon ½ cup filling onto bottom

half of bun. Top with a sprinkle of scallions, if using. Cover with top half of bun. To serve open-faced, spoon ¼ cup filling over each half of bun.

Chef's Notes

Prepared barbecue sauces can vary widely in the amount of sugar and fat they can contain. Be sure to check the nutritional information on the label, and look for a barbecue sauce with less than 5 grams of sugar and less than 3 grams of fat per serving, without hydrogenated fats or highly saturated fats such as coconut oil. Ideally, choose brands that do not include high-fructose corn syrup, preservatives, or artificial colors. One example is Annie's Organic BBQ Sauce, which contains 4 grams of sugar and 1 gram of fat per serving.

Nutrition Facts

Serving Size: 1 sandwich
Servings: 6

AMOUNT PER SERVING
Calories: 255
Calories from Fat: 18

	AMOUNT PER SERVING	% DAILY VALUE
Total Fat:	2 g	3%
Saturated Fat:	0 g	0%
Trans Fat:	0 g	
Cholesterol:	0 mg	0%
Sodium:	638 mg	27%
Total Carbohydrate:	45 g	15%
Dietary Fiber:	11 g	44%
Sugars:	8 g	
Protein:	19 g	38%

EXCELLENT SOURCE OF: fiber, vitamins B_1, B_2, B_3, B_6, B_{12}, iron, zinc
GOOD SOURCE OF: potassium, calcium

Mushroom Stroganoff

Studded with chunks of flavorful cremini mushrooms, this creamy vegan pasta dish makes a perfect fall or winter entrée. Cannellini beans add protein, while fresh thyme, dry sherry, and paprika add flavor. An inexpensive, domestic dry sherry works fine for this recipe. Avoid any product labeled "sherry cooking wine," as it is heavily salted to make it unpalatable for drinking.

Serves: 4
  Serving Size: 1½ cups
  Prep Time: 10 minutes
  Cook Time: 40 minutes
  Ready Time: 50 minutes

  2 cups coarsely chopped onion
  8 ounces cremini mushrooms, quartered
  ⅔ cup dry sherry
  2 tablespoons Bragg Liquid Aminos or reduced-sodium tamari
  2 tablespoons fresh lemon juice
  1 tablespoon chopped fresh thyme or 1 teaspoon dried
  2 teaspoons paprika
  1 teaspoon freshly ground pepper
  3 cups unsweetened soy milk
  2 teaspoons sweet rice flour, arrowroot, or cornstarch
  1 can (15 ounces) no-salt-added cannellini beans, rinsed and drained
     (1½ cups)
  8 ounces whole-grain or gluten-free penne or fettuccini
  2 tablespoons minced chives or flat-leaf parsley, for garnish (optional)

1. In a large heavy-bottomed sauté pan over medium-high heat, bring onions, mushrooms, sherry, liquid aminos or tamari, lemon juice, thyme, paprika, and pepper to a boil. Reduce heat to medium and cook, stirring frequently, until the liquid has reduced, 15–20 minutes.
2. Stir in soy milk and cook, stirring occasionally, for 5 minutes.
3. In a small bowl, whisk the sweet rice flour, arrowroot, or corn-

starch with 1 tablespoon water until smooth. Add to mushroom mixture. Simmer until the mixture thickens, 2–3 minutes. Stir in cannellini beans. Remove from heat and set aside for flavors to meld.

4. In a large pot over high heat, bring about 4 quarts of water to a boil. Add pasta and cook, stirring occasionally to prevent sticking, according to package directions. While pasta is cooking, gently rewarm mushroom sauce, if necessary.

5. Drain pasta. Toss pasta with mushroom sauce. Garnish with chives or parsley, if desired.

Chef's Notes

Sweet rice flour, made from finely ground glutinous or "sticky" rice, adds thickness and body to sauces and soups. Check the label before purchasing, as sweet rice flour is not the same as regular rice flour. ("Sweet rice" refers to the type of rice; it does not contain added sugar.) Look for it in the Asian products, gluten-free, or specialty flours section of your supermarket. We've had good results using Koda Farms' Mochiko Blue Star brand as well as Bob's Red Mill Sweet Rice Flour. Arrowroot or cornstarch can be substituted if you can't find sweet rice flour.

Nutrition Facts

Serving Size: 1½ cups
Servings: 4

AMOUNT PER SERVING
Calories: 321
Calories from Fat: 45

	AMOUNT PER SERVING	% DAILY VALUE
Total Fat:	5 g	8%
Saturated Fat:	0 g	0%
Trans Fat:	0 g	
Cholesterol:	0 mg	0%
Sodium:	441 mg	18%
Total Carbohydrate:	49 g	16%
Dietary Fiber:	9 g	36%
Sugars:	7 g	
Protein:	16 g	32%

EXCELLENT SOURCE OF: fiber, vitamin A, magnesium
GOOD SOURCE OF: vitamin C, B vitamins, potassium, iron

Pasta Carbonara

Skip the high fat while you enjoy the satisfying flavors of this Ornish Kitchen pasta dish. Hearty whole-grain penne is bathed in a creamy sauce with a kick of smoke and spice and plenty of bright, sweet green peas and fresh broccoli (or substitute asparagus tips for the broccoli). It's easy to make your own oil-free roasted garlic puree, but you can also look for prepared roasted garlic puree in specialty grocery stores.

Serves: 4
Serving Size: 1¼ cups
Prep Time: 10 minutes
Cook Time: 20 minutes
Ready Time: 30 minutes

6 ounces uncooked whole-grain or gluten-free penne (2 cups)
⅔ cup frozen baby peas
2 cups broccoli florets (5 ounces)
¼ cup dried tomatoes (not oil-packed)
2 cups unsweetened low-fat soy milk
¼ cup Roasted Garlic puree (page 410)
2 tablespoons white miso
1½ tablespoons nutritional yeast
1½ teaspoons finely chopped fresh oregano or ½ teaspoon dried
1 teaspoon chopped canned chipotles in adobo sauce
1 teaspoon paprika
2 teaspoons arrowroot, cornstarch, or sweet rice flour
Fine sea salt to taste
Freshly ground pepper to taste

1. Fill a large saucepan two-thirds full of water. Bring to boil over high heat. Cook pasta according to package directions. One minute before pasta is ready, add peas. Drain pasta and peas in a colander and set aside.
2. While pasta is cooking, place a vegetable steamer basket in a saucepan and add water to just below bottom of steamer basket. Over high heat, bring water to a boil. Add broccoli. Cover and

steam until broccoli is just tender but still bright green, 4 to 5 minutes. Remove basket from steamer and set aside.

3. In a small bowl, cover dried tomatoes with hot water. Let stand until tomatoes are softened, about 5 minutes. Drain. Slice tomatoes into strips.

4. In a medium heavy-bottomed saucepan over medium heat, whisk together soy milk, roasted garlic, miso, nutritional yeast, oregano, chipotles, and paprika. Add drained tomato and bring mixture to a simmer. Cook, whisking frequently, until mixture starts to thicken, 4–5 minutes.

5. In a small bowl, whisk arrowroot, cornstarch, or sweet rice flour with 1 tablespoon water to make a smooth paste. Whisk paste into sauce and cook until mixture thickens, 1–2 minutes.

6. Just before serving, stir pasta, peas, and broccoli into sauce. Cook, stirring, until mixture is heated through. Taste for seasoning, adding salt and/or pepper as needed. Serve immediately.

Chef's Notes

Miso is a thick, tangy paste typically made from fermented soybeans. White miso, also called shiro or sweet miso, is fermented for a shorter time than yellow or red miso. It is mild in flavor and less salty. If you are reducing your soy intake, look for miso made from chickpeas.

Nutrition Facts

Serving Size: 1¼ cups
Servings: 4

AMOUNT PER SERVING
Calories: 293
Calories from Fat: 36

	AMOUNT PER SERVING	% DAILY VALUE
Total Fat:	4 g	6%
Saturated Fat:	0 g	0%
Trans Fat:	0 g	
Cholesterol:	0 mg	0%
Sodium:	479 mg	20%
Total Carbohydrate:	51 g	17%
Dietary Fiber:	11 g	44%
Sugars:	6 g	
Protein:	16 g	32%

EXCELLENT SOURCE OF: fiber, vitamin A, thiamin, riboflavin, niacin, vitamins B_6, B_{12}, vitamin C, folate, iron
GOOD SOURCE OF: potassium

Lavash Veggie Wrap

Lavash is a thin, rectangular Middle Eastern flatbread that's perfect for rolling into sandwich wraps. Choose whole-grain lavash or use a large whole-grain tortilla for the wrap. For variety, substitute other vegetable combinations for the cucumber, red bell pepper, and romaine lettuce called for here. Try grated carrots, baby spinach, baby kale, sliced tomatoes, and/or sprouts. A base of hummus adds protein and fiber without added fat; it can be made 2–3 days in advance.

Serves: 4

Serving Size: 1 wrap
Prep Time: 30 minutes
Cook Time: N/A
Ready Time: 30 minutes

1 large cucumber
1 large red bell pepper
4 sheets whole-wheat lavash
2 cups Hummus (page 412)
2 cups chopped romaine lettuce
4 teaspoons capers, chopped
¼ cup chopped red onion

1. Peel and seed the cucumber. Cut into 16 strips, each about 4 inches long and ½ inch wide. Slice red pepper in half and remove stem, seeds, and ribs. Slice into 16 strips, each about ½ inch wide.
2. Lay out a sheet of lavash on a clean work surface with the short edge facing you. Spread a thin layer of hummus (about ½ cup) over the lavash, leaving a ½-inch margin around all four edges.
3. Distribute 4 pieces of the cucumbers horizontally along the lower third of the lavash. Stack 4 of the red pepper strips on top of the cucumbers. Finally, stack ½ cup romaine on top of the red peppers. Sprinkle 1 teaspoon capers and 1 tablespoon red onion over the hummus on the remaining two-thirds of the lavash.
4. Starting at the short end closest to you, roll the lavash into a tight

cylinder. Set aside, seam side down. Repeat process with remaining lavash sheets and remaining vegetables.

5. Slice ¼ inch off the ends of each lavash and discard. Then slice each lavash roll into about five 1½-inch rounds and serve. These can be made 1–2 hours in advance.

Nutrition Facts

Serving Size: 1 wrap
Servings: 4

AMOUNT PER SERVING
Calories: 308
Calories from Fat: 27

	AMOUNT PER SERVING	% DAILY VALUE
Total Fat:	3 g	5%
Saturated Fat:	0 g	0%
Trans Fat:	0 g	
Cholesterol:	0 mg	0%
Sodium:	477 mg	20%
Total Carbohydrate:	58 g	19%
Dietary Fiber:	11 g	44%
Sugars:	5 g	
Protein:	14 g	28%

EXCELLENT SOURCE OF: fiber, vitamin A, vitamin C, vitamin K, copper

GOOD SOURCE OF: iron, calcium, iodine, magnesium, phosphorus, potassium, zinc

Hearty Three-Bean Veggie Stew

This easy, hearty meatless stew makes a perfect warm-up on a cold winter's day, thanks to a medley of protein-rich beans, tasty veggies, and Italian herbs. Pair it with a warm slice of whole-grain bread and a tossed salad, or spoon it over a serving of polenta or quinoa. Like many bean dishes, this stew is even better if made a day ahead so the flavors have a chance to meld. Let stew cool after cooking, transfer to a covered container, and refrigerate for up to 3 days. Reheat just before serving.

Serves: 6

Serving Size: 1¼ cups
Prep Time: 10 minutes
Cook Time: 30 minutes
Ready Time: 40 minutes

2 cups coarsely chopped onion
2 cups coarsely chopped red bell pepper
2 cups coarsely chopped zucchini
1 tablespoon finely minced garlic
1 tablespoon finely chopped fresh thyme or 1½ teaspoons dried
2 teaspoons finely chopped fresh marjoram or oregano or 1 teaspoon dried
½ teaspoon fine sea salt
¼ teaspoon freshly ground black pepper
3½ cups low-sodium vegetable juice
1 can (15 ounces) no-salt-added red kidney beans, rinsed and drained (1½ cups)
1 can (15 ounces) no-salt-added cannellini, rinsed and drained (1½ cups)
1 can (15 ounces) no-salt-added black beans, rinsed and drained (1½ cups)
2 teaspoons lemon zest
2 tablespoons lemon juice
1 tablespoon pure maple syrup
¼ teaspoon crushed red pepper flakes (optional)
3 cups chopped destemmed kale

1. In a large heavy-bottomed pot over medium heat, sauté onions, red pepper, zucchini, ¼ cup water, garlic, thyme, marjoram or oregano, salt, and black pepper, stirring frequently, until onions are translucent and vegetables have softened, about 10 minutes.
2. Add vegetable juice, kidney beans, cannellini beans, black beans, lemon zest, lemon juice, maple syrup, and red pepper flakes, if using. Bring to a simmer and let cook, stirring frequently, for 15 minutes.
3. Fold in kale and cook another 3–4 minutes. If you want a soupier consistency, add a little more vegetable juice. Taste for seasoning, adding additional black pepper, red pepper flakes, and/or herbs as needed.

Nutrition Facts

Serving Size: 1¼ cups
Servings: 6

AMOUNT PER SERVING
Calories: 250
Calories from Fat: 18

	AMOUNT PER SERVING	% DAILY VALUE
Total Fat:	2 g	3%
Saturated Fat:	0 g	0%
Trans Fat:	0 g	
Cholesterol:	0 mg	0%
Sodium:	536 mg	22%
Total Carbohydrate:	47 g	16%
Dietary Fiber:	13 g	52%
Sugars:	13 g	
Protein:	13 g	26%

EXCELLENT SOURCE OF: fiber, vitamin A, vitamin B$_6$, vitamin C, potassium, iron, phosphorus, magnesium
GOOD SOURCE OF: folate, calcium, zinc

Tempeh Enchiladas

Tempeh's delicious, dense texture makes it a perfect replacement for meat in these Mexican-style enchiladas. You can also make them with cooked pinto beans or your favorite vegetarian ground meat alternative, or use the filling in tacos or tostadas. For a quick and easy option, use a healthy pre-made enchilada sauce without added oils or prepare in advance this delicious Red Enchilada Sauce (page 414) using flavorful, mild dried chili peppers.

Serves: 4
  Serving Size: 2 enchiladas
  Prep Time: 30 minutes
  Cook Time: 1 hour
  Ready Time: 1 hour 30 minutes

2 cups chopped seeded fresh pasilla or poblano peppers (4 peppers)
1½ cups chopped onion
2 teaspoons chopped fresh oregano or 1 teaspoon dried
¾ teaspoon ground cumin
¼ teaspoon fine sea salt, divided
8 ounces tempeh, diced
1 cup corn kernels, fresh or frozen
3½ cups Red Enchilada Sauce (page 414)
⅔ cup chopped cilantro, divided
8 corn tortillas, 6½-inch diameter
1 lime, cut in wedges, for garnish

1. Preheat oven to 350°F. To make the filling, combine fresh peppers, onions, oregano, cumin, ⅛ teaspoon salt, and ¼ cup water in a large saucepan over medium heat. Bring to a simmer and cook, stirring occasionally, until onions are soft and translucent, 7–10 minutes.
2. Add tempeh, corn, remaining ⅛ teaspoon salt, and 1 cup enchilada sauce. Simmer, stirring frequently, for 5 minutes. Remove from heat and stir in ⅓ cup cilantro.
3. Wrap tortillas in aluminum foil. Place in oven until tortillas are

heated through, about 10 minutes. (Or, to heat in microwave, place tortillas between 2 damp paper towels. Microwave on high until warmed, about 1 minute.)

4. To assemble the enchiladas, spread 1 cup enchilada sauce over the bottom of a 15 × 10 × 2-inch baking pan. Dip each tortilla in the remaining enchilada sauce, letting any extra run back into the saucepan. Place tortilla on a plate. Spoon ½ cup filling down the center of the tortilla. Roll up the sides of the tortilla over the filling. Flip over and place filled tortilla, seam side down, in the prepared baking pan. Repeat with remaining tortillas.

5. Spoon 1 cup enchilada sauce over the enchiladas. (Recipe can be prepared to this point up to 8 hours ahead. Cover pan and refrigerate until needed.) Bake enchiladas until golden brown around the edges, about 20 minutes. Reheat remaining enchilada sauce. Garnish each serving with 2 tablespoons enchilada sauce, remaining chopped cilantro, and a lime wedge.

Chef's Notes

Pasilla and poblano peppers are dark green, medium-sized, mildly spicy chili peppers. They have a flattened conical shape and pointed ends.

Nutrition Facts

Serving Size: 2 enchiladas
Servings: 4

AMOUNT PER SERVING
Calories: 356
Calories from Fat: 54

	AMOUNT PER SERVING	% DAILY VALUE
Total Fat:	6 g	9%
Saturated Fat:	1 g	5%
Trans Fat:	0 g	
Cholesterol:	0 mg	0%
Sodium:	331 mg	14%
Total Carbohydrate:	56 g	19%
Dietary Fiber:	16 g	64%
Sugars:	15 g	
Protein:	21 g	42%

EXCELLENT SOURCE OF: fiber, vitamin A, vitamin B$_6$, vitamin C
GOOD SOURCE OF: folate, iron, calcium, potassium

BBQ Tempeh Sandwich

Looking for a versatile meat-free option that's low in fat but high in fiber and plant protein? Try our barbecue-sauced "TLT" made with tempeh, lettuce, and tomato. Tempeh, made from fermented, cultured whole soybeans, has a mild, versatile flavor and a firm texture. Some brands of barbecue sauce can be surprisingly high in sugar and/or fat. Look for a brand with 5 grams or less of sugar and 3 grams or less of fat per serving. To top these sandwiches, whip up a batch of oil-free Vegan Mayo (page 400).

Serves: 4
Serving Size: 1 sandwich
Prep Time: 30 minutes
Cook Time: 45 minutes
Ready Time: 1 hour 15 minutes

For barbecued tempeh:
½ cup prepared barbecue sauce (less than 5 g sugar and 3 g fat per serving)
1 tablespoon apple cider vinegar, preferably raw, organic, and unfiltered
⅛ teaspoon chipotle powder or 2 dashes hot sauce
12 ounces tempeh

For sandwiches:
8 whole-grain sandwich thins
4 slices tomato
4 thin slices red onion
4 romaine lettuce leaves
8–12 fresh basil leaves
2 teaspoons Vegan Mayo (page 400)

1. In a 9 × 13-inch Pyrex glass baking pan, combine the barbecue sauce, ½ cup water, vinegar, and chipotle powder or hot sauce.
2. Slice the tempeh in half horizontally to a ¼-inch thickness. Add the sliced tempeh to the baking pan, turning to coat both sides.

Marinate the tempeh for at least 15 minutes and up to 8 hours. (If marinating for more than 1 hour, cover with plastic wrap and refrigerate.)

3. Preheat oven to 350°F. Line a baking sheet with parchment paper. Transfer the tempeh to the baking sheet, reserving the extra marinade. Bake for 20 minutes.

4. Turn tempeh over, basting with reserved marinade. Bake for an additional 15–25 minutes, until edges are lightly brown and barbecue sauce looks glazed. (The cooking time can vary based on different brands of tempeh and barbecue sauce, so check frequently to prevent burning.)

5. Remove the tempeh from the oven. Divide tempeh into four portions, slicing to match the size of the sandwich thins. Arrange tempeh on 4 sandwich thins. Top with tomato, onion, lettuce, and basil leaves. Drizzle with remaining marinade, if desired. Spread ½ teaspoon Vegan Mayo on each of the remaining sandwich thins. Top tempeh with mayo-spread sandwich thins.

Chef's Notes

Barbecue sauces can vary widely in the amount of sugar and fat they can contain. Be sure to check the nutritional information on the label, and look for a barbecue sauce with less than 5 grams of sugar and less than 3 grams of fat per serving with no hydrogenated fats or highly saturated fats such as coconut oil. Ideally, choose brands that avoid high-fructose corn syrup, preservatives, and/or artificial coloring. One suggested brand is Annie's Organic BBQ Sauce, which has 4 grams of sugar and 1 gram of fat per serving.

Nutrition Facts

Serving Size: 1 sandwich
Servings: 4

AMOUNT PER SERVING
Calories: 333
Calories from Fat: 81

	AMOUNT PER SERVING	% DAILY VALUE
Total Fat:	9 g	14%
Saturated Fat:	1 g	5%
Trans Fat:	0 g	
Cholesterol:	0 mg	0%
Sodium:	417 mg	17%
Total Carbohydrate:	43 g	14%
Dietary Fiber:	15 g	60%
Sugars:	8 g	
Protein:	23 g	46%

EXCELLENT SOURCE OF: fiber, vitamin A, vitamin C, vitamin K, folate, iron

GOOD SOURCE OF: potassium, calcium

Tex-Mex Tortilla Pie

We've updated this layered Tex-Mex family favorite with a filling of poblano peppers and black beans instead of the typical ground beef. For an extra boost of flavor, try a drizzle of Smoky Chipotle Sauce (page 406) on top.

Serves: 8

Serving Size: 1 wedge
Prep Time: 30 minutes
Cook Time: 30 minutes
Ready Time: 1 hour

Nonstick cooking spray
2 cups chopped onion
2 cups finely chopped seeded poblano peppers (4 peppers; 1 pound)
1 tablespoon minced garlic
1½ teaspoons ground cumin, divided
2 teaspoons chopped fresh oregano or 1 teaspoon dried, divided
1 can (14.5 ounces) no-salt-added diced fire-roasted tomatoes
1 can (15 ounces) no-salt-added black beans, rinsed and drained
   (1½ cups)
1 cup corn kernels, fresh or frozen
1 teaspoon chopped canned chipotles in adobo sauce, plus more to
   taste (see Chef's Notes)
⅓ cup finely chopped cilantro, plus more for garnish
1 tablespoon lime juice
5 whole-wheat tortillas, 10-inch diameter
1 jar (24 ounces) low-fat, low-sodium marinara sauce (2½ cups)

1. Preheat oven to 375°F. Line a baking sheet with parchment paper and spray lightly with cooking spray.
2. In a large, 12-inch heavy-bottomed sauté pan, combine onions, peppers, garlic, ¾ teaspoon cumin, 1 teaspoon fresh oregano (or ½ teaspoon dried), and ½ cup water. Bring to a boil over high heat. Reduce heat to medium and simmer, stirring occasionally, until

onions are translucent and water has evaporated, about 10 minutes.

3. Add tomatoes (including juice), black beans, corn, and chipotles. Cook, stirring frequently, until liquids evaporate, about 10 minutes. Remove from heat and allow to cool slightly.

4. Stir in the remaining ¾ teaspoon cumin and remaining 1 teaspoon fresh oregano (or ¼ teaspoon dried). Add cilantro and lime juice. Taste for seasoning. Using a large spoon or a potato masher, mash the mixture roughly so it will stick together and be easier to spread.

5. Measure out 1 cup marinara sauce and place in a small bowl. To assemble pie, place one tortilla in the center of the prepared baking sheet. Using the marinara sauce in the bowl, spread 3 tablespoons sauce evenly over the tortilla. (Use a pastry brush if you have one.) Spread 1 cup bean mixture evenly over the tortilla, making sure to spread it out to the edges.

6. Top with a second tortilla. Spread with 3 more tablespoons marinara and 1 cup filling. Repeat with 2 more tortillas, sauce, and beans for a total of 4 layers.

7. Top with remaining tortilla. Spread remaining marinara sauce in the bowl over the top of the tortilla. Bake until golden brown on top and warmed through, 15–20 minutes.

8. While tortilla pie is baking, heat remaining 1½ cups marinara sauce in a small saucepan until warm.

9. When pie is ready, pick up both sides of the parchment paper and transfer pie, still on parchment, to a cutting board. Cut into 8 wedges. Serve each portion topped with 2–3 tablespoons warm marinara sauce. Garnish with cilantro.

Chef's Notes

Canned chipotles in adobo sauce are a great (and inexpensive) staple to have in your pantry, useful for boosting heat and flavor in many Mexican- and Southwestern-inspired dishes. When jalapeño peppers are smoked and dried, they become chipotles, with a medium spiciness and a pleasant smokiness. Adobo sauce is a smooth, piquant mixture of dried chili peppers, herbs, and vinegar. Look for canned chipotles in adobo in the Latin American/Hispanic foods section of your supermarket; we like the widely available Embasa brand. For ease of use, puree the contents of a small (7 ounces) can in the blender. Transfer the puree to a small, closed container. Refrigerate and use as needed. Marinara sauces can be surprisingly high in fat and/or sodium, so check labels carefully before buying. Choose one with 3 grams or less of fat and 140 milligrams or less of sodium per serving.

Nutrition Facts

Serving Size: 1 wedge
Servings: 8

AMOUNT PER SERVING
Calories: 250
Calories from Fat: 36

	AMOUNT PER SERVING	% DAILY VALUE
Total Fat:	4 g	6%
Saturated Fat:	1 g	5%
Trans Fat:	0 g	
Cholesterol:	0 mg	0%
Sodium:	609 mg	25%
Total Carbohydrate:	44 g	15%
Dietary Fiber:	18 g	72%
Sugars:	8 g	
Protein:	10 g	20%

EXCELLENT SOURCE OF: fiber, vitamin C
GOOD SOURCE OF: vitamin A, iron

Tempeh Chili Verde

Black beans and roasted tempeh add healthy plant protein to this tangy Mexican-style stew of peppers, tomatillos, and corn. Serve over brown rice or quinoa, or scoop it up with a warm corn tortilla.

Serves: 4
Serving Size: 1 cup
Prep Time: 35 minutes
Cook Time: 25 minutes
Ready Time: 1 hour

8 ounces tempeh, diced
3 poblano peppers (12 ounces) (see Chef's Notes)
12 ounces tomatillos, husks removed and roughly chopped
2 cups roughly chopped onion
1 tablespoon minced garlic
¼ teaspoon fine sea salt, divided
½ cup chopped cilantro, plus more for garnish
1½ tablespoons fresh lime juice, plus more as needed
1 teaspoon pure maple syrup
½ teaspoon ground cumin
1 teaspoon finely chopped jalapeño pepper (optional)
1 cup corn kernels, fresh or frozen
1 can (15 ounces) no-salt-added black beans, rinsed and drained
   (1½ cups)
2⅔ cups cooked brown rice or quinoa for serving (optional)

1. Preheat oven to 400°F. Line a baking sheet with parchment paper. Spread diced tempeh over prepared baking sheet and bake until golden brown, about 20 minutes.
2. To roast the poblano peppers, char the peppers directly over a gas flame or under a broiler until blackened on all sides. If charring the peppers over a gas flame, use high heat and rotate frequently using tongs, for 4–5 minutes. If using broiler, arrange peppers on a broiler pan and broil about 2 inches from heat, turning occasionally with tongs, for 20–30 minutes. Transfer charred peppers

to a bowl, cover with a plate, and let steam for 10 minutes. Remove skins and seeds from peppers. Chop peppers and set aside.

3. In a medium heavy-bottomed saucepan over medium heat, combine the tomatillos, onions, garlic, ½ cup water, and ⅛ teaspoon salt. Cook until tomatillos are soft and onions are translucent, 10–15 minutes. Let cool slightly.

4. Transfer two-thirds of the tomatillo mixture (about 1½ cups) to a blender. Add roasted poblano peppers, cilantro, lime juice, maple syrup, cumin, ½ cup water, and remaining ⅛ teaspoon salt. Blend on high speed until smooth. Taste for seasoning; add chopped jalapeño to taste if you want a spicier sauce.

5. Pour the puree back into the saucepan with the remaining unblended tomatillo mixture. Stir in the baked tempeh, corn, and black beans. Over low heat, bring to a simmer and let cook for 10 minutes. If mixture seems too thick, add more water.

6. Taste for seasoning and add more lime juice if needed. Divide into bowls, spooning each serving over ⅔ cup cooked rice or quinoa, if desired. Garnish with cilantro.

Chef's Notes

Although poblano peppers are typically described as only mildly hot, some poblanos can, in fact, be quite spicy. If you want to reduce a pepper's heat, remove the seeds and interior ribs of the pepper before cooking it. You can also taste a small bite of each pepper to gauge its heat before using. Poblano peppers typically weigh about 4 ounces per pepper.

Nutrition Facts

Serving Size: 1 cup
Servings: 4

AMOUNT PER SERVING
Calories: 340
Calories from Fat: 63

	AMOUNT PER SERVING	% DAILY VALUE
Total Fat:	7 g	9%
Saturated Fat:	1 g	5%
Trans Fat:	0 g	
Cholesterol:	0 mg	0%
Sodium:	180 mg	8%
Total Carbohydrate:	51 g	19%
Dietary Fiber:	10 g	36%
Sugars:	12 g	
Protein:	21 g	42%

EXCELLENT SOURCE OF: fiber, vitamin C, potassium, iron, magnesium

GOOD SOURCE OF: vitamin A, thiamin, riboflavin, vitamin B_6, calcium, phosphorus

Grilled Portobello Mushroom Burgers

Summer's here and it's time to fire up the grill for these satisfying porto-bello mushroom burgers, topped with grilled onions and peppers and a lively, vibrant green Basil Mayo (page 402). Made from silken tofu, this mayonnaise makes a great sandwich spread or vegetable dip. It's best used within a day of being made.

Serves: 4
Serving Size: 1 burger
Prep Time: 30 minutes
Cook Time: 20 minutes
Ready Time: 50 minutes

¼ cup balsamic vinegar
1 tablespoon plus 1 teaspoon Bragg Liquid Aminos (see Chef's Notes)
1 teaspoon fresh rosemary
½ teaspoon minced garlic
⅛ teaspoon freshly ground black pepper
4 portobello mushrooms (4 ounces each), stems removed
4 slices red onion, ½ inch thick
2 red bell peppers, quartered
4 whole-grain buns, sliced
4 tablespoons Basil Mayo (page 402)
4 lettuce leaves

1. Prepare the grill at medium-high heat or preheat oven to 400°F. Line a baking sheet with parchment paper.
2. To make the marinade, in a small bowl whisk together vinegar, liquid aminos, 1 tablespoon water, rosemary, garlic, and black pepper.
3. Wipe the mushroom caps with a damp paper towel. Place mush-rooms, red onion slices, and bell peppers on prepared baking sheet. Brush the marinade on both sides of the vegetables.
4. If using the grill, grill the mushrooms, onions, and peppers until tender and lightly browned, 10–15 minutes. Turn and baste with marinade after 5–7 minutes. Remove the vegetables from the grill

and baste again with remaining marinade. (Alternatively, bake the vegetables in the oven for 10 minutes, baste, and continue baking for another 10 minutes, until tender and golden brown. Remove from the oven and baste again with remaining marinade.)

5. Slice red peppers into strips. Separate onion slices into rings.
6. Toast buns until golden brown. To assemble, place the bottom half of each bun on a plate. Spread 1 tablespoon Basil Mayo over the bun. (Save remaining mayonnaise for another use.) Top with a mushroom, red pepper slices, onion rings, and a lettuce leaf. Cover with the top of the bun. Serve immediately.

Chef's Notes

Bragg Liquid Aminos can be substituted with low-sodium tamari or soy sauce.

Nutrition Facts

Serving Size: 1 burger
Servings: 4

AMOUNT PER SERVING
Calories: 270
Calories from Fat: 36

	AMOUNT PER SERVING	% DAILY VALUE
Total Fat:	4 g	6%
Saturated Fat:	0 g	0%
Trans Fat:	0 g	
Cholesterol:	0 mg	0%
Sodium:	470 mg	20%
Total Carbohydrate:	51 g	17%
Dietary Fiber:	13 g	52%
Sugars:	15 g	
Protein:	14 g	28%

EXCELLENT SOURCE OF: vitamin A, vitamin C, vitamin K, selenium, copper, iron
GOOD SOURCE OF: vitamin B_6, thiamin, manganese, potassium, phosphorus, folate, riboflavin, pantothenic acid, calcium

Moroccan Vegetable Stew

This autumn vegetable stew shines with the glowing hues and fragrant aromas of a Moroccan bazaar. It's full of powerful cell-protecting antioxidants and health-promoting ingredients such as inflammation-fighting turmeric, heart-healthy squash, and protein-packed chickpeas. Golden raisins add a touch of natural sweetness. Accompany the stew with high-protein quinoa. If you can find it, black quinoa makes an especially dramatic backdrop for these vivid colors, but any type of quinoa will do.

Serves: 6

Serving Size: 1½ cups stew, ¼ cup cooked quinoa
Prep Time: 20 minutes
Cook Time: 50 minutes
Ready Time: 1 hour 10 minutes

2 cups diced onion
2 teaspoons minced garlic
1½ teaspoons finely chopped ginger
2 teaspoons ground coriander, divided
1 cinnamon stick, about 3 inches long
½ teaspoon turmeric
¼ teaspoon fine sea salt
3½ cups low-sodium vegetable broth
3 cups butternut squash, peeled and cubed (12 ounces)
1 can (14.5 ounces) no-salt-added diced fire-roasted tomatoes
8 ounces green beans, cut into 1-inch lengths
1½ cups cooked or 1 can (15 ounces) chickpeas, no salt added, rinsed and drained
½ cup firmly packed golden raisins
Zest of 1 lemon
½ cup coarsely chopped cilantro
1½ cups warm cooked quinoa

1. In a large saucepan over medium heat, combine onions, garlic, ginger, 1½ teaspoons coriander, cinnamon stick, turmeric, and

salt with ½ cup vegetable broth. Sauté, stirring frequently, until onions are softened and translucent, 7–10 minutes.

2. Add remaining 3 cups vegetable broth, squash, and tomatoes. Raise heat to high and bring to a boil. Reduce heat to medium and simmer for about 30 minutes, until squash is just barely cooked through.

3. Add green beans, chickpeas, raisins, and lemon zest. Cook for 7–10 minutes, until green beans are tender. Stir in remaining ½ teaspoon coriander.

4. Just before serving, stir in cilantro. Serve warm, over quinoa.

Nutrition Facts

Serving Size: 1½ cups stew, ¼ cup cooked quinoa
Servings: 6

AMOUNT PER SERVING
Calories: 259
Calories from Fat: 18

	AMOUNT PER SERVING	% DAILY VALUE
Total Fat:	2 g	3%
Saturated Fat:	0 g	0%
Trans Fat:	0 g	
Cholesterol:	0 mg	0%
Sodium:	344 mg	14%
Total Carbohydrate:	51 g	17%
Dietary Fiber:	8 g	32%
Sugars:	18 g	
Protein:	9 g	18%

EXCELLENT SOURCE OF: fiber, vitamin A, vitamin C, iron, phosphorus, magnesium, copper
GOOD SOURCE OF: riboflavin, folate, potassium, calcium, zinc

Greek Tabbouleh Pita Pocket

Roasted eggplant puree and quinoa-based tabbouleh salad are tucked together in a whole-grain pita pocket to make this satisfying meatless meal. Perfect for lunch or dinner, this combination of crunchy fresh vegetables and high-protein whole grains is rich in fiber, phytochemicals, and vitamin C. For additional plant protein, add a spoonful of Hummus (page 412) to each pita pocket.

Serves: 6

Serving Size: 1 pita pocket
Prep Time: 20 minutes
Cook Time: 40 minutes
Ready Time: 1 hour

2 medium eggplants, sliced into ½-inch-thick rounds
1 teaspoon minced garlic
¾ teaspoon ground cumin
¾ teaspoon fine sea salt, divided
⅛ teaspoon plus ½ teaspoon freshly ground pepper, divided
1 cup quinoa
2 cups cherry tomatoes, quartered
2 cucumbers, peeled, seeded, and finely chopped (2 cups)
½ cup thinly sliced scallions
½ cup coarsely chopped mint
3 tablespoons fresh lemon juice
3 whole-grain pita breads, 7-inch diameter

1. Preheat oven to 350°F. Line two baking sheets with parchment paper.
2. To roast the eggplant, arrange eggplant slices on prepared baking sheets. Bake until soft, 20–25 minutes.
3. Transfer eggplant slices to a food processor fitted with a metal blade. Add garlic, cumin, ¼ teaspoon salt, and ⅛ teaspoon pepper. Process until chunky-smooth, stopping to scrape down bowl with a rubber spatula as needed. Set aside.
4. Prepare quinoa according to package directions. Once cooked, transfer quinoa to a medium bowl to cool. (Spread quinoa up the sides of the bowl; this will speed the cooling process and keep it from getting too moist.)

5. When quinoa has cooled to room temperature, add tomatoes, cucumber, scallions, mint, lemon juice, remaining ½ teaspoon salt, and ½ teaspoon pepper. Toss to combine. Taste for seasoning and add more lemon juice, salt, and/or pepper as needed.
6. To prepare the pita pockets, cut pita breads in half to create two pockets. Wrap pockets in foil. Place in a 350°F oven for 15 minutes, until soft and warmed through.
7. Remove pita pockets from foil. Spread ⅓ cup eggplant mixture inside each pita pocket. Spoon in 1 cup tabbouleh.

Chef's Notes

Pita breads come in various sizes. For this recipe, we suggest looking for pita breads about 7 inches in diameter. If you can only find smaller pita breads, you may want to serve two pita pockets instead of one. It's helpful to have an extra pita bread or two on hand when making this recipe, as sometimes it's tricky to open the "pockets" without tearing the breads. If you have leftover pita scraps, make pita chips. Preheat oven to 350°F. Cut pita scraps into triangles, arrange on a baking sheet, and bake until crisp, about 8 minutes. If you have any leftover eggplant puree, serve it alongside the pita chips.

Nutrition Facts

Serving Size: 1 pita pocket
Servings: 6

AMOUNT PER SERVING
Calories: 257
Calories from Fat: 27

	AMOUNT PER SERVING	% DAILY VALUE
Total Fat:	3 g	5%
Saturated Fat:	0 g	0%
Trans Fat:	0 g	
Cholesterol:	0 mg	0%
Sodium:	468 mg	20%
Total Carbohydrate:	50 g	17%
Dietary Fiber:	10 g	40%
Sugars:	7 g	
Protein:	11 g	22%

EXCELLENT SOURCE OF: fiber, vitamin A, vitamin C, folate, potassium, phosphorus, magnesium, copper
GOOD SOURCE OF: vitamins B_1, B_2, B_3, B_6, iron, zinc

Swiss Chard and Sweet Potato Burrito

Got a burrito craving? Satisfy it with this hearty, colorful recipe full of high-fiber, nutrient-rich greens, beans, red bell peppers, and sweet potatoes. This tasty mixture also works well as a filling for soft tacos. If you'd like a spicier kick, add some chipotles in adobo sauce, or a few dashes of your favorite hot sauce.

Serves: 4
    Serving Size: 1 burrito
    Prep Time: 20 minutes
    Cook Time: 30 minutes
    Ready Time: 50 minutes

4 whole-grain tortillas, 10-inch diameter
1 sweet potato, peeled and chopped into ½-inch pieces (2 cups)
1 cup chopped red onion
1 cup chopped red bell pepper
1¼ cups low-sodium vegetable broth, plus more if needed
1½ teaspoons ground cumin, divided
1½ teaspoons ground coriander, divided
1 teaspoon chili powder, divided
⅛ teaspoon fine sea salt
freshly ground pepper
3 cups roughly chopped Swiss chard
1 can (15 ounces) no-salt-added white beans, rinsed and drained
    (1½ cups)
½ cup chopped cilantro
1 tablespoon fresh lime juice

1. Preheat oven to 400°F. Wrap tortillas in foil and set aside.
2. In a medium, 12-inch sauté pan over medium heat, combine sweet potato, red onions, red peppers, vegetable broth, ¾ teaspoon cumin, ¾ teaspoon coriander, ½ teaspoon chili powder, salt, and pepper. Cook over medium heat, stirring frequently, until sweet potatoes are cooked through, onions are soft, and liquid has evaporated, 12–15 minutes. If liquid evaporates be-

fore sweet potatoes are soft, add additional vegetable broth as needed.

3. Stir in the Swiss chard, adding more broth if mixture seems dry. Cook until chard has wilted and broth has evaporated, about 1 minute. Remove from heat.

4. Fold in beans, cilantro, and lime juice. Add remaining ¾ teaspoon cumin, ¾ teaspoon coriander, and ½ teaspoon chili powder. Mix well and taste for seasoning, adding more salt or pepper as needed.

5. Place foil-wrapped tortillas in the preheated oven and heat until tortillas are flexible and warmed through, 5–7 minutes. Reheat vegetable mixture if needed while tortillas are warming.

6. Unwrap tortillas. On a dry work surface, lay out a tortilla and fill the bottom third of the tortilla with approximately 1 cup vegetable mixture. Fold outside edges inward and roll up from the bottom, away from you, to form a tight cylinder. Repeat with remaining tortillas and vegetables.

7. Place burritos seam side down. Cut each burrito in half and serve.

Chef's Notes

There are two other ways to warm tortillas: over a gas flame or in a non-stick skillet. To use a gas flame, turn a stovetop burner to high and place tortilla directly over the flame. Let tortilla cook for 2–3 seconds, then turn, using tongs. Repeat, turning the tortilla every 2–3 seconds, until warmed through and browned along the edges. To use a skillet, place one tortilla at a time in a large nonstick skillet over medium-high heat. Heat until warmed through on both sides, 20–30 seconds per side, turning with tongs as needed.

Nutrition Facts

Serving Size: 1 burrito
Servings: 4

AMOUNT PER SERVING
Calories: 278
Calories from Fat: 36

	AMOUNT PER SERVING	% DAILY VALUE
Total Fat:	4 g	6%
Saturated Fat:	0 g	0%
Trans Fat:	0 g	
Cholesterol:	0 mg	0%
Sodium:	678 mg	28%
Total Carbohydrate:	58 g	19%
Dietary Fiber:	22 g	88%
Sugars:	8 g	
Protein:	15 g	30%

EXCELLENT SOURCE OF: fiber, vitamin A, vitamin B_1, vitamin C, vitamin K, iron, magnesium, manganese
GOOD SOURCE OF: vitamins B_2, B_6, calcium, molybdenum, phosphorus, potassium, zinc

Hawaiian-Style Chili

Move over, Texas and Cincinnati. The Hawaiian take on America's favorite stew brings pineapple and Maui onion into the mix for an unforgettable sweet counterpoint to the chili's heat. Already packed with lots of fiber from the pineapple and plant protein from the kidney beans, island-style chili gets an additional healthy twist in the Ornish test kitchen, when we replace the greasy ground beef and bacon with heart-protective veggie crumbles. With so many delicious flavors mingling in one bowl, you'll never miss the meat! Don't just take our word for it. Invite some carnivorous friends over to share and see if they detect the swap.

Serves: 6
> Serving Size: 1¼ cups chili over ⅔ cup rice
> Prep Time: 30 minutes
> Cook Time: 15 minutes
> Ready Time: 45 minutes

4 cups brown rice
2 cups roughly chopped sweet Maui or Vidalia onion
1½ cups chopped red bell pepper
1½ tablespoons chili powder, divided
1 can (14.5 ounces) no-salt-added diced fire-roasted tomatoes
2½ cups veggie crumbles or cubed tempeh
1 can (15 ounces) no-salt-added kidney beans (1½ cups)
1 can (15 ounces) low-sodium tomato sauce
2 cups finely chopped pineapple
¾ teaspoon dried oregano
¼ teaspoon fine sea salt
Hot sauce or crushed red pepper flakes, for garnish (optional)
⅓ cup chopped cilantro and/or scallions (optional)

1. Prepare brown rice according to package directions. Set aside 4 cups cooked rice for this recipe, and save the rest for another use. (One and a half cups uncooked rice will yield about 4 cups cooked.)

2. In a large heavy-bottomed sauté pan, combine onions, bell peppers, ½ tablespoon chili powder, and ½ cup water. Place over high heat and bring mixture to a boil. Reduce heat to a simmer and cook until onions are tender and liquid has evaporated, 8–10 minutes.

3. Add tomatoes with juice, veggie crumbles or tempeh, kidney beans with their liquid (or an additional ½ cup water if using home-cooked beans), tomato sauce, chopped pineapple, remaining 1 tablespoon chili powder, oregano, and salt. Bring to a boil, then reduce heat to medium-low and simmer, uncovered, until flavors meld, about 5 minutes. Remove from heat and fold in ¼ cup cilantro and/or scallions just before serving, reserving the rest for garnish.

4. Serve chili warm over cooked rice with a dash of hot sauce or a pinch of red pepper flakes (if using) and 2 teaspoons cilantro and/or scallions per serving if desired.

Chef's Notes

Veggie crumbles, also known as veggie ground, are the vegetarian cook's secret weapon for replicating meaty dishes in a healthier way. We use Yves Veggie Cuisine Meatless Ground in the test kitchen, but lots of brands are available, so experiment and find your favorite. Tempeh is a great whole-food swap for veggie ground crumbles. Tempeh is a fermented form of soy with a similar meaty texture, packed with health-promoting prebiotic and probiotic compounds.

For the tastiest chili bowl, make sure your dried spices are up to date, ideally not more than 6 months old. If you can't recall how long your chili powder or dried oregano has been hanging around in your cupboard, pick up a fresh bottle. You'll be surprised at the difference it makes!

This chili does great when reheated, so it's perfect for do-ahead entertaining. You can even freeze it.

Nutrition Facts

Serving Size: 1¼ cups chili over ⅔ cup rice
Servings: 6

AMOUNT PER SERVING
Calories: 270
Calories from Fat: 18

	AMOUNT PER SERVING	% DAILY VALUE
Total Fat:	2 g	3%
Saturated Fat:	0 g	0%
Trans Fat:	0 g	
Cholesterol:	0 mg	0%
Sodium:	410 mg	17%
Total Carbohydrate:	50 g	17%
Dietary Fiber:	11 g	44%
Sugars:	15 g	
Protein:	19 g	38%

EXCELLENT SOURCE OF: fiber, vitamin A, thiamin, vitamin C, iron

GOOD SOURCE OF: vitamin B$_{12}$, manganese, vitamin K, calcium, magnesium, phosphorus, potassium

Veggie Lentil Loaf

Deliciously rich in fiber, thanks to a blend of brown rice, lentils, and vegetables, this easy meatless dish is a versatile comfort-food staple. The Smoky Chipotle Sauce (page 406) gives it a delectable smoky-sweet glaze on top.

Serves: 6
   Serving Size: 1½-inch slice
   Prep Time: 1 hour
   Cook Time: 1 hour
   Ready Time: 2 hours

Smoky Chipotle Sauce (page 406)
1 cup uncooked short-grain brown rice
1 cup uncooked green lentils
8 ounces frozen spinach, thawed
1½ cups diced onion
1½ cups grated carrot
1 tablespoon minced garlic
2 tablespoons Bragg Liquid Aminos, divided
1 tablespoon fresh thyme or 1½ teaspoons dried thyme, divided
1 teaspoon dried oregano
½ teaspoon freshly ground pepper, divided

1. Prepare chipotle sauce and refrigerate until ready to use.
2. Preheat oven to 375°F. Prepare rice and lentils according to package instructions. (The rice and lentils can be prepared up to 2 days ahead of time and refrigerated until needed.)
3. Place thawed spinach in a colander in the sink or over a deep bowl. Using your hands, squeeze or press spinach vigorously to remove excess liquid. Continue to squeeze and press spinach until it is almost dry; excess liquid left in the spinach will make a soggy loaf. Once drained, you should have about ¾ cup spinach. Set aside.
4. In a large sauté pan over medium-low heat, sauté the onions, carrots, garlic, 1 tablespoon liquid aminos, 1½ teaspoons of the fresh thyme, oregano, ¼ teaspoon pepper, and ½ cup water. Stirring frequently, sauté until onions are translucent, 7–10 minutes.

5. In a large bowl, combine the cooked rice and the lentils with the onion mixture. Add the remaining 1 tablespoon liquid aminos, 1¼ teaspoons fresh thyme, and ¼ teaspoon pepper. Mix well.
6. Spoon half of the rice mixture (about 3½ cups) into a food processor. Pulse until a thick paste forms, scraping down the bowl with a spatula. The mixture will be fairly dry. Mix the paste into the remaining lentil mixture. Add the spinach and stir well to combine.
7. Line a baking sheet with parchment paper. Form lentil mixture into a tightly packed loaf 2 inches high and 9 inches long. Cut into six 1½-inch slices, leaving about an inch of space between portions so heat and air can circulate. Bake for about 30 minutes, or until slices are lightly brown and crisp on all sides. Remove from oven and spread a heaping tablespoon of chipotle sauce evenly on top of each slice. Let cook for an additional 10 minutes. Remove from oven. Let rest 10 minutes before serving. Serve with chipotle sauce on the side, if desired.

Nutrition Facts

Serving Size: one 1½-inch slice
Servings: 6

AMOUNT PER SERVING
Calories: 290
Calories from Fat: 9

	AMOUNT PER SERVING	% DAILY VALUE
Total Fat:	1 g	2%
Saturated Fat:	0 g	0%
Trans Fat:	0 g	
Cholesterol:	0 mg	0%
Sodium:	390 mg	16%
Total Carbohydrate:	55 g	18%
Dietary Fiber:	8 g	32%
Sugars:	5 g	
Protein:	14 g	28%

EXCELLENT SOURCE OF: fiber, vitamin A, vitamin K, iron, folate,
GOOD SOURCE OF: vitamin C, thiamin, potassium, calcium, magnesium, phosphorus, manganese

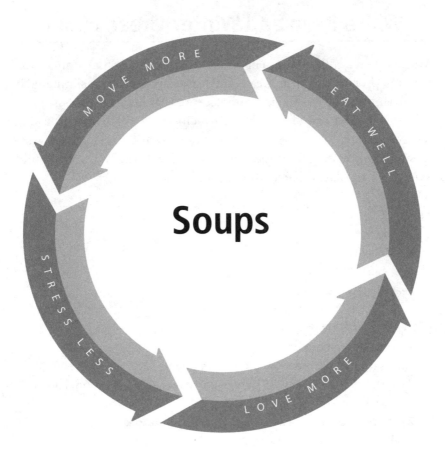

MOVE MORE

EAT WELL

LOVE MORE

STRESS LESS

Soups

White Bean and Winter Greens Soup

Warm up on a chilly autumn or winter night with this nourishing soup. Creamy, protein-rich white beans and leafy dark greens are simmered in a nutrient-packed vegetable broth accented with garlic, onions, miso, and thyme. You can also make this recipe with rutabagas instead of sweet potatoes. Rutabagas look like jumbo-sized turnips, with a waxy, creamy skin shading to purple and pale yellow flesh. They have a mild, sweetly earthy flavor that lends itself well to soups.

Serves: 6
Serving Size: 1 cup
Prep Time: 10 minutes
Cook Time: 30 minutes
Ready Time: 40 minutes

1½ cups coarsely chopped onion
2 teaspoons minced garlic
4 cups low-sodium vegetable broth, divided
3 cups cooked or 2 cans (15 ounces each) no-salt-added cannellini or navy beans, rinsed and drained
2 cups peeled and coarsely chopped sweet potatoes
3 tablespoons sweet white miso
2 teaspoons chopped fresh thyme, divided
¼ teaspoon fine sea salt
¼ teaspoon freshly ground pepper
2 cups destemmed chopped kale or chard (1.5 ounces)
Crushed red pepper flakes (optional)

1. In a medium saucepan over medium heat, combine onions, garlic, and ½ cup broth. Cook, stirring frequently, until onions are softened and transparent, about 10 minutes.
2. Add the remaining 3½ cups broth, beans, sweet potatoes, miso, 1½ teaspoons of the thyme, salt, and pepper. Bring to a simmer and cook until sweet potatoes are tender and flavors have melded, 10–15 minutes.
3. Add kale and remaining ½ teaspoon thyme. Simmer until kale is

tender, 3–4 minutes. Taste for seasoning, adding more miso or pepper as needed. Sprinkle with red pepper flakes before serving, if desired.

Chef's Notes

This soup is best made 1–2 days in advance, allowing flavors to mingle and develop together; cover and refrigerate until needed.

Nutrition Facts

Serving Size: 1 cup
Servings: 6

AMOUNT PER SERVING
Calories: 189
Calories from Fat: 9

	AMOUNT PER SERVING	% DAILY VALUE
Total Fat:	1 g	2%
Saturated Fat:	0 g	0%
Trans Fat:	0 g	
Cholesterol:	0 mg	0%
Sodium:	508 mg	21%
Total Carbohydrate:	36 g	12%
Dietary Fiber:	9 g	36%
Sugars:	7 g	
Protein:	9 g	18%

EXCELLENT SOURCE OF: fiber, vitamin A, thiamin, vitamin C, magnesium
GOOD SOURCE OF: riboflavin, potassium, iron, phosphorus, zinc, copper

---

Thai Coconut Soup

This light, sophisticated soup is similar to a Thai tom yum goong—tart and tangy with fresh lime juice, spicy with serrano pepper, and full of heart-healthy winter squash, zucchini, and mushrooms. Kabocha squash is a drum-shaped winter squash, green or orange-skinned, with a dense orange flesh. Look for it in well-stocked produce stores, farmers' markets, or online; butternut squash makes a good substitute.

Serves: 4

Serving Size: 2¼ cups
Prep Time: 10 minutes
Cook Time: 15 minutes
Ready Time: 25 minutes

4 ounces soba (Japanese buckwheat noodles)
6 cups pure coconut water
½ cup thinly sliced shallots
2 kaffir lime leaves or ¾ teaspoon lime zest
¼ cup fresh lime juice
1 tablespoon plus 1 teaspoon Bragg Liquid Aminos or reduced-sodium tamari
2 tablespoons minced lemongrass
1 tablespoon finely chopped ginger
1 teaspoon finely chopped, seeded red serrano pepper, plus more if desired
1 teaspoon minced garlic, optional
4 cups unpeeled kabocha or peeled butternut squash, seeded and chopped (1¼ pounds)
1 cup thinly sliced shiitake or white button mushroom caps
1 small zucchini, halved and sliced into half-moons (1 cup)
¼ cup thinly sliced fresh basil, for garnish

1. Cook soba noodles according to package directions. Drain and set aside.
2. In a medium heavy-bottomed pot over medium heat, combine coconut water, shallots, kaffir lime leaves or lime zest, lime juice,

liquid aminos or tamari, lemongrass, ginger, 1 teaspoon minced serrano pepper, and garlic, if using. Bring to a gentle simmer.

3. Add the squash and simmer for 6–8 minutes, until tender. Add mushrooms and zucchini. Simmer for another 5 minutes, until vegetables are tender.

4. Taste for seasoning, adding additional lime juice or minced serrano pepper if desired. Add cooked soba noodles. Divide soup among 4 bowls and garnish with basil.

Chef's Notes

If you are new to kabocha squash, also known as Japanese pumpkin, it is versatile and has a wonderful sweet chestnut-like taste. One of the trickiest parts about this large squash is cutting it. Be careful! Use a large, heavy knife and, using a steady hand with significant pressure, cut unpeeled squash in half. Remove seeds, then quarter and chop into smaller pieces. Butternut squash makes a fine substitute if you can't locate kabocha squash.

Lemongrass is a stalky plant with a lemony essence. Look for firm stalks; the lower stalk should be pale yellow, almost white, while upper stalks are green. To prepare, remove the root end as well as the tough outer leaves, leaving just the whiter and more tender part. Bruise the lower ends by bending several times, or pounding with a mallet (or rolling pin, or small saucepan), and finely chop.

Shortcut: If you are not in the mood to battle lemongrass, or you can't find it, look for prepared lemongrass paste in a tube in the produce section at most grocery stores.

Nutrition Facts

Serving Size: 2¼ cups
Servings: 4

AMOUNT PER SERVING
Calories: 270
Calories from Fat: 9

	AMOUNT PER SERVING	% DAILY VALUE
Total Fat:	1 g	1%
Saturated Fat:	0 g	0%
Trans Fat:	0 g	
Cholesterol:	0 mg	0%
Sodium:	510 mg	22%
Total Carbohydrate:	54 g	18%
Dietary Fiber:	3g	16%
Sugars:	25 g	
Protein:	9 g	19%

EXCELLENT SOURCE OF: vitamin A, vitamin C
GOOD SOURCE OF: fiber, vitamin B$_6$, calcium

Indian Lentil Soup

Tomatoes and red lentils give this soup a glowing sunset hue. This recipe is inspired by dhal (also spelled dal or daal), a staple of Indian cuisine. A fragrant, gently spiced puree made from a variety of lentils and dried peas, dhal is typically served alongside rice and vegetables to make a simple yet filling meal. If you can't find red lentils, substitute orange or yellow lentils.

Serves: 5
    Serving Size: 1 cup
    Prep Time: 15 minutes
    Cook Time: 45 minutes
    Ready Time: 1 hour

1 teaspoon whole cumin seeds
2 cups coarsely chopped onion
1¼ cups red lentils
1 cup seeded and diced Roma (plum) tomatoes
1 tablespoon finely chopped ginger
2 teaspoons minced garlic
¼ teaspoon fine sea salt
¾ teaspoon turmeric
¾ teaspoon ground coriander
⅛ teaspoon cayenne
¼ cup plus 1 tablespoon chopped cilantro, divided

1. In a medium heavy-bottomed saucepan over medium heat, toast the cumin seeds, shaking the pan frequently, until they smell lightly toasted and fragrant, 2–3 minutes.
2. Add 4 cups water, onions, lentils, tomatoes, ginger, garlic, salt, turmeric, coriander, and cayenne. Stir over high heat until mixture is combined. Bring to a boil.
3. Reduce heat to low, partially cover, and simmer, stirring frequently, until lentils are soft, about 35 minutes.
4. Just before serving, stir in ¼ cup cilantro. Season to taste with more cayenne and salt, if needed. Garnish with remaining cilantro.

Nutrition Facts

Serving Size: 1 cup
Servings: 5

AMOUNT PER SERVING
Calories: 221
Calories from Fat: 18

	AMOUNT PER SERVING	% DAILY VALUE
Total Fat:	2 g	3%
Saturated Fat:	0 g	0%
Trans Fat:	0 g	
Cholesterol:	0 mg	0%
Sodium:	139 mg	6%
Total Carbohydrate:	38 g	13%
Dietary Fiber:	9 g	36%
Sugars:	5 g	
Protein:	14 g	28%

EXCELLENT SOURCE OF: fiber, vitamin C, iron

GOOD SOURCE OF: vitamin B$_1$, potassium

Miso Soup with Soba

This soothing, nourishing soup, full of nutrient-rich sea vegetables, tofu cubes, and whole-grain buckwheat noodles, is a perfect pick-me-up at any time of day. In fact, since it's high in protein and easily digestible, miso soup is a popular breakfast item in Japan. Look for dried wakame (pronounced *wah-KA-may*) or arame (*AH-rah-may*)—two types of seaweed prized for their high fiber, nutrient, and mineral content, as well as their sweet, mild flavor—in specialty grocery or natural foods stores. Most sea vegetables are soaked before using.

Serves: 8
  Serving Size: 1 cup
  Prep Time: 10 minutes
  Cook Time: 15 minutes
  Ready Time: 25 minutes

  4 pieces (1 × 6 inches) dry wakame or arame sea vegetable (½ ounce)
  ½ cup white (shiro) miso paste
  2 tablespoons finely chopped ginger
  2 teaspoons reduced-sodium tamari
  8 ounces shiitake mushrooms, stems removed, thinly sliced
  2 ounces soba (Japanese buckwheat noodles)
  1 cup cubed soft to medium-firm tofu
  ⅓ cup thinly sliced scallions

1. Place wakame or arame in a medium bowl. Fill with warm water to cover by 1 inch. Let soak for 15 minutes. Drain. Chop roughly and set aside.
2. In a small bowl, stir miso with ½ cup water to loosen.
3. In a medium saucepan over medium heat, combine miso mixture, 6 cups water, ginger, tamari, and shiitakes. Bring to a gentle simmer. Reduce heat if needed and simmer for 10 minutes.
4. Add soba noodles and cook according to package directions.
5. When soba noodles are done, add tofu, wakame or arame, and scallions. Taste for seasoning and add more tamari if needed. Serve hot.

Chef's Notes

Miso is a thick, tangy paste typically made from fermented soybeans. White miso, also called shiro or sweet miso, is fermented for a shorter time than yellow or red miso. It is mild in flavor and less salty. For a soy alternative, look for miso made from chickpeas at some natural foods stores.

Nutrition Facts

Serving Size: 1 cup
Servings: 8

AMOUNT PER SERVING
Calories: 88
Calories from Fat: 9

	AMOUNT PER SERVING	% DAILY VALUE
Total Fat:	1 g	2%
Saturated Fat:	0 g	0%
Trans Fat:	0 g	
Cholesterol:	0 mg	0%
Sodium:	767 mg	32%
Total Carbohydrate:	15 g	5%
Dietary Fiber:	4 g	16%
Sugars:	4 g	
Protein:	7 g	14%

EXCELLENT SOURCE OF: iodine

GOOD SOURCE OF: fiber, iron

Quick Lentil Chili

Red lentils make a fast and easy chili, perfect for warming up after a day of frosty winter sports. This simple one-pot meal is excellent for holiday crowds or for a no-fuss dinner with family and friends. (It's even better the next day.) Butternut squash is easy to find, but we also like green- or orange-skinned kabocha squash, which has a rich, chestnutty flavor that makes it worth searching out. A dollop of Smoky Chipotle Sauce (page 406) makes a wonderful topping.

Serves: 6
Serving Size: 1 cup
Prep Time: 15 minutes
Cook Time: 55 minutes
Ready Time: 1 hour 10 minutes

1½ cups coarsely chopped onion
1½ cups diced red bell pepper
4 cups low-sodium vegetable broth, divided
1 tablespoon minced jalapeño
1 tablespoon minced garlic
¼ teaspoon fine sea salt
¼ teaspoon freshly ground black pepper
4 cups peeled and cubed butternut squash (1¼ pounds)
1 cup red lentils
1 tablespoon fresh lime juice, plus more to taste
2 teaspoons chili powder
2 teaspoons ground cumin
1 teaspoon smoked paprika
1 teaspoon dried oregano
½ cup chopped cilantro, divided (optional)
6 small corn or whole-wheat tortillas (optional)

1. In a large heavy-bottomed pot over medium heat, combine onions, red pepper, ½ cup broth, jalapeño, garlic, salt, and black pepper. Cook, stirring frequently, until liquid is evaporated and onions are translucent, about 10 minutes.

2. Add remaining 3½ cups broth, squash, lentils, lime juice, chili powder, cumin, smoked paprika, and oregano. Bring to a boil.
3. Reduce heat, cover, and simmer for 15 minutes, stirring occasionally. Remove lid and cook, stirring frequently, for an additional 15–20 minutes, until lentils are thoroughly cooked and squash is tender but still holds its shape. If mixture seems too thick, add a little water as needed. Chili is done when most of the liquid has been absorbed.
4. Stir in ¼ cup cilantro, if using. Taste for seasoning and add more lime juice and/or spices as needed.
5. Divide into 6 bowls. Garnish each bowl with a sprinkle of the remaining cilantro, if desired. Serve each bowl with a warmed corn or whole-wheat tortilla, if desired.

Nutrition Facts

Serving Size: 1 cup
Servings: 6

AMOUNT PER SERVING
Calories: 196
Calories from Fat: 9

	AMOUNT PER SERVING	% DAILY VALUE
Total Fat:	1 g	2%
Saturated Fat:	0 g	0%
Trans Fat:	0 g	
Cholesterol:	0 mg	0%
Sodium:	235 mg	10%
Total Carbohydrate:	35 g	12%
Dietary Fiber:	8 g	32%
Sugars:	7 g	
Protein:	11 g	22%

EXCELLENT SOURCE OF: fiber, vitamin A, vitamin C
GOOD SOURCE OF: potassium, iron

Butternut Squash Soup with Corn and Green Chiles

This deep orange, nutrient-rich soup is at its best in the autumn, when you can find freshly harvested butternut and other similar hard-skinned winter squashes at local farmers' markets. If your squash isn't sweet enough, add a dash of maple syrup to balance out the lime juice and spices. Like a little heat? Serve with your favorite hot sauce.

Serves: 8
Serving Size: 1 cup
Prep Time: 15 minutes
Cook Time: 15 minutes
Ready Time: 30 minutes

5 cups peeled, cubed butternut squash (1½ pounds)
2 cups chopped onion
1½ teaspoons ground cumin, divided
1 teaspoon ground coriander, divided
1 teaspoon chili powder, divided
½ teaspoon fine sea salt, divided
2 cups fresh or frozen corn kernels
1 can (7 ounces) diced green chiles, drained
1 cup unsweetened soy milk
¼ cup chopped cilantro, plus cilantro sprigs for garnish
1 tablespoon fresh lime juice

1. In a large heavy-bottomed pot, combine the butternut squash, onions, ¾ teaspoon cumin, ½ teaspoon coriander, ½ teaspoon chili powder, ¼ teaspoon salt, and 4 cups water. Bring to a boil over high heat.
2. Reduce heat to medium. Simmer until squash is tender, about 10 minutes. Add corn, green chiles, soy milk, the remaining ¾ teaspoon cumin, ½ teaspoon coriander, ½ teaspoon chili powder, and ½ teaspoon salt. Simmer until corn has cooked and flavors have melded, about 5 minutes.

3. Remove from heat and let cool slightly. Measure out half the soup (about 4 cups) and place in a blender. Blend until smooth.
4. Stir the pureed mixture back into the remaining soup in the pot. Add cilantro and lime juice and stir to combine. Season to taste with more salt and lime juice, if desired. Reheat if necessary. Serve hot, garnished with cilantro sprigs.

Nutrition Facts

Serving Size: 1 cup
Servings: 8

AMOUNT PER SERVING
Calories: 107
Calories from Fat: 9

	AMOUNT PER SERVING	% DAILY VALUE
Total Fat:	1 g	2%
Saturated Fat:	0 g	0%
Trans Fat:	0 g	
Cholesterol:	0 mg	0%
Sodium:	236 mg	10%
Total Carbohydrate:	25 g	8%
Dietary Fiber:	4 g	16%
Sugars:	5 g	
Protein:	3 g	6%

EXCELLENT SOURCE OF: vitamin A, vitamin C
GOOD SOURCE OF: fiber, folate, calcium, magnesium, manganese, phosphorus, potassium

Curried Yellow Split Pea Soup

This filling, nourishing soup is high in both protein and fiber, thanks to a blend of dried yellow split peas and lots of kale and vegetables. Like many bean soups, this keeps well in the refrigerator and gets even tastier a day or two after it's made.

Serves: 9

> Serving Size: 1 cup
> Prep Time: 15 minutes
> Cook Time: 60–75 minutes
> Ready Time: 1 hour 15 minutes–1 hour 30 minutes

1½ tablespoons curry powder
1½ tablespoons ground coriander
1½ tablespoons cumin seeds
¾ teaspoon fine sea salt
½ teaspoon freshly ground pepper
1½ tablespoons minced garlic
1½ cups roughly chopped carrot
2 cups roughly chopped onion
¾ cup dried yellow split peas
1 can (14.5 ounces) no-salt-added diced fire-roasted tomatoes
3 cups finely chopped destemmed kale
1½ tablespoons pure maple syrup
1½ tablespoons lemon juice
Pinch cayenne or dash of hot sauce (optional)

1. In a small bowl, mix curry powder and ground coriander. Set aside.
2. In a large pot over medium-low heat, toast the cumin seeds until fragrant, 1½–2 minutes. To prevent burning, stir frequently or shake the pan to keep the seeds moving.
3. Add curry mixture. Stirring constantly, toast in the pan until aromatic, about 30 seconds. Remove from heat and immediately pour spices into a small, shallow bowl to cool. When spices are cool, add salt and pepper, stir to mix, and set aside.

4. In the same pan over high heat, combine garlic, carrots, onions, and ¾ cup water. Stir in one-third of the toasted spice mixture. Bring to a boil. Reduce heat to medium and simmer until onions are tender and translucent and liquid has evaporated, 8–10 minutes.
5. Add 6 cups water, split peas, and another one-third of the spice mixture. Simmer, stirring occasionally, until peas are soft, 45–60 minutes (see Chef's Notes).
6. Add tomatoes, kale, remaining spice mixture, maple syrup, and lemon juice and stir until incorporated. Raise heat to high and bring mixture back to a boil. Reduce heat to medium and simmer until kale is tender, about 5 minutes. Taste for seasoning, adding more salt, pepper, lemon juice and/or maple syrup as desired. Like a spicy soup? Add a pinch of cayenne or a dash of hot sauce.

Chef's Notes

The cooking time of split peas will vary depending on their age and dryness. Some will be tender in 45 minutes or less, and some may take over an hour. We typically cook them until they are soft and tender but still keep their shape. However, if you want a thicker, less brothy soup, you can keep cooking them until they break down more fully.

Nutrition Facts

Serving Size: 1 cup
Servings: 9

AMOUNT PER SERVING
Calories: 119
Calories from Fat: 9

	AMOUNT PER SERVING	% DAILY VALUE
Total Fat:	1 g	2%
Saturated Fat:	0 g	0%
Trans Fat:	0 g	
Cholesterol:	0 mg	0%
Sodium:	334 mg	14%
Total Carbohydrate:	22 g	7%
Dietary Fiber:	7 g	28%
Sugars:	7 g	
Protein:	5 g	10%

EXCELLENT SOURCE OF: fiber, vitamin A, vitamin C, vitamin K
GOOD SOURCE OF: manganese

Traditional Split Pea Soup

After a brisk hike on a winter day, nourish both body and spirit with this warm and savory vegetable soup. It keeps well and even tastes better a day or two after it's made. Sherry vinegar, which has a deep complexity with a hint of natural sweetness, really makes the flavors pop, so it's worth adding to your pantry. If you're used to the smokiness of ham in pea soup, try adding a small amount of natural liquid smoke flavor for a pleasant tinge of smokiness without the fat. If using dried herbs, crumble them between your fingertips to release their aromas before adding.

Serves: 6
Serving Size: 1¼ cups
Prep Time: 15 minutes
Cook Time: 45 minutes
Ready Time: 1 hour

1½ cups split peas, green or yellow
2 cups coarsely chopped red-skinned potatoes
2 cups coarsely chopped onion
1 cup coarsely chopped carrot
1 cup coarsely chopped celery
2 tablespoons minced garlic
1 tablespoon chopped fresh rosemary or 1 teaspoon dried
1 tablespoon chopped fresh thyme or 1 teaspoon dried
1 tablespoon sherry vinegar
½ teaspoon natural liquid smoke flavoring (optional)
1 teaspoon fine sea salt
¼ teaspoon freshly ground pepper

1. In a large heavy-bottomed pot over high heat, combine all ingredients. Add 7 cups water and bring to a boil.
2. Reduce heat to medium and simmer, stirring occasionally, until peas are very soft and vegetables are tender, 35–45 minutes. Taste for seasoning, adding additional vinegar, salt, and/or pepper as needed.

Nutrition Facts

Serving Size: 1¼ cups
Servings: 6

AMOUNT PER SERVING
Calories: 266
Calories from Fat: 9

	AMOUNT PER SERVING	% DAILY VALUE
Total Fat:	1 g	2%
Saturated Fat:	0 g	0%
Trans Fat:	0 g	
Cholesterol:	0 mg	0%
Sodium:	463 mg	19%
Total Carbohydrate:	48 g	16%
Dietary Fiber:	15 g	60%
Sugars:	8 g	
Protein:	14 g	28%

EXCELLENT SOURCE OF: fiber, vitamin A, vitamin C, folate, potassium, phosphorus, magnesium

GOOD SOURCE OF: vitamins B_2, B_3, B_6, zinc

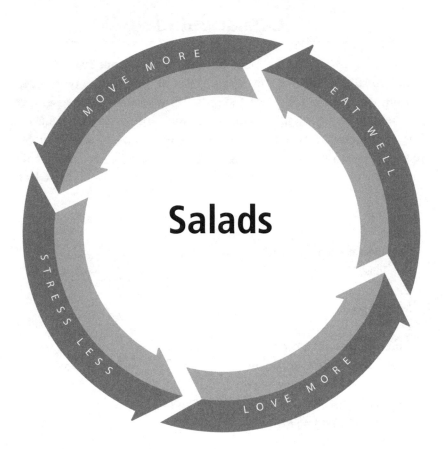

MOVE MORE

EAT WELL

LOVE MORE

STRESS LESS

Salads

Caesar Salad

The swagger of this healthy Caesar salad comes from its deliciously tangy dressing. Here, nutrient-rich silken tofu replaces the typical eggs and oil, while nutritional yeast stands in for Parmesan cheese. Garlic, lemon juice, horseradish, capers, and mustard punch up the flavors. This outstanding dressing also makes a delicious party dip or spread. Be creative with the greens: romaine lettuce is classic, but many chefs are now replacing it with nutrient-packed kale or other dark leafy greens.

Serves: 8
Serving Size: 1 cup
Prep Time: 15 minutes
Cook Time: 20 minutes
Ready Time: 35 minutes

6 ounce silken tofu, drained
2 tablespoons fresh lemon juice
1 tablespoon red wine vinegar
1 tablespoon capers, rinsed and drained (optional)
1½ teaspoon Worcestershire sauce
1 teaspoon minced garlic
2 tablespoons nutritional yeast
1 teaspoon dry mustard
½ teaspoon onion powder
¼ teaspoon fine sea salt
⅛ teaspoon freshly ground pepper
4 slices whole-grain bread or 1½ cups packaged fat-free croutons
8 ounces romaine, torn or roughly chopped
2 carrots, peeled and thinly sliced
½ cup thinly sliced radishes

1. To make the dressing, in a blender, combine tofu, 2 tablespoons water, lemon juice, red wine vinegar, capers if using, Worcestershire sauce, garlic, nutritional yeast, dry mustard, onion powder, salt, and pepper. Blend on high speed for about 10 seconds, until

mixture is smooth. (Dressing can be prepared several days in advance and refrigerated until needed.)

2. If making croutons, preheat oven to 250°F. Line a rimmed baking sheet with parchment paper. Trim crusts from bread slices. Cut bread into 1-inch cubes (or preferred crouton size). Spread on prepared baking sheet. Bake until crisp throughout, 15–20 minutes. Let cool.

3. In a large bowl, combine romaine lettuce, carrots, radishes, and croutons, if using. Add half of the dressing. Toss and taste for seasoning. Add additional dressing as needed. Serve immediately.

Chef's Notes

This rich-tasting, creamy Caesar dressing will keep in the refrigerator for at least a week. Besides tasting great on salads, it also makes a wonderful dip for vegetable crudités. Try making a veggie snack tray with carrot slices, red bell pepper wedges, and jicama sticks. Worcestershire sauce typically contains a small amount of anchovy. If you are exclusively plant-based, look for vegan Worcestershire sauce in natural foods stores.

For a kale Caesar, substitute kale for half or all of the romaine lettuce. Massage kale leaves well with dressing.

Nutrition Facts

Serving Size: 1 cup
Servings: 8

AMOUNT PER SERVING
Calories: 88
Calories from Fat: 18

	AMOUNT PER SERVING	% DAILY VALUE
Total Fat:	2 g	3%
Saturated Fat:	0 g	0%
Trans Fat:	0 g	
Cholesterol:	0 mg	0%
Sodium:	255 mg	11%
Total Carbohydrate:	14 g	5%
Dietary Fiber:	3 g	12%
Sugars:	6 g	
Protein:	6 g	12%

EXCELLENT SOURCE OF: vitamin A, vitamins B_1, B_2, B_3, B_6, vitamin C
GOOD SOURCE OF: fiber, vitamin B_{12}, folate, iron

Citrus Confetti Salad

This crunchy salad is bursting with brilliant colors and summery flavors. With a mix of sweet cherry tomatoes, crisp red bell peppers, sweet oranges, and crunchy jicama in a tangy orange-mustard dressing, it's abundant in health-promoting nutrients and cardioprotective antioxidants. If clementines or tangerines are not in season, feel free to substitute navel oranges, peeled and sliced into segments.

Serves: 4
Serving Size: 2 cups
Prep Time: 20 minutes
Cook Time: N/A
Ready Time: 20 minutes

3 tablespoons frozen orange juice concentrate, thawed
1 tablespoon fresh lime juice
1½ tablespoons finely chopped shallots
1½ teaspoons Dijon mustard
⅛ teaspoon fine sea salt
¼ teaspoon freshly ground black pepper
¼ teaspoon ground cumin
¼ cup thinly sliced red onion
4 ounces jicama, peeled and cut into matchsticks (1 cup)
1 cup clementine or tangerine segments, or one can (15 ounces) mandarin orange segments, drained
½ cup cherry tomatoes, halved or quartered
¼ cup finely diced red bell pepper
8 ounces romaine lettuce, torn into bite-sized pieces (2 small heads)
¼ cup coarsely chopped cilantro

1. To make dressing, in a medium bowl, whisk together orange juice concentrate, lime juice, shallots, mustard, salt, black pepper, and cumin. Set aside to let flavors blend.
2. Place onion slices in a small bowl and cover with cold water. Let stand for 10 minutes. (Soaking takes some of the "bite" out of raw onion.) Drain and pat dry.

3. In a large salad bowl, toss jicama, orange segments, cherry tomatoes, red onions, red bell peppers, romaine lettuce, and cilantro together.
4. Add three-quarters of the dressing. Toss gently until vegetables are lightly coated. Taste for seasoning. Add additional dressing as needed. Serve immediately.

Chef's Notes

Jicama (pronounced *HICK-ah-ma*) is the round, tuberous root of a Mexican vine. It has a papery, pale brown skin that is always removed before eating. Inside, the flesh is white, crisp, and juicy, with a mild, earthy flavor and slight sweetness. Typically eaten raw, it is high in fiber and contains both potassium and vitamin C. In Mexico, sticks of peeled jicama are sprinkled with lime juice and chili pepper and served as a popular snack.

Nutrition Facts

Serving Size: 2 cups
Servings: 4

AMOUNT PER SERVING
Calories: 86
Calories from Fat: 0

	AMOUNT PER SERVING	% DAILY VALUE
Total Fat:	0 g	0%
Saturated Fat:	0 g	0%
Trans Fat:	0 g	
Cholesterol:	0 mg	0%
Sodium:	212 mg	9%
Total Carbohydrate:	21 g	7%
Dietary Fiber:	4 g	16%
Sugars:	14 g	
Protein:	3 g	6%

EXCELLENT SOURCE OF: vitamin A, vitamin C
GOOD SOURCE OF: fiber

Wild Rice and Quinoa Waldorf Salad

Rich in fiber and packed with vitamins C and B, protective antioxidants, and health-promoting phytochemicals, this filling main-dish salad is inspired by the classic Waldorf salad. We've skipped the high-fat mayonnaise dressing for a tangy citrus vinaigrette and added a hearty blend of wild rice and protein-rich quinoa to a mixture of sweet apples, celery, and greens. Try garnishing with fresh pomegranate seeds when they're in season.

Serves: 6
Serving Size: 1 cup
Prep Time: 15 minutes
Cook Time: 45 minutes
Ready Time: 1 hour

½ cup wild rice
¾ teaspoon fine sea salt, divided
½ cup white quinoa
2 tablespoons apple cider vinegar
2 tablespoons fresh lemon juice
1½ teaspoons pure maple syrup
1 teaspoon whole-grain mustard
⅛ teaspoon freshly ground pepper
2 cups thinly sliced apple
⅔ cup diced celery
¼ cup dried currants
¼ cup thinly sliced scallions
2 cups baby spinach, baby kale, or baby arugula

1. In a small heavy-bottomed saucepan, cook wild rice according to package directions, adding ¼ teaspoon salt.
2. In a separate small heavy-bottomed saucepan, cook quinoa according to package directions, adding ¼ teaspoon salt.
3. In a small bowl, whisk together vinegar, lemon juice, maple syrup, mustard, the remaining ¼ teaspoon salt, and pepper. Set aside.
4. When wild rice and quinoa are cooked, combine the grains in a

large bowl and let cool to room temperature. (Spread the grains out along the sides of the bowl; they will cool faster when spread out this way, rather than heaped in a central pile.)

5. When grains are cool, add apples, celery, currants, scallions, and spinach, kale, or arugula. Add dressing and toss to coat.

Nutrition Facts

Serving Size: 1 cup
Servings: 6

AMOUNT PER SERVING
Calories: 150
Calories from Fat: 9

	AMOUNT PER SERVING	% DAILY VALUE
Total Fat:	1 g	2%
Saturated Fat:	0 g	0%
Trans Fat:	0 g	
Cholesterol:	0 mg	0%
Sodium:	320 mg	13%
Total Carbohydrate:	32 g	11%
Dietary Fiber:	3 g	12%
Sugars:	10 g	
Protein:	5 g	10%

GOOD SOURCE OF: fiber, folate, iron, phosphorus, magnesium

Kale and Brussels Sprout Salad

This power-packed salad is a beautiful and delicious mix of the top heart-healthy ingredients including kale, brussels sprouts, red cabbage, carrots, and edamame, all held together with a simple citrus zest. A bowl of this colorful salad is also abundant in fiber. It makes the perfect addition to any meal or is satisfying enough to enjoy on its own.

Serves: 4
  Serving Size: 1 cup
  Prep Time: 15 minutes
  Cook Time: N/A
  Ready Time: 15 minutes

  8 ounces brussels sprouts
  3 cups chopped destemmed curly kale
  3 cups shredded red cabbage
  1 cup julienned or shredded carrots
  1 teaspoon lemon zest
  1 tablespoon lemon juice
  ¼ teaspoon fine sea salt or to taste (optional)
  ¼ cup cooked edamame

1. Pull any yellow outer leaves off the brussels sprouts. Slice brussels sprouts thinly.
2. Mix all the ingredients except edamame in a large bowl mix; massage the salad well to infuse all the flavors.
3. Mix in the edamame when you are ready to serve.

Chef's Notes
  This salad holds well for a couple of days covered in refrigerator.

Nutrition Facts

Serving Size: 1 cup
Servings: 4

AMOUNT PER SERVING
Calories: 80
Calories from Fat: 9

	AMOUNT PER SERVING	% DAILY VALUE
Total Fat:	1 g	2%
Saturated Fat:	0 g	0%
Trans Fat:	0 g	
Cholesterol:	0 mg	0%
Sodium:	210 mg	9%
Total Carbohydrate:	15 g	5%
Dietary Fiber:	5 g	20%
Sugars:	6 g	
Protein:	5 g	10%

EXCELLENT SOURCE OF: vitamin A, folate, vitamin K,
vitamin C
GOOD SOURCE OF: fiber, iron

Mediterranean Salad with Pita Crisps

Tired of the same old green salads? Wake up your lunchtime with this delicious alternative. We've taken our inspiration from a popular eastern Mediterranean salad known as fattoush, which mixes raw vegetables like cucumbers, lettuce, and tomatoes with pieces of toasted pita bread. Two special ingredients, pomegranate molasses and sumac, jazz up the crunch with tantalizingly bright, tangy, fruity flavors. Little Gem, a miniature version of romaine lettuce, offers great sweetness and crunch; you can also use baby romaine or hearts of romaine.

Serves: 4
> Serving Size: 2 cups
> Prep Time: 15 minutes
> Cook Time: 15 minutes
> Ready Time: 30 minutes

1 whole-wheat pita bread, split horizontally

2 teaspoons ground sumac

2 tablespoons fresh lemon juice

2 tablespoons pomegranate molasses

⅛ teaspoon fine sea salt

⅛ teaspoon freshly ground pepper

¼ cup thinly sliced red onion

½ teaspoon minced garlic

5 cups roughly chopped or torn baby romaine, hearts of romaine, or Little Gem lettuce

2 cups cherry tomatoes, halved

1 English or hothouse cucumber, peeled, seeded, and diced (1½ cups)

1 cup flat-leaf parsley leaves

½ cup fresh mint leaves

1. Preheat oven to 325°F. Line a small baking pan with parchment paper or use a nonstick baking pan. Place split pita rounds on pan. Bake until dry and crisp, about 15 minutes. Remove from oven and let cool. Break pita into bite-sized pieces.
2. In a small bowl, cover sumac with 1 tablespoon hot water. Let

steep for 5 minutes. Whisk in lemon juice, pomegranate molasses, salt, and pepper. Add onions and garlic. Set aside for 5 minutes to let onion soften and mellow.

3. In a large bowl, toss together romaine lettuce, cherry tomatoes, cucumber, parsley, and mint. Add pita pieces, soaked onions, and half the dressing. Toss and taste for seasoning, adding additional salt and/or remaining dressing, as needed.

Chef's Notes

Made from fresh pomegranate juice cooked down to a thick, tangy syrup, pomegranate molasses is a versatile condiment with a tart, fruity flavor. Look for it in shops specializing in Middle Eastern foods, in a well-stocked supermarket, or online at kalustyans.com. To make homemade pomegranate molasses, simmer ½ cup unsweetened pomegranate juice in a small saucepan over medium heat until reduced to 1½ tablespoons, 10–15 minutes. Watch carefully so it doesn't burn. Remove from heat and stir in 1½ teaspoons pure maple syrup. Sumac, made from the dried berries of the sumac bush, is a crumbly reddish-purple powder with a bright, lemony taste. Look for it in shops specializing in Middle Eastern foods, in a well-stocked supermarket, or online at kalustyans.com. If you can't find sumac, substitute 1 teaspoon each ground cumin and coriander and omit the hot water.

Nutrition Facts

Serving Size: 2 cups
Servings: 4

AMOUNT PER SERVING
Calories: 122
Calories from Fat: 9

	AMOUNT PER SERVING	% DAILY VALUE
Total Fat:	1 g	2%
Saturated Fat:	0 g	0%
Trans Fat:	0 g	
Cholesterol:	0 mg	0%
Sodium:	286 mg	12%
Total Carbohydrate:	21 g	7%
Dietary Fiber:	4 g	16%
Sugars:	7 g	
Protein:	9 g	18%

EXCELLENT SOURCE OF: vitamin A, vitamin C
GOOD SOURCE OF: fiber, folate, potassium, calcium, iron

Spinach, Apple, and Fennel Salad

Want to brighten up your fall and winter meals? This crisp, refreshing salad will do the trick. Fresh fennel bulbs have a crunchy, celery-like texture and a light, clean licorice flavor. To prepare, remove any tough stalks from the top of the bulb. Cut bulb into quarters lengthwise. Using a sharp knife, cut out the triangular core in the center of each quarter and discard. Thinly slice each quarter lengthwise.

Serves: 4
Serving Size: 2 cups
Prep Time: 10–15 minutes
Cook Time: N/A
Ready Time: 10–15 minutes

4 tablespoons apple cider vinegar, preferably raw, unfiltered, and organic
½ teaspoon orange zest
1 tablespoon fresh orange juice
1½ teaspoons pure maple syrup
1 teaspoon whole-grain mustard
½ teaspoon ground fennel seeds
½ teaspoon curry powder
¼ teaspoon fine sea salt
¼ teaspoon freshly ground pepper
8 cups baby spinach
2 apples, such as Braeburn, Honeycrisp, or Pink Lady, cored and thinly sliced
1 medium fennel bulb, cored and thinly sliced (2 cups)
⅓ cup dry-roasted soy nuts (see Chef's Notes)
¼ cup chopped scallions

1. To make the vinaigrette, in a small bowl whisk together vinegar, orange zest, orange juice, maple syrup, mustard, ground fennel seeds, curry powder, salt, and pepper. Set aside.
2. In a large bowl, toss the spinach with the apples, fennel, soy nuts, and scallions. Season lightly with additional salt and pepper, if

desired. Toss with three-quarters of the vinaigrette. Taste for seasoning. Add remaining vinaigrette as necessary. Serve immediately.

Chef's Notes

Dry-roasted soybeans, known as soy nuts, are a crunchy high-protein snack packed with essential amino acids. They can take the place of nuts or croutons in any salad.

Nutrition Facts

Serving Size: 2 cups
Servings: 4

AMOUNT PER SERVING
Calories: 119
Calories from Fat: 18

	AMOUNT PER SERVING	% DAILY VALUE
Total Fat:	2 g	3%
Saturated Fat:	0 g	0%
Trans Fat:	0 g	
Cholesterol:	0 mg	0%
Sodium:	317 mg	13%
Total Carbohydrate:	23 g	8%
Dietary Fiber:	6 g	24%
Sugars:	10 g	
Protein:	5 g	10%

EXCELLENT SOURCE OF: fiber, vitamin A, vitamin C
GOOD SOURCE OF: iron

Coleslaw

No, this isn't your grammy's coleslaw—it's still yummy, but a whole lot healthier. We've slashed the fat and enhanced the nutrition by using deliciously creamy vegan mayo. A must-have at your next summer's day picnic!

Serves: 6

Serving Size: 1 cup
Prep Time: 30 minutes
Cook Time: N/A
Ready Time: 30 minutes

½ cup Vegan Mayo (page 400)
2 tablespoons champagne vinegar (see Chef's Notes)
1½ tablespoons pure maple syrup
1 teaspoon freshly squeezed lemon juice
1 teaspoon celery seed
6 cups shredded cabbage (preferably a mix of green and purple)
1 medium to large carrot, peeled and shredded
⅓ cup chopped scallions
¼ teaspoon fine sea salt
¼ teaspoon freshly ground black pepper

1. Combine mayo with vinegar, maple syrup, lemon juice, and celery seed in a large bowl. Add the cabbage, carrot, and scallions. Season with salt and pepper. Mix well and serve at once, or chill before serving.

Chef's Notes

The coleslaw can made 1 day in advance and refrigerated.

If you don't have champagne vinegar on hand, apple cider vinegar would make a fine substitute.

Nutrition Facts

Serving Size: 1 cup
Servings: 6

AMOUNT PER SERVING
Calories: 58
Calories from Fat: 9

	AMOUNT PER SERVING	% DAILY VALUE
Total Fat:	1 g	2%
Saturated Fat:	0 g	0%
Trans Fat:	0 g	
Cholesterol:	0 mg	0%
Sodium:	159 mg	7%
Total Carbohydrate:	11 g	4%
Dietary Fiber:	3 g	12%
Sugars:	7 g	
Protein:	3 g	6%

EXCELLENT SOURCE OF: vitamin A, vitamin C, vitamin K

GOOD SOURCE OF: fiber, manganese

Arugula Salad with Beets and Oranges

Deep jewel-colored beets, brilliant oranges, dark green arugula, and an optional pearly dusting of snowy white feta makes this elegant salad a stunning addition to any holiday table. Not only does this salad make a beautiful presentation, it offers an outstanding package of health-promoting nutrients that are rich in antioxidants and essential vitamins and minerals.

Serves: 4
   Serving Size: 1 cup
   Prep Time: 15 minutes
   Cook Time: 1 hour
   Ready Time: 1 hour 15 minutes

12 ounces beets (about 1½ medium beets, greens removed)
1 tablespoon sherry vinegar
1 tablespoon frozen orange juice concentrate, thawed
½ teaspoon Dijon mustard
Pinch fine sea salt
Pinch freshly ground black pepper
3 tablespoons thinly sliced red onion
4 cups baby arugula
⅔ cup navel orange segments (about 2 oranges), or one can
   (15 ounces) mandarin orange segments, drained

1. Preheat oven to 400°F. Wash beets and wrap individually with aluminum foil. Cook until beets are tender when pierced with a fork, 50–60 minutes. Remove from the oven. Unwrap and allow beets to cool.
2. While beets are roasting, make the vinaigrette. In a small bowl, whisk together vinegar, orange juice concentrate, 1 tablespoon water, mustard, salt, and pepper. Add the red onions and let marinate for 10 minutes.
3. Once beets are cool enough to handle, peel and roughly chop.
4. Place the arugula in a large bowl. Add the beets and the orange segments. Lift red onions from the vinaigrette and sprinkle them

on the salad. Toss with half of the vinaigrette. Taste for seasoning, and add remaining vinaigrette and/or pepper to taste.

5. Divide among 4 serving plates.

Nutrition Facts

Serving Size: 1 cup
Servings: 4

AMOUNT PER SERVING
Calories: 77
Calories from Fat: 0

	AMOUNT PER SERVING	% DAILY VALUE
Total Fat:	.25 g	0%
Saturated Fat:	0 g	0%
Trans Fat:	0 g	
Cholesterol:	0 mg	0%
Sodium:	90.5 mg	4%
Total Carbohydrate:	16.5 g	5%
Dietary Fiber:	3 g	12%
Sugars:	13 g	
Protein:	2 g	4%

EXCELLENT SOURCE OF: fiber, vitamin A, vitamin C
GOOD SOURCE OF: calcium, iron

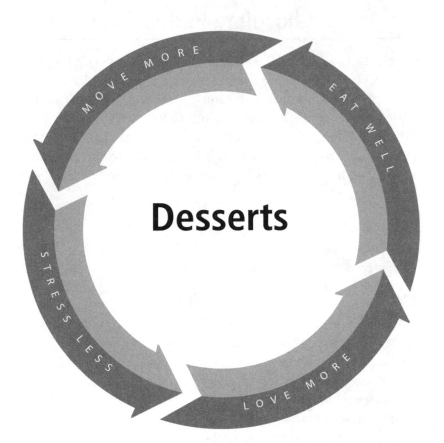

Desserts

MOVE MORE
EAT WELL
LOVE MORE
STRESS LESS

Chocolate Pudding

The secret ingredient in this deliciously easy and practically instant chocolate pudding? Silken tofu. Once blended together with cocoa powder, maple syrup, vanilla, and naturally sweet stevia, this custard-textured form of tofu is transformed into an intensely chocolaty dessert that's full of valuable phytonutrients, flavonoids, and natural plant protein. Make sure you use unsweetened cocoa powder, not prepared cocoa mix. The pudding can be kept in the refrigerator for up to 3 days.

Serves: 6

Serving Size: ⅓ cup
Prep Time: 5 minutes
Cook Time: N/A
Ready Time: 5 minutes

16 ounces firm silken tofu (2 cups)
¾ cup unsweetened cocoa powder
¼ cup pure maple syrup
1 tablespoon vanilla extract
1½ teaspoons powdered stevia
Pinch fine sea salt
1 cup raspberries or chopped strawberries, for garnish (optional)

1. In a food processor fitted with a metal blade, combine tofu, cocoa powder, maple syrup, ¼ cup water, vanilla, stevia, and salt. Process until mixture is smooth and creamy, stopping as necessary to scrape down the bowl with a rubber spatula. Taste and adjust seasoning as needed with more maple syrup and/or vanilla. Adjust consistency with a little more water as needed.
2. Divide pudding mixture among 6 small serving dishes. Refrigerate until chilled, about least 30 minutes. Top each portion with berries, if using.

Chef's Notes

Widely used for vegan desserts, silken tofu has a delicate, custardy texture that's very different from regular tofu. Different brands of silken tofu can vary greatly in flavor and texture. We've had best results using Morinaga's Mori-Nu firm silken tofu. Look for it in aseptic (non-refrigerated) packages in the Asian foods section of your grocery store. You can also order it directly from Morinaga or other online retailers.

Nutrition Facts

Serving Size: ⅓ cup
Servings: 6

AMOUNT PER SERVING
Calories: 108
Calories from Fat: 27

	AMOUNT PER SERVING	% DAILY VALUE
Total Fat:	3 g	5%
Saturated Fat:	0 g	0%
Trans Fat:	0 g	
Cholesterol:	0 mg	0%
Sodium:	54 mg	2%
Total Carbohydrate:	17 g	6%
Dietary Fiber:	4 g	16%
Sugars:	9 g	
Protein:	7 g	14%

GOOD SOURCE OF: riboflavin, fiber, manganese

Chocolate Raspberry Cupcakes

These dense, fudgy cupcakes are a chocolate lover's dream, with no added sugar and no added fat. Fresh raspberries add sophistication, making them a perfect special-occasion dessert. Whole-wheat pastry flour is milled more finely and made from lower-protein wheat, so it's more delicate and better for baking muffins, cakes, cookies, and quick breads while still offering all the benefits of a whole grain. These are best served the day they're made.

Serves: 12

    Serving Size: 1 cupcake
    Prep Time: 20 minutes
    Cook Time: 15 minutes
    Ready Time: 35 minutes

Nonstick cooking spray
1 cup pitted Medjool dates (6 ounces; 8–10 dates)
1 cup whole-wheat pastry flour
½ cup unsweetened cocoa powder
1 teaspoon baking powder
½ teaspoon baking soda
¼ teaspoon fine sea salt
1 cup unsweetened almond milk
¼ cup pure maple syrup
2 teaspoons vanilla extract
1 teaspoon apple cider vinegar
1 cup fresh raspberries (4 ounces)

1. Preheat oven to 350°F. Lightly spray a 12-cup muffin pan with nonstick cooking spray, or line muffin cups with paper liners and lightly spray liners.
2. Place dates in a small bowl. Cover with ¾ cup hot water. Cover bowl and let sit until dates are soft, 10–15 minutes.
3. In a food processor fitted with a metal blade, process softened dates and any remaining soaking liquid until smooth. Set aside.

4. In a large bowl, whisk together flour, cocoa powder, baking powder, baking soda, and salt.
5. In a medium bowl, whisk together date puree, almond milk, maple syrup, vanilla, and vinegar.
6. Stir wet ingredients into dry ingredients, mixing gently just until smooth. Fold in raspberries.
7. Spoon ¼ cup batter into each muffin cup. Bake until a toothpick inserted in the center of a cupcake comes out clean, 10–15 minutes. Place muffin pan on a rack and let cupcakes cool in the pan for 10 minutes, until cupcakes pull away slightly from the edges of the muffin cups. Remove cupcakes from pan. Serve warm or let cool to room temperature.

Nutrition Facts

Serving Size: 1 cupcake
Servings: 12

AMOUNT PER SERVING
Calories: 108
Calories from Fat: 9

	AMOUNT PER SERVING	% DAILY VALUE
Total Fat:	1 g	2%
Saturated Fat:	0 g	0%
Trans Fat:	0 g	
Cholesterol:	0 mg	0%
Sodium:	164 mg	7%
Total Carbohydrate:	27 g	9%
Dietary Fiber:	4 g	16%
Sugars:	17 g	
Protein:	2 g	4%

GOOD SOURCE OF: fiber

Cinnamon Oatmeal Bites

These simple-to-make little bites use the natural sweetness of dates instead of refined sugar and are packed with health-promoting ingredients such as oatmeal, cinnamon, and quinoa. Great for a healthy sweet snack and even breakfast.

Serves: 15
    Serving Size: 1 bite
    Prep: 30 minutes
    Cook: 5 minutes
    Ready: 35 minutes

    3 tablespoons cooked quinoa
    ⅔ cup firmly packed pitted Medjool dates (about 4 ounces) (see Chef's Notes)
    1½ teaspoons vanilla extract
    1 teaspoon ground cinnamon
    ¼ teaspoon ground nutmeg
    ⅛ teaspoon fine sea salt
    1 cup rolled oats

1. Rinse the quinoa and drain thoroughly. Place in a small heavy sauté pan over medium-high heat and toast, stirring frequently, until all moisture has evaporated and the quinoa is golden brown, 3–5 minutes. Transfer to a shallow bowl to cool.
2. Place the dates, 1 tablespoon water, vanilla, cinnamon, nutmeg, and salt in a food processor. Process until a paste forms. Using a rubber spatula, scrape down the sides of the bowl. Add the oats and process until a ball forms. If the mixture seems dry, add 1 more tablespoon water and process again.
3. Transfer to a bowl. If the mixture is sticky, chill well before rolling into balls. Using 1 tablespoon mixture for each ball, roll between the palms of your hands. After shaping, roll each ball in the toasted quinoa. Serve at room temperature.

Chef's Notes

For best results, use soft, moist dates. If the dates are not pliable, place in a small bowl, add hot water to cover, and soak for 15 minutes. Drain and pat dry before proceeding with the recipe.

Freshly grated nutmeg has an especially vibrant flavor, though of course you can use pre-ground nutmeg. If you have a whole nutmeg, use a Microplane or special nutmeg grater.

Prep ahead: These bites can be made up to 3 days in advance and refrigerated in an airtight container.

Nutrition Facts

Serving Size: 1 bite
Servings: 15

AMOUNT PER SERVING
Calories: 80
Calories from Fat: 0

	AMOUNT PER SERVING	% DAILY VALUE
Total Fat:	0 g	0%
Saturated Fat:	0 g	0%
Trans Fat:	0 g	
Cholesterol:	0 mg	0%
Sodium:	25 mg	1%
Total Carbohydrate:	17 g	6%
Dietary Fiber:	2 g	8%
Sugars:	10 g	
Protein:	5 g	10%

Carrot Cupcakes

These cupcakes offer all the spicy-sweet pleasure of carrot cake, with no added fat and plenty of whole-grain fiber and plant-based nutrition. Like most nonfat baked goods, these are best enjoyed the day they are made.

Serves: 12
Serving Size: 1 cupcake
Prep Time: 30 minutes
Cook Time: 30–35 minutes
Ready Time: 1 hour 5 minutes

Nonstick cooking spray
2¼ cups whole-wheat pastry flour
⅓ cup packed brown sugar
2 teaspoons baking powder
1 teaspoon powdered stevia
1½ teaspoons ground cinnamon
¾ teaspoon fine sea salt
¼ teaspoon ground nutmeg
⅛ teaspoon ground cloves
1 tablespoon flaxseed meal
1½ cups grated carrot (about 3 medium)
¾ cup unsweetened almond milk
½ cup unsweetened applesauce
2 teapoons vanilla extract

1. Preheat oven to 375°F. Lightly spray a muffin pan with nonstick cooking spray, or line cups with paper liners and lightly spray liners.
2. In a large bowl, mix together flour, brown sugar, baking powder, stevia, cinnamon, salt, nutmeg, and cloves.
3. In a medium bowl, mix flaxseed meal with 1 tablespoon water. Let sit until water is absorbed, 1–2 minutes. Add carrots, almond milk, applesauce, and 2 teaspoons vanilla extract.
4. Stir the carrot mixture into the flour mixture. Mix well.

5. Spoon ¼ cup batter into each muffin cup. Bake for 30 to 35 minutes, until a toothpick inserted in the center comes out clean. Remove from oven and let cool on a rack. Place muffin pan on a rack and let cupcakes cool in the pan for 10 minutes, until cupcakes pull away slightly from the edges of the muffin cups. Remove cupcakes from pan and let cool completely on a rack.

Nutrition Facts

Serving Size: 1 cupcake
Servings: 12

AMOUNT PER SERVING
Calories: 70
Calories from Fat: 0

	AMOUNT PER SERVING	% DAILY VALUE
Total Fat:	0 g	0%
Saturated Fat:	0 g	0%
Trans Fat:	0 g	
Cholesterol:	0 mg	0%
Sodium:	210 mg	9%
Total Carbohydrate:	17 g	6%
Dietary Fiber:	3 g	11%
Sugars:	8 g	
Protein:	1 g	2%

EXCELLENT SOURCE OF: vitamin A

Apple Crisp

Bring the taste of autumn into your kitchen! This delectable apple crisp is rich in fiber and flavor but low in added sugar and fat. For best results, use a mixture of sweet, mellow apples, like Golden Delicious, McIntosh, Gala, Pink Lady, or Honeycrisp. A handful of dark or golden raisins in the filling can add an additional boost of fiber, iron, and natural sweetness.

Serves: 8

Serving Size: ⅓ cup
Prep Time: 15 minutes
Cook Time: 60 minutes
Ready Time: 1 hour 15 minutes

6 apples, peeled, cored, and chopped into ¾-inch pieces (6 cups)
¾ cup unsweetened apple juice or fresh apple cider
2 teaspoons lemon juice
2 teaspoons vanilla extract
2 teaspoons ground cinnamon
2 teaspoons arrowroot or cornstarch
¼ teaspoon ground nutmeg
Pinch plus ¼ teaspoon fine sea salt
1 cup old-fashioned rolled oats
¼ cup whole-wheat flour or gluten-free flour
3 tablespoons coconut sugar or turbinado (raw) sugar (see Chef's Notes)
2 tablespoons pure maple syrup

1. Preheat oven to 350°F. In a large bowl, combine apples, apple juice, lemon juice, vanilla, cinnamon, arrowroot or cornstarch, nutmeg, and a pinch of salt. Stir until apples are well coated. Spread apple mixture evenly in an 8 × 8-inch glass baking dish.
2. In a medium bowl, combine oats, flour, sugar, maple syrup, and the remaining ¼ teaspoon salt. Mix until syrup is fully incorporated; mixture will be dry.
3. Spread oat mixture evenly over apples. Cover baking dish with

aluminum foil. Bake for 45 minutes. Remove foil and continue to bake for another 10–15 minutes, until apples are tender and topping is lightly browned. Serve warm or at room temperature.

Chef's Notes

Coconut sugar (also called coconut palm sugar), a longtime staple in Southeast Asian kitchens, is derived from the sap of the cut flower buds of the coconut palm. Look for it in natural foods stores or among the "alternative sugars" in your supermarket's baking aisle. If you can't find coconut sugar, substitute a fine-grain turbinado (raw) sugar.

Nutrition Facts

Serving Size: ⅓ cup
Servings: 8

AMOUNT PER SERVING
Calories: 161
Calories from Fat: 9

	AMOUNT PER SERVING	% DAILY VALUE
Total Fat:	1 g	2%
Saturated Fat:	0 g	0%
Trans Fat:	0 g	
Cholesterol:	0 mg	0%
Sodium:	75 mg	3%
Total Carbohydrate:	35 g	12%
Dietary Fiber:	4 g	16%
Sugars:	19 g	
Protein:	2 g	4%

GOOD SOURCE OF: fiber

Cocoa Truffles

Chocolate lovers, rejoice! Finally, a moist, fudgy, delicious truffle that's good for you, too. Sweet, nutrient-dense Medjool dates take the place of sugar here, while unsweetened cocoa powder is rich in flavonoids (antioxidant compounds that help ward off inflammation and lower blood pressure) as well as in health-boosting minerals like iron and zinc. These can be made 2–3 days in advance and stored in the refrigerator until needed.

Serves: 16

Serving Size: 1 truffle

Prep Time: 15 minutes

Cook Time: N/A

Ready Time: 15 minutes

1 cup firmly packed pitted Medjool dates (6 ounces; 8–10 dates) (see Chef's Notes)

½ cup unsweetened cocoa powder, plus ¼ cup for rolling (optional)

1½ teaspoons vanilla extract

¼ teaspoon fine sea salt

1. Place dates in a food processor fitted with a metal blade. Pulse dates several times to make a paste. Add ½ cup cocoa powder, 2 tablespoons warm water, vanilla, and salt. Pulse until mixture is smooth and forms a ball. (If mixture needs a little more moisture to come together, add 1–2 more teaspoons of water.)
2. Remove chocolate mixture from processor and transfer to a bowl.
3. Using 1 tablespoon truffle mixture for each ball, shape balls between the palms of your hands. Place truffles on a plate. (If mixture seems sticky, refrigerate until well chilled before rolling.)
4. To coat (optional), put ¼ cup cocoa powder in a shallow bowl. Roll each ball in cocoa powder after shaping and return to plate. Cover and refrigerate until serving.

Chef's Notes

For best results, use soft, moist dates for this recipe. If you can only find firm, dry ones, soak them in hot water to cover for 15 minutes. Drain and pat dry before proceeding with the recipe.

Variations

For Mexican Truffles, add ½ teaspoon ground cinnamon and, optionally, ⅛ teaspoon cayenne with the cocoa powder in step 1.

For flavor variations, add a few drops of peppermint or coconut extract to the date mixture before rolling into balls.

Nutrition Facts

Serving Size: 1 truffle
Servings: 16

AMOUNT PER SERVING
Calories: 40
Calories from Fat: 0

	AMOUNT PER SERVING	% DAILY VALUE
Total Fat:	0 g	0%
Saturated Fat:	0 g	0%
Trans Fat:	0 g	
Cholesterol:	0 mg	0%
Sodium:	35 mg	2%
Total Carbohydrate:	11 g	4%
Dietary Fiber:	3 g	11%
Sugars:	4 g	
Protein:	1 g	2%

Raspberry Thumbprint Cookies

This flexible recipe packs a lot of fiber and nutrition into a tasty, whole-some, bite-sized package. Because they contain no eggs, these cookies can be enjoyed raw, making them a fun kitchen project for all ages. However, if you like a crunchier texture, you can also bake them. Baked or raw, these cookies freeze very well. To use, thaw frozen cookies and store in the refrigerator for up to 3 days.

Serves: 20
    Serving Size: 1 cookie
    Prep Time: 20 minutes
    Cook Time: 20 minutes
    Ready Time: 40 minutes

1 cup firmly packed pitted Medjool dates (6 ounces; 8–10 dates)
¼ cup flaxseed meal
1½ cups crispy rice cereal, preferably brown rice
1¼ cups old-fashioned rolled oats
1½ teaspoons vanilla extract
1 teaspoon ground cinnamon
¼ teaspoon almond extract
⅛ teaspoon fine sea salt
¾ cup frozen raspberries (3 ounces), measured while frozen
¼ teaspoon almond extract

1. To make the cookies, place dates and flaxseed meal in a small bowl. Cover with ½ cup boiling water. Cover bowl and set aside until dates are soft and hydrated and liquid has thickened, 10–15 minutes.
2. Using a food processor fitted with a metal blade, pulse rice cereal and oats for 3 seconds. Repeat two or three times, until mixture is coarsely ground. Transfer mixture to a small bowl and set aside.
3. Place the date mixture into the food processor. Add vanilla, cinnamon, almond extract, and salt. Puree until smooth, stopping to scrape down the sides with a rubber spatula as needed. Measure

out ¼ cup date puree and set aside for use in the raspberry filling.

4. Pour oat and rice mixture onto the remaining date puree in the food processor. Pulse together until mixture is smooth and date puree is thoroughly incorporated. Taste and season with additional vanilla, cinnamon, almond extract, or salt if necessary. Mixture should be firm enough to roll into a ball. If it seems too wet, add a little more crushed rice cereal; if too dry, add a small amount of water.

5. To make the filling, thaw raspberries until they are soft enough to mash. In a medium bowl, whisk together the thawed raspberries, reserved ¼ cup date puree, and almond extract. Mixture should look like a bright red jam.

6. Line a baking sheet with parchment paper. To make raw cookies, roll dough into balls, using a rounded tablespoon of cookie dough for each ball. Arrange balls on prepared baking sheet. Make a 1-inch indentation in the center of each ball by pressing down with your thumb. Spoon 1 teaspoon raspberry filling into each cookie. Cover and chill in the refrigerator for at least 1 hour before serving.

7. To make baked cookies, follow the above instructions, but do not chill. Preheat oven to 350°F. Bake filled cookies for 20 minutes.

Nutrition Facts

Serving Size: 1 cookie
Servings: 20

AMOUNT PER SERVING
Calories: 69
Calories from Fat: 9

	AMOUNT PER SERVING	DAILY VALUE
Total Fat:	1 g	2%
Saturated Fat:	0 g	0%
Trans Fat:	0 g	
Cholesterol:	0 mg	0%
Sodium:	27 mg	1%
Total Carbohydrate:	15 g	5%
Dietary Fiber:	2 g	8%
Sugars:	7 g	
Protein:	2 g	4%

Pumpkin Pie

There's plenty to be thankful for in this classic holiday dessert, now updated with lots of health-promoting ingredients, less sugar, and no saturated fat or cholesterol. A slice of this robustly flavorful pie is rich in antioxidants, omega-3s, and phytonutrients, making it a perfect ending to a meal full of gratitude for good health and happiness. Want to take the stress out of your holiday dessert preparations? Make this pie a day in advance and warm slightly just before serving. And if you feel like making a variation on the traditional pumpkin pie, try substituting 1¾ cups sweet potato puree in place of the pumpkin and reduce the maple syrup by half.

Serves: 12
   Serving Size: 1 slice
   Prep Time: 30 minutes
   Cook Time: 50 minutes
   Ready Time: 1 hour 20 minutes, plus 2 hours to cool

   3 tablespoons flaxseed meal, divided (see Chef's Notes)
   ½ teaspoon ground ginger
   8 ounces low-fat graham crackers (about 12 crackers)
   1 can (15 ounces) unsweetened pumpkin puree
   1 cup unsweetened soy milk or oat milk
   3½ tablespoons pure maple syrup
   2 tablespoons cornstarch
   1 tablespoon vanilla extract
   1¼ teaspoons ground cinnamon
   ½ teaspoon stevia powder
   ½ teaspoon fine sea salt
   ½ teaspoon ground ginger
   ⅛ teaspoon ground nutmeg
   Pinch ground cloves

   1. Preheat oven to 325°F. For the crust, stir together 1½ tablespoons flaxseed meal, ginger, and ⅓ cup plus 1 tablespoon water in a small bowl. For the filling, stir together the remaining 1½ table-

spoons flaxseed meal and ¼ cup water in a separate bowl. Set both "flax eggs" (a spiced "flax egg" and a plain "flax egg") aside until mixtures have thickened, about 10 minutes.

2. To make the crust, crumble graham crackers into a food processor fitted with the metal blade. Pulse until crackers form fine crumbs. Add spiced "flax egg" mixture and pulse until mixture holds its form when pressed.

3. Using your fingers, press the mixture evenly over the bottom and sides of a nonstick 9-inch pie pan. Keep in mind that the crust will shrink slightly when cooked, so press crust just beyond the top of the pie plate, onto the edge if possible. Bake until crust is lightly browned, about 10 minutes. Remove from oven and set on a rack to cool slightly. Raise oven temperature to 350°F.

4. To make the filling, place pumpkin, soy milk, maple syrup, cornstarch, vanilla, cinnamon, stevia, salt, ginger, nutmeg, cloves, and remaining plain "flax egg" in a blender. Blend until smooth.

5. Pour filling into prepared crust. (You may not need all the filling. It will depend upon the depth of your pie plate.) Bake for 35–45 minutes, until mixture appears set in the center and/or the internal temperature is 170° F. Check after 30 minutes. Remove pie from oven and cool on wire rack for at least 2 hours. Serve at room temperature.

Chef's Notes

Flaxseed meal absorbs liquid readily and helps take the place of eggs as a binder in low-fat baked goods. It can be found in many natural foods stores. If you can't find flaxseed meal, grind whole flaxseeds in a clean spice or coffee grinder or blender to make your own.

Nutrition Facts

Serving Size: 1 slice
Servings: 12

AMOUNT PER SERVING
Calories: 155
Calories from Fat: 18

	AMOUNT PER SERVING	% DAILY VALUE
Total Fat:	2 g	3%
Saturated Fat:	0 g	0%
Trans Fat:	0 g	
Cholesterol:	0 mg	0%
Sodium:	250 mg	0%
Total Carbohydrate:	33 g	11%
Dietary Fiber:	4 g	16%
Sugars:	16 g	
Protein:	3 g	6%

EXCELLENT SOURCE OF: vitamin A

GOOD SOURCE OF: fiber, calcium

Minted Pineapple

Fresh fruit is the healthiest way to end a meal. Why not have fun and dress it up a little, without adding fat or sugar? We've turned fresh pineapple into something special by tossing it with a frothy, tangy pineapple sauce made with fresh mint and lime juice. Be sure to choose a sweet, ripe pineapple. The bottom should have a little "give" to it, and the skin near the base should smell tropically sweet.

Serves: 4
   Serving Size: 1 cup
   Prep Time: 10 minutes
   Cook Time: N/A
   Ready Time: 10 minutes

1 ripe pineapple, peeled, cored, cut into cubes, and chilled (about
    5 cups)
¾ cup firmly packed fresh mint leaves
1 tablespoon lime juice, plus more to taste
Liquid or powdered stevia to taste (optional)
2 tablespoons chopped fresh mint, for garnish

1. Place chilled pineapple in a medium bowl.
2. Measure out 1 cup pineapple cubes. Place in a blender with mint leaves, ¼ cup water, and lime juice. Puree on high speed until smooth. Taste; if pineapple isn't very sweet, add a small amount of liquid or powdered stevia to taste.
3. Pour pineapple puree over the remaining pineapple cubes. Toss to coat. Serve immediately, or chill until ready to serve. Divide into bowls and garnish with additional chopped mint.

Nutrition Facts

Serving Size: 1 cup
Servings: 4

AMOUNT PER SERVING
Calories: 100
Calories from Fat: 0

	AMOUNT PER SERVING	% DAILY VALUE
Total Fat:	0 g	0%
Saturated Fat:	0 g	0%
Trans Fat:	0 g	
Cholesterol:	0 mg	0%
Sodium:	0 mg	0%
Total Carbohydrate:	26 g	9%
Dietary Fiber:	3 g	12%
Sugars:	20 g	
Protein:	1 g	2%

EXCELLENT SOURCE OF: vitamin C, fiber
GOOD SOURCE OF: folate, copper, vitamins B_1, B_6

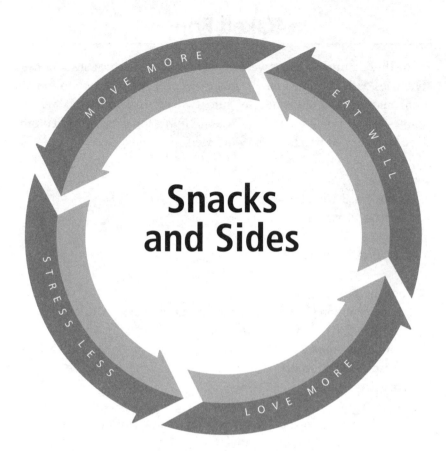

MOVE MORE

EAT WELL

Snacks
and Sides

LOVE MORE

STRESS LESS

Baked Fries

Enjoy these crunchy potato wedges, our version of robust steak house–style fries with no added fat. To make wedges, cut each potato in half, then quarters. Cut each quarter into two or three wedges. We love yellow-fleshed potatoes, such as Yukon Golds, for these, but medium-sized red-skinned potatoes also work well.

Serves: 6
　　Serving Size: 5–6 wedges
　　Prep Time: 10 minutes
　　Cook Time: 30–35 minutes
　　Ready Time: 40–45 minutes

Nonstick cooking spray
3 medium Yukon Gold or red-skinned potatoes (about 1½ pounds),
　　unpeeled, cut into ¾-inch wedges
1 teaspoon chopped fresh rosemary
⅛ teaspoon fine sea salt
⅛ teaspoon freshly ground pepper

1. Preheat oven to 450°F. Lightly spray a large rimmed baking sheet with nonstick cooking spray.
2. Spread potatoes evenly on the baking sheet. Sprinkle with rosemary, salt, and pepper.
3. Bake, turning once halfway through, until wedges are golden brown and crisp, 30–35 minutes. Serve hot.

Nutrition Facts

Serving Size: 5–6 wedges
Servings: 6

AMOUNT PER SERVING
Calories: 130
Calories from Fat: 0

	AMOUNT PER SERVING	% DAILY VALUE
Total Fat:	0 g	0%
Saturated Fat:	0 g	0%
Trans Fat:	0 g	
Cholesterol:	0 mg	0%
Sodium:	80 mg	3%
Total Carbohydrate:	29 g	10%
Dietary Fiber:	3 g	12%
Sugars:	2 g	
Protein:	3 g	6%

EXCELLENT SOURCE OF: vitamin C, potassium

GOOD SOURCE OF: vitamins B_3, B_6, copper, manganese, magnesium, phosphorus

Roasted Roots

Warm up with this colorful, easy combination of roasted root vegetables. Feel free to experiment with other similar vegetables, such as sweet potatoes, turnips, rutabagas, and/or winter squash. It's important to cut all the roasting vegetables into uniformly sized pieces so that the cooking time will be the same for all. Aim for small, bite-sized chunks or cubes about ¾ inch in size.

Serves: 4
Serving Size: 1 cup
Prep Time: 10 minutes
Cook Time: 20–25 minutes
Ready Time: 30–35 minutes

1 medium shallot, peeled and roughly chopped
1 tablespoon chopped fresh rosemary or 1 teaspoon dried, crumbled
¼ teaspoon fine sea salt, divided
¼ teaspoon pepper, divided
2 cups unpeeled chopped Yukon Gold potatoes
2 cups peeled, chopped beets
2 cups chopped carrots

1. Preheat oven to 425°F. Line a rimmed baking sheet with parchment paper.
2. In a blender, combine ¼ cup water, shallot, rosemary, ⅛ teaspoon salt, and ⅛ teaspoon pepper. Blend until smooth
3. Combine the potatoes, beets, and carrots on the prepared baking sheet. Add the shallot mixture. Season with remaining ⅛ teaspoon salt and ⅛ teaspoon pepper. Toss until well mixed. Spread vegetables evenly over the baking sheet.
4. Bake until vegetables are tender and lightly browned, 20–25 minutes. Serve warm.

Nutrition Facts

Serving Size: 1 cup
Servings: 4

AMOUNT PER SERVING
Calories: 140
Calories from Fat: 0

	AMOUNT PER SERVING	% DAILY VALUE
Total Fat:	0 g	0%
Saturated Fat:	0 g	0%
Trans Fat:	0 g	
Cholesterol:	0 mg	0%
Sodium:	260 mg	1%
Total Carbohydrate:	30 g	10%
Dietary Fiber:	6 g	24%
Sugars:	11 g	
Protein:	4 g	8%

EXCELLENT SOURCE OF: fiber, vitamin A, vitamin C, folate, iron, manganese

GOOD SOURCE OF: vitamin B_6, potassium

Garlic Roasted Potatoes

Rosemary and garlic are the perfect flavor partners for these classic roasted potatoes. Yukon Gold potatoes have thin skins and a naturally buttery-tasting yellow flesh that makes them particularly good in a low-fat, heart-healthy diet. Make sure to chop your potatoes into uniformly sized pieces so they will cook evenly.

Serves: 6
Serving Size: ¾ cup
Prep Time: 10 minutes
Cook Time: 30 minutes
Ready Time: 40 minutes

Nonstick cooking spray
2 pounds Yukon Gold potatoes, unpeeled, cut into 1-inch pieces (about 6 cups)
1 tablespoon chopped fresh rosemary or 1 teaspoon dried, crumbled
1 teaspoon garlic powder
1 teaspoon onion powder
¼ teaspoon fine sea salt
¼ teaspoon freshly ground pepper

1. Preheat oven to 425°F. Lightly spray a rimmed baking sheet with nonstick cooking spray.
2. In a large bowl, toss potatoes with rosemary, garlic powder, onion powder, salt, and pepper.
3. Spread potatoes in an even layer over the prepared baking sheet. Bake for 20 minutes. Using a spatula, stir potatoes to ensure even browning. Bake for an additional 5–10 minutes, until potatoes are tender and browned.
4. Remove from oven. Taste for seasoning and add additional salt if desired. Serve warm.

Nutrition Facts

Serving Size: ¾ cup
Servings: 6

AMOUNT PER SERVING
Calories: 110
Calories from Fat: 0

	AMOUNT PER SERVING	% DAILY VALUE
Total Fat:	0 g	0%
Saturated Fat:	0 g	0%
Trans Fat:	0 g	
Cholesterol:	0 mg	0%
Sodium:	144 mg	6%
Total Carbohydrate:	27 g	9%
Dietary Fiber:	3 g	12%
Sugars:	1 g	
Protein:	3 g	6%

GOOD SOURCE OF: fiber, calcium

Glazed Acorn Squash with Orange and Ginger

Need a fresh vegetable side for your holiday menus? Try this flavorful roasted winter squash, glazed with citrusy sweetness and sparked with fresh ginger and a hint of nutmeg. It's a wonderful addition to any holiday table, but it's also easy—and healthy enough—for any weeknight meal. Acorn squash is easy to find in supermarket produce sections. They have a deeply indented skin that can be blue-green, orange, or cream, along with a distinctive acorn-like shape and fibrous yellow-orange flesh.

Serves: 4
Serving Size: 1 squash half
Prep Time: 10 minutes
Cook Time: 40 minutes
Ready Time: 50 minutes

2 medium acorn squash
¼ teaspoon orange zest
¼ cup freshly squeezed orange juice
1 tablespoon pure maple syrup
1 teaspoon grated fresh ginger
Pinch cayenne
Pinch fine sea salt
Freshly ground black pepper, to taste
Freshly ground nutmeg, to taste

1. Preheat oven to 425° F. Place squash on its side. Cut the squash in half at its widest point. Scrape out seeds and discard. Cut across to remove a thin layer of the bottom tip so squash half will sit upright. Cut across stem end to remove stem so second squash half will sit upright. (Be very careful not to cut off too much, creating a hole in the squash). Repeat with remaining squash.
2. Place squash halves upright in a 9 × 13-inch baking dish. Pour water around the squash halves, enough to cover the bottom of the baking dish by ⅛ inch.

3. In a small bowl, whisk together orange zest, orange juice, maple syrup, ginger, cayenne, and salt. Place 1 tablespoon of the mixture into the cavity of each squash half. Using a pastry brush, brush mixture over squash. Season squash with black pepper and nutmeg.
4. Cover baking pan with aluminum foil. Bake until squash is tender, about 30 minutes. Uncover, baste squash with any accumulated juices, and bake uncovered until squash is lightly glazed and golden brown, about 10 minutes.

Nutrition Facts

Serving Size: 1 squash half
Servings: 4

AMOUNT PER SERVING
Calories: 107
Calories from Fat: 0

	AMOUNT PER SERVING	% DAILY VALUE
Total Fat:	0 g	0%
Saturated Fat:	0 g	0%
Trans Fat:	0 g	
Cholesterol:	0 mg	0%
Sodium:	80 mg	3%
Total Carbohydrate:	28 g	9%
Dietary Fiber:	3 g	12%
Sugars:	5 g	
Protein:	2 g	4%

EXCELLENT SOURCE OF: vitamin B_1, vitamin C, potassium
GOOD SOURCE OF: vitamin A, vitamin B_6, magnesium

Farro with Mushrooms

"Farro" is an Italian term that can refer to any one of three ancient grains—emmer, einkorn, or spelt—that are precursors to modern wheat. Farro has a nutty flavor and satisfyingly chewy texture, and is high in B vitamins and magnesium. It makes a deliciously different substitute for brown rice in pilafs and hearty soups. Whole farro, which has the most fiber and nutrients, must be soaked overnight in water to cover before using.

Serves: 6
Serving Size: ½ cup
Prep Time: 10 minutes
Cook Time: 25–40 minutes
Ready Time: 35–50 minutes

1 cup uncooked farro, preferably whole or semi-perlato (see Chef's Notes)
¼ teaspoon fine sea salt
1 bay leaf
8 ounces cremini mushrooms
1 cup diced onion
1 tablespoon chopped fresh thyme or 1 teaspoon dried, divided
2 teaspoons minced garlic
2 teaspoons Bragg Liquid Aminos
⅛ teaspoon freshly ground pepper

1. If using whole farro, pour into a medium bowl, add cold water to cover, and let soak at least 8 hours or overnight. Drain well before using. Do not toast soaked farro (step 2); instead, combine farro with water, salt, and bay leaf as instructed in step 3. Bring to a simmer, cover, and proceed as directed.
2. If using semi-perlato or perlato farro, in a medium heavy-bottomed saucepan over medium-high heat, toast the dry farro, shaking occasionally, until it begins to look and smell toasted and nutty, about 3 minutes.
3. Carefully add 1¾ cups water, salt, and bay leaf (mixture will sput-

ter) and stir. Cover pan and simmer until the farro is tender but still chewy. This can take anywhere from 25 to 40 minutes, depending on the type of farro used. Check after 15 minutes, and again after 25 minutes. If liquid evaporates before the grain is tender, add more water as necessary.

4. While farro is cooking, prepare the mushrooms. In a large skillet over high heat, combine the mushrooms, onions, 1½ teaspoons fresh thyme (or ½ teaspoon dried), garlic, liquid aminos, pepper, and ¼ cup water over high heat. Bring to a boil, reduce heat to medium-high, and cook until onions and mushrooms are tender and slightly brown and moisture has evaporated, about 10 minutes.

5. Reduce the heat to a simmer. Stir in the cooked farro. Cook for 2–3 minutes. Add remaining 1½ teaspoons thyme (or ½ teaspoon dried). Taste for seasoning, adding more liquid aminos and/or pepper to taste. Serve warm.

Chef's Notes

Whole farro has the most fiber and nutrients but must be soaked overnight in water before using. Faster options include semi-perlato (semi-pearled) and perlato (pearled), which are polished to remove some or all of the outer bran covering and need no presoaking. Semi-perlato will take longer to cook than perlato.

Nutrition Facts

Serving Size: ½ cup
Servings: 6

AMOUNT PER SERVING
Calories: 118
Calories from Fat: 0

	AMOUNT PER SERVING	% DAILY VALUE
Total Fat:	0 g	0%
Saturated Fat:	0 g	0%
Trans Fat:	0 g	
Cholesterol:	0 mg	0%
Sodium:	226 mg	9%
Total Carbohydrate:	25 g	8%
Dietary Fiber:	3 g	12%
Sugars:	2 g	
Protein:	5 g	10%

GOOD SOURCE OF: fiber, ribolflavin, copper, selenium

Mashed Cauliflower

Looking for warm winter comfort food that's a little more exciting than plain old mashed potatoes? Scented with nutmeg and thyme, this creamy cauliflower puree offers a generous dose of cell-protective antioxidants and powerful phytochemicals, including cancer-protective isothiocyanates and indoles. If you can find golden cauliflower (sometimes called "cheddar" cauliflower), it will make a beautifully tinted mash. For a cheese-like accent, try garnishing the puree with a sprinkle of nutritional yeast.

Serves: 4
  Serving Size: ¾ cup
  Prep Time: 15 minutes
  Cook Time: 30 minutes
  Ready Time: 45 minutes

1 cup chopped onion
1 cup unsweetened soy milk
½ teaspoon garlic powder
1 teaspoon chopped fresh thyme or ½ teaspoon dried thyme
⅛ teaspoon fine sea salt
⅛ teaspoon freshly ground pepper
Pinch freshly ground nutmeg
1 tablespoon cornstarch
6 cups cauliflower florets (about 3 pounds from 1 large head cauliflower)
1 tablespoon finely chopped chives or nutritional yeast for garnish (optional)

1. In a large sauté pan, combine onions with ¼ cup water over high heat. Bring to a boil. Reduce heat to medium. Cook, stirring frequently, until onions are tender and liquid has evaporated, about 10 minutes. Add soy milk, garlic powder, thyme, salt, pepper, and nutmeg. Bring soy milk to a simmer. Be careful not to boil. Combine cornstarch in 1 tablespoon water in a small bowl. Whisk cornstarch mixture into the onion mixture. Cook about 2 min-

utes, whisking frequently, until mixture is thick and creamy. Remove from heat. Set aside.

2. Place a vegetable steamer basket in a saucepan and add water to just below bottom of steamer basket. Over high heat, bring water to a boil. Add cauliflower florets, cover, and steam until tender, 8–10 minutes. (You may need to steam cauliflower in batches, depending on the size of your steamer.) Remove strainer basket. Discard steaming water from the pot.

3. Place steamed cauliflower back into the empty pot. Add the sauce to the cauliflower. Using a hand masher, sturdy whisk, or immersion blender, mash the cauliflower to desired consistency. Alternatively, blend in a food processor fitted with the metal blade.

4. Taste for seasoning, adding more thyme, salt, pepper, or nutmeg as needed. Serve warm with a sprinkle of chives and/or nutritional yeast, if desired.

Nutrition Facts

Serving Size: ¾ cup
Servings: 4

AMOUNT PER SERVING
Calories: 70
Calories from Fat: 9

	AMOUNT PER SERVING	% DAILY VALUE
Total Fat:	1 g	2%
Saturated Fat:	0 g	0%
Trans Fat:	0 g	
Cholesterol:	0 mg	0%
Sodium:	221 mg	9%
Total Carbohydrate:	12 g	4%
Dietary Fiber:	5 g	20%
Sugars:	4 g	
Protein:	6 g	12%

EXCELLENT SOURCE OF: fiber, vitamins B_1, B_2, B_3, B_6, B_{12}, vitamin C, folate, potassium
GOOD SOURCE OF: phosphorus

Quinoa and Cauliflower Tabbouleh

Tabbouleh, a popular Mediterranean salad, is typically made with cracked bulgur wheat mixed with plenty of parsley and mint. We've updated it here by using red quinoa, a high-protein "superfood" that's naturally gluten-free. Raw cauliflower, cherry tomatoes, and diced red onion turn it into a satisfying main-dish meal, perfect over a bed of tender butter lettuce or mixed spring greens.

Serves: 6

Serving Size: 1 cup
Prep Time: 10 minutes
Cook Time: 20 minutes
Ready Time: 30 minutes

1 cup red quinoa
4 cups cauliflower florets (about 2 pounds from 1 medium cauliflower)
1 cup cherry tomatoes, quartered
½ cup chopped flat-leaf parsley
½ cup chopped fresh mint
¼ cup capers, coarsely chopped
¼ cup diced red onion
¼ cup freshly squeezed lemon juice
¼ cup freshly squeezed orange juice
1 teaspoon ground cumin
½ teaspoon freshly ground pepper
¼ teaspoon fine sea salt (optional)

1. Prepare the quinoa according to package instructions.
2. While the quinoa is cooking, prepare the cauliflower. Chop into smaller florets. Place in a food processor fitted with a metal blade. Pulse several times to mince cauliflower until it has a granular texture similar to couscous.
3. In a medium bowl, combine cauliflower with tomatoes, parsley, mint, capers, onions, lemon juice, orange juice, cumin, pepper, and salt, if using.

4. Fold cooled quinoa into cauliflower mixture. Taste for seasoning, adding additional salt and pepper to taste.

Nutrition Facts

Serving Size: 1 cup
Servings: 6

AMOUNT PER SERVING
Calories: 147
Calories from Fat: 18

	AMOUNT PER SERVING	% DAILY VALUE
Total Fat:	2 g	3%
Saturated Fat:	0 g	0%
Trans Fat:	0 g	
Cholesterol:	0 mg	0%
Sodium:	409 mg	17%
Total Carbohydrate:	27 g	9%
Dietary Fiber:	5 g	20%
Sugars:	6 g	
Protein:	7 g	14%

EXCELLENT SOURCE OF: fiber, vitamin A, vitamin C
GOOD SOURCE OF: folate, potassium

Baked Sweet Potato Fries

These baked sweet potato wedges make a great accompaniment to any of our sandwiches or vegetarian burgers. Sweet potatoes are rich in vitamin A, fiber, and potassium.

Serves: 6

Serving Size: 5–6 wedges
Prep Time: 15 minutes
Cook Time: 35 minutes
Ready Time: 50 minutes

Nonstick cooking spray (optional)
2 medium sweet potatoes (about 1½ pounds)
¼ teaspoon fine sea salt
¼ teaspoon freshly ground pepper
⅛ teaspoon ground cinnamon (optional)

1. Preheat oven to 450°F. Line a large rimmed baking sheet with parchment paper or lightly spray with nonstick cooking spray.
2. Cut each sweet potato in half, then into quarters. Cut each quarter into approximately 4 wedges, each about ¾ inch wide. To promote even cooking, try to make the potato wedges uniform in size. If needed, trim wedges slightly to achieve similar sizing.
3. Spread wedges evenly on the baking sheet in a single layer, skin-side up. Sprinkle with salt, pepper, and cinnamon, if using.
4. Bake until wedges are tender, 20–30 minutes. Turn the oven to broil. Broil until browned and crisp, 3–5 minutes. Watch carefully to avoid burning.
5. Remove from oven. Cool wedges in pan for 5 minutes before serving. Serve warm.

Nutrition Facts

Serving Size: 5–6 wedges
Servings: 6

AMOUNT PER SERVING
Calories: 98
Calories from Fat: 0

	AMOUNT PER SERVING	% DAILY VALUE
Total Fat:	0 g	0%
Saturated Fat:	0 g	0%
Trans Fat:	0 g	
Cholesterol:	0 mg	0%
Sodium:	159 mg	7%
Total Carbohydrate:	23 g	8%
Dietary Fiber:	3 g	12%
Sugars:	5 g	
Protein:	2 g	4%

EXCELLENT SOURCE OF: vitamin A

GOOD SOURCE OF: fiber, vitamin B_6, manganese, potassium

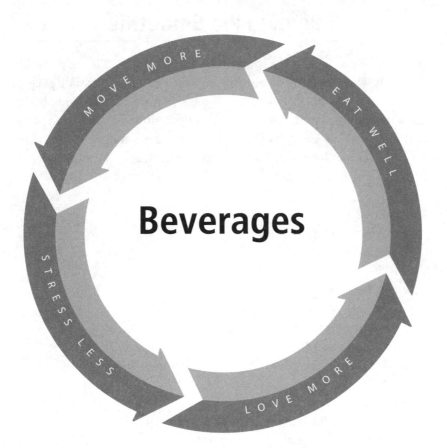

MOVE MORE

EAT WELL

Beverages

STRESS LESS

LOVE MORE

Pumpkin Pie Smoothie

This creamy pumpkin spice smoothie is like drinking a slice of pumpkin pie—only with loads of health-promoting benefits. One tall glass is packed with cell-protective antioxidants, vitamins, and minerals, including carotene, lutein, vitamin A, and potassium. Thanks to the flaxseed meal and soy milk, it's also a good source of omega-3s. Enjoy this delicious seasonal smoothie as an energy-boosting afternoon snack or as a tasty way to start a healthy day!

Serves: 2
   Serving Size: 1¼ cups
   Prep Time: 5 minutes
   Cook Time: N/A
   Ready Time: 5 minutes

   ½ cup unsweetened pumpkin puree
   1 cup unsweetened soy milk
   1 small ripe banana, peeled, broken into chunks, and frozen
   ¾ cup ice (about 6 ice cubes)
   1 tablespoon flaxseed meal
   1 teaspoon pumpkin pie spice (see Chef's Notes)
   ¾ teaspoon finely chopped fresh ginger
   ½ teaspoon vanilla extract
   Few drops liquid stevia (optional)

1. Place all ingredients in a blender. Blend on high speed until frothy and smooth.
2. Taste and add additional spices or stevia, if using. The flaxseed meal will thicken the smoothie as it stands; add more soy milk to thin it if necessary.

Chef's Notes

We love the convenience of pumpkin pie spice, a warm, autumn-y blend of cinnamon, ginger, and cloves (and sometimes allspice, nutmeg, and/or mace, too) that's sold in the spice section of most supermarkets. It's great for adding a dash of sweet spice to apple, pear, and pumpkin desserts and baked goods. If you don't have it on hand, you can make your own using ½ teaspoon ground cinnamon, ¼ teaspoon ground ginger, ⅛ teaspoon nutmeg, and ⅛ teaspoon allspice.

Nutrition Facts

Serving Size: 1¼ cups
Servings: 2

AMOUNT PER SERVING
Calories: 153
Calories from Fat: 36

	AMOUNT PER SERVING	% DAILY VALUE
Total Fat:	4 g	6%
Saturated Fat:	0 g	0%
Trans Fat:	0 g	
Cholesterol:	0 mg	0%
Sodium:	49 mg	2%
Total Carbohydrate:	27 g	9%
Dietary Fiber:	5 g	20%
Sugars:	16 g	
Protein:	6 g	12%

EXCELLENT SOURCE OF: fiber, vitamin A, riboflavin, vitamin B_{12}
GOOD SOURCE OF: potassium, calcium

Ginger-Lemon Spritzer

This cool, crisp, and refreshing drink is the perfect way to stay healthy, hydrated, and happy in warm weather. The ginger and citrus with a hint of natural sweetness not only offers a truly delicious energizing beverage but also provides an abundance of health-promoting benefits. Ginger has been shown to have a positive impact on digestion and powerful anti-inflammatory, antioxidant, and immune-boosting agents. The lemon adds an additional boost of cell-protecting vitamin C.

Serves: 4

Serving Size: 1 cup
Prep Time: 5 minutes
Cook Time: N/A
Ready Time: 5 minutes

1 pound ginger, as fresh, plump, and moist as possible
1 quart seltzer or still water
½ cup freshly squeezed lemon juice
1 teaspoon stevia powder

1. To make ginger juice, cut the ginger into pieces about the size of a cherry. Combine ginger with 3 cups water in a blender and blend until the mixture is smooth, without any solid pieces.
2. Pour this mixture into a cheesecloth-lined sieve over a bowl.
3. Separate the juice from the pulp and put the pulp aside for the compost.
4. Combine ½ cup ginger juice with 1 quart seltzer water or still water, lemon juice, and stevia.
5. Place leftover ginger juice in a small container and refrigerate; use within a week. You may also pour the leftover ginger juice into ice cube trays, freeze, and then place the cubes in a freezer bag for future use.

Nutrition Facts

Serving Size: 1 cup
Servings: 4

AMOUNT PER SERVING
Calories: 35
Calories from Fat: 0

	AMOUNT PER SERVING	% DAILY VALUE
Total Fat:	0 g	0%
Saturated Fat:	0 g	0%
Trans Fat:	0 g	
Cholesterol:	0 mg	0%
Sodium:	5 mg	0%
Total Carbohydrate:	8 g	3%
Dietary Fiber:	1 g	4%
Sugars:	1 g	
Protein:	1 g	<1%

GOOD SOURCE OF: vitamin C

Tropical Green Smoothie

Looking for a fast, vitally energizing breakfast or afternoon pick-me-up? This refreshing smoothie combines nutrient-rich spinach with sweet fresh pineapple and cooling cucumber and mint. Pureeing rather than juicing these ingredients preserves all their valuable natural fiber, so you'll feel satisfied the healthy way.

Serves: 2
    Serving Size: 1 cup
    Prep Time: 5 minutes
    Cook Time: N/A
    Ready Time: 5 minutes

    2 cups firmly packed fresh spinach
    1½ cups peeled and chopped pineapple
    ¾ cup peeled and chopped cucumber
    ¾ cup lightly packed fresh mint
    ¾ cup ice (about 6 ice cubes)
    1 teaspoon lemon juice
    Liquid or powdered stevia (optional)

1. Combine spinach, pineapple, cucumber, mint, ½ cup water, ice, and lemon juice in a blender. Blend on high speed until smooth. Taste and add a small amount of stevia for sweetening if necessary.

Nutrition Facts

Serving Size: 1 cup
Servings: 2 servings

AMOUNT PER SERVING
Calories: 90
Calories from Fat: 36

	AMOUNT PER SERVING	% DAILY VALUE
Total Fat:	4 g	6%
Saturated Fat:	0 g	0%
Trans Fat:	0 g	
Cholesterol:	0 mg	0%
Sodium:	51 mg	2%
Total Carbohydrate:	21 g	7%
Dietary Fiber:	4 g	16%
Sugars:	13 g	
Protein:	3 g	6%

EXCELLENT SOURCE OF: vitamin C, vitamin A, vitamin K, folate

GOOD SOURCE OF: fiber, calcium, iron, magnesium, copper

Caffree Mocha

Love creamy coffee-shop drinks? This Caffree Mocha offers warm choc-olaty pleasure without the jitters of caffeine. Instead, you'll get healthy plant-based nutrition from soy milk, cocoa powder, and just a hint of stevia, maple syrup, or turbinado sugar for sweetening. Look in the natural-foods section of your favorite grocery store for caffeine-free roasted-grain beverage powders.

Serves: 2

Serving Size: 1 cup
Prep Time: 1 minutes
Cook Time: 4 minutes
Ready Time: 5 minutes

2 cups unsweetened soy milk
1 tablespoon unsweetened cocoa powder
1 tablespoon roasted-grain beverage powder (such as Kaffree Roma)
¾ teaspoon vanilla extract
Pinch stevia powder or turbinado sugar, or a few drops pure maple syrup

1. In a small heavy-bottomed pot over medium-low heat, whisk soy milk, cocoa powder, roasted-grain beverage powder, vanilla, and stevia, sugar, or maple syrup together. Cook, whisking frequently, until mixture is smooth and hot. Remove from heat just before it reaches a simmer.

Nutrition Facts

Serving Size: 1 cup
Servings: 2

AMOUNT PER SERVING
Calories: 90
Calories from Fat: 36

	AMOUNT PER SERVING	% DAILY VALUE
Total Fat:	4 g	6%
Saturated Fat:	0 g	0%
Trans Fat:	0 g	
Cholesterol:	0 mg	0%
Sodium:	477 mg	20%
Total Carbohydrate:	6 g	2%
Dietary Fiber:	2 g	8%
Sugars:	1 g	
Protein:	8 g	16%

EXCELLENT SOURCE OF: vitamins B_1, B_{12}, calcium
GOOD SOURCE OF: vitamin A

Caffreecino

Enjoy a warm cup of this caffeine-free coffee alternative at any time of day. Since it contains no caffeine or sugar, this caffreecino is great served after dinner or even just before bed. Using soy milk and your favorite roasted-grain beverage powder, you can have this creamy, vanilla-scented hot drink ready in minutes.

Serves: 2
   Serving Size: 1 cup
   Prep Time: 1 minute
   Cook Time: 4 minutes
   Ready Time: 5 minutes

   2 cups unsweetened soy milk
   2 teaspoons roasted-grain beverage powder (such as Kaffree Roma)
   ¼ teaspoon vanilla extract
   ¼ teaspoon powdered stevia

1. In a small heavy-bottomed pot over medium-low heat, combine soy milk, roasted-grain beverage powder, vanilla, and stevia. Cook, stirring frequently, until mixture is warm; remove from heat just before it reaches a simmer. Taste and adjust with additional beverage powder, vanilla, and/or stevia.

Variation

For a Hot Chocolate Caffreecino, whisk into the soy milk mixture 2 teaspoons unsweetened cocoa powder along with an additional ¼ teaspoon vanilla extract and ¼ teaspoon stevia. Heat as directed.

Nutrition Facts

Serving Size: 1 cup
Servings: 2

AMOUNT PER SERVING
Calories: 82
Calories from Fat: 36

	AMOUNT PER SERVING	% DAILY VALUE
Total Fat:	4 g	6%
Saturated Fat:	0 g	0%
Trans Fat:	0 g	
Cholesterol:	0 mg	0%
Sodium:	85 mg	4%
Total Carbohydrate:	5 g	2%
Dietary Fiber:	1 g	4%
Sugars:	1 g	
Protein:	7 g	14%

EXCELLENT SOURCE OF: vitamins B_2, B_{12}, calcium
GOOD SOURCE OF: vitamin A

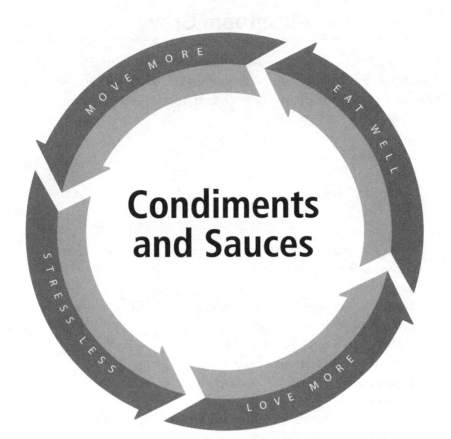

Condiments
and Sauces

MOVE MORE

EAT WELL

STRESS LESS

LOVE MORE

Mushroom Gravy

Enjoy all the creamy goodness of traditional mushroom gravy, without the fat! If creminis are not available, you can use white button mushrooms, or a mixture of your favorite wild mushrooms.

Serves: 8
Serving Size: ¼ cup
Prep Time: 5 minutes
Cook Time: 20 minutes
Ready Time: 25 minutes

4 cups (8 ounces) thinly sliced cremini mushrooms (or use any combination of mushrooms)
⅓ cup finely chopped shallots
2 tablespoons Bragg Liquid Aminos or reduced-sodium tamari
2 cups unsweetened soy milk
1 tablespoon chopped fresh thyme
¼ teaspoon freshly ground pepper
1½ tablespoons sweet rice flour, arrowroot, or cornstarch

1. In a heavy-bottomed saucepan over medium-low heat, sauté the mushrooms, shallots, liquid aminos or tamari, and 2 tablespoons water, stirring frequently, until mushrooms have released their liquid and the liquid has evaporated, 7–10 minutes.
2. Add soy milk, thyme, and pepper. Raise heat to medium, bring to a simmer, and cook for 10 minutes.
3. In a small bowl, whisk sweet rice flour, arrowroot, or cornstarch with 2½ tablespoons water until smooth. Whisk this mixture into mushrooms. Cook, stirring constantly, until mixture thickens and loses any raw starch taste, 2–3 minutes. If mixture becomes too thick, thin with a little more soy milk.
4. Taste for seasoning, adding more liquid aminos or tamari and/or pepper to taste. Serve warm.

Nutrition Facts

Serving Size: ¼ cup
Servings: 8

AMOUNT PER SERVING
Calories: 35
Calories from Fat: 9

	AMOUNT PER SERVING	% DAILY VALUE
Total Fat:	1 g	2%
Saturated Fat:	0 g	0%
Trans Fat:	0 g	
Cholesterol:	0 mg	0%
Sodium:	260 mg	11%
Total Carbohydrate:	5 g	2%
Dietary Fiber:	1 g	4%
Sugars:	1 g	
Protein:	3 g	6%

GOOD SOURCE OF: vitamin B_2

Lemon Miso Dressing

This tangy, Asian-inspired dressing uses high-protein, high-fiber white beans in place of oil. It's best made a few hours in advance, so it can be fully infused with the flavors of the ginger and garlic.

Serves: 8
Serving Size: 2 tablespoons
Prep Time: 5 minutes
Cook Time: N/A
Ready Time: 5 minutes

⅓ cup canned white beans, rinsed and drained
⅓ cup water
3 tablespoons sweet or mellow white miso (such as Miso Master)
3 tablespoons lemon juice
2 teaspoons pure maple syrup
1 teaspoon finely chopped fresh ginger
½ teaspoon minced garlic
⅛ teaspoon freshly ground pepper

1. Place all ingredients in a blender. Starting on low speed and gradually increasing speed to high, blend until smooth. Taste for seasoning and add more garlic or ginger as needed.

Chef's Notes

Miso is a thick, tangy paste typically made from fermented soybeans. White miso is fermented for a shorter time than yellow or red miso, so it is milder in flavor and less salty. However, sodium levels can vary depending on the brand. We recommend starting with 3 tablespoons and adjusting to suit your taste. If you prefer a milder flavor, add another tablespoon of white beans along with an additional tablespoon of water.

Nutrition Facts

Serving Size: 2 tablespoons
Servings: 8

AMOUNT PER SERVING
Calories: 27
Calories from Fat: 0

	AMOUNT PER SERVING	**% DAILY VALUE**
Total Fat:	0 g	0%
Saturated Fat:	0 g	0%
Trans Fat:	0 g	
Cholesterol:	0 mg	0%
Sodium:	156 mg	7%
Total Carbohydrate:	5 g	2%
Dietary Fiber:	0.5 g	0%
Sugars:	2 g	
Protein:	1 g	2%

Chipotle Mayo

Made with silken tofu, this voluptuous, vegan mayonnaise is both oil- and egg-free. Chipotle peppers are jalapeño peppers that have been smoked and dried. They are readily available canned in tangy, vinegar-based adobo sauce. They add a smoky kick and a tingle of heat.

Serves: 16
Serving Size: 1 tablespoon
Prep Time: 5 minutes
Cook Time: N/A
Ready Time: 5 minutes

12 ounces firm silken tofu
2 tablespoons lime juice plus more to taste
1 tablespoon pure maple syrup
1 teaspoon chipotles in adobo sauce, plus more to taste
½ teaspoon minced garlic
½ teaspoon chili powder
¼ teaspoon fine sea salt
¼ teaspoon smoked paprika

1. In a food processor fitted with a metal blade, combine all the ingredients and 1 tablespoon water. Process until creamy. Taste for seasoning, adding more lime juice, chipotles, and/or salt if desired. If too thick, add a little more water.

Nutrition Facts

Serving Size: 1 tablespoon
Servings: 16

AMOUNT PER SERVING
Calories: 20
Calories from Fat: 9

	AMOUNT PER SERVING	% DAILY VALUE
Total Fat:	1 g	2%
Saturated Fat:	0 g	0%
Trans Fat:	0 g	
Cholesterol:	0 mg	0%
Sodium:	87 mg	4%
Total Carbohydrate:	2 g	1%
Dietary Fiber:	0 g	0%
Sugars:	1 g	
Protein:	2 g	4%

Vegan Mayo

This recipe transforms this classic condiment into a heart-healthy spread. By substituting firm silken tofu for the usual egg yolk and oil, the saturated fat and cholesterol drop away, leaving heart-healthy plant protein and a mix of cardioprotective antioxidants.

Serves: 12

Serving Size: 1 tablespoon
Prep: 5 minutes
Ready: 5 minutes

12 ounces firm silken tofu
2 tablespoons fresh lemon juice
1½ teaspoons Dijon mustard
1 teaspoon onion powder
½ teaspoon garlic powder
⅛ teaspoon powdered stevia, or ¾ teaspoon pure maple syrup
⅛ teaspoon fine sea salt
⅛ teaspoon freshly ground pepper

1. In a food processor fitted with a metal blade, blend all ingredients until creamy. Taste for seasoning and add more lemon juice and/or salt as needed.

Chef's Notes

Silken tofu has a delicate, custardy texture that's very different from regular tofu. Different brands of silken tofu can vary greatly in flavor and texture. We've had very good results using Morinaga's Mori-Nu firm silken tofu. Look for it in aseptic (non-refrigerated) packages in the Asian foods section of your grocery store. You can also order it directly from Morinaga or other online retailers.

Nutrition Facts

Serving Size: 1 tablespoon
Servings: 12

AMOUNT PER SERVING
Calories: 20
Calories from Fat: 9

	AMOUNT PER SERVING	% DAILY VALUE
Total Fat:	1 g	2%
Saturated Fat:	0 g	0%
Trans Fat:	0 g	0%
Cholesterol:	0 mg	0%
Sodium:	50 mg	2%
Total Carbohydrate:	1 g	0%
Dietary Fiber:	0 g	0%
Sugars:	0 g	0%
Protein:	2 g	4%

EXCELLENT SOURCE OF: vitamin C

GOOD SOURCE OF: vitamin A, iron

Basil Mayo

Made from a base of silken tofu, this vibrantly green, flavorful vegan mayonnaise has no added fat and makes a great sandwich spread or vegetable dip. It's best used within a day of being made.

Serves: 28
Serving Size: 1 tablespoon
Prep: 5 minutes
Ready: 5 minutes

12 ounces firm silken tofu
2 tablespoons fresh lemon juice
1 teaspoon Dijon mustard
⅛ teaspoon stevia
1 teaspoon onion powder
¾ teaspoon garlic powder
¼ teaspoon fine sea salt
⅛ teaspoon freshly ground pepper
¾ cup firmly packed fresh basil

1. Place tofu, lemon juice, mustard, stevia, onion powder, garlic powder, salt, and pepper in a blender or in a food processor fitted with a metal blade. Blend on medium speed until mixture is creamy.
2. Add basil and blend or process again until basil is completely pureed and mixture is bright green. If mayonnaise seems too thick, add 2–3 tablespoons water. Cover and refrigerate until needed.

Chef's Notes

Widely used for vegan desserts, dips, and spreads, silken tofu has a delicate, custardy texture that's very different from regular tofu. Different brands of silken tofu can vary greatly in flavor and texture. We've had best results using Morinaga's Mori-Nu firm silken tofu. Look for it in aseptic (non-refrigerated) packages in the Asian foods section of your grocery store. You can also order it directly from Morinaga or other online retailers.

Nutrition Facts

Serving Size: 1 tablespoon
Servings: 28

AMOUNT PER SERVING
Calories: 10
Calories from Fat: 0

	AMOUNT PER SERVING	% DAILY VALUE
Total Fat:	0 g	9%
Saturated Fat:	0 g	5%
Trans Fat:	0 g	
Cholesterol:	0 mg	0%
Sodium:	30 mg	6%
Total Carbohydrate:	1 g	15%
Dietary Fiber:	0 g	36%
Sugars:	0 g	
Protein:	1 g	36%

Tofu Hollandaise Sauce

Planning a festive brunch? With this lemony-bright, cholesterol-free sauce on hand, you're ready to turn any breakfast dish into a special occasion. Try using it to dress up an egg-white scramble or frittata; it's also wonderful as an accompaniment to steamed asparagus or broccoli. Add a few sprigs of fresh tarragon, dill, and/or basil to make a vibrant herbed hollandaise.

Serves: 8

Serving Size: 3 tablespoons
Prep: 10 minutes
Cook: 2 minutes
Ready: 12 minutes

16 ounces silken tofu, drained and patted dry
2 tablespoons nutritional yeast
1 tablespoon white miso or chickpea miso (see Chef's Notes)
½ teaspoon lemon zest
1½ tablespoons fresh lemon juice
¼ teaspoon dry mustard
¼ teaspoon fine sea salt
¼ teaspoon freshly ground pepper
¼ teaspoon turmeric
Pinch cayenne or dash of hot sauce (optional)

1. Break tofu into chunks. Using a food processor fitted with a metal blade, pulse tofu, nutritional yeast, 2 tablespoons water, miso, lemon zest, lemon juice, dry mustard, salt, pepper, and turmeric until mixture is smooth and creamy. Taste for seasoning and add cayenne or hot sauce, if desired. Refrigerate until needed. (Mixture can be prepared up to this point and refrigerated for up to 3 days before serving.)
2. Just before serving, spoon the sauce into a double boiler or small heavy-bottomed saucepan. Over low heat, warm the sauce, stirring frequently. Remove from heat as soon as sauce is warmed. Thin with additional water if necessary.

Chef's Notes

Miso is a thick, tangy paste typically made from fermented soybeans. White miso, also called shiro or sweet miso, is fermented for a shorter time than yellow or red miso. It is mild in flavor and less salty. If you are reducing your soy intake, look for miso made from chickpeas at some natural foods stores.

Nutrition Facts

Serving Size: 3 tablespoons
Servings: 8

AMOUNT PER SERVING
Calories: 40
Calories from Fat: 9

	AMOUNT PER SERVING	% DAILY VALUE
Total Fat:	1 g	2%
Saturated Fat:	0 g	0%
Trans Fat:	0 g	
Cholesterol:	0 mg	0%
Sodium:	141 mg	6%
Total Carbohydrate:	2 g	1%
Dietary Fiber:	1 g	4%
Sugars:	0 g	
Protein:	4 g	8%

EXCELLENT SOURCE OF: vitamins B_1, B_2, B_3, B_6
GOOD SOURCE OF: vitamin B_{12}

Smoky Chipotle Sauce

This versatile, no-cook sauce adds punchy flavor to so many dishes. It's sweet, spicy, and smoky, thanks to a mixture of chipotle peppers, roasted red peppers, and prunes, and it keeps well in the refrigerator. Chipotle peppers are dried and smoked jalapeños; look for them canned in adobo, a tangy, vinegar-based sauce, in the Latino/Hispanic foods section of your supermarket. An easy, oil-free roasted garlic puree adds complexity, while prunes bring sweetness, body, and heart-healthy fiber and nutrients.

Serves: 18
    Serving Size: 2 tablespoons
    Prep Time: 5 minutes
    Cook Time: N/A
    Ready Time: 5 minutes

1 cup roasted red peppers, drained
¾ cup pitted prunes
¼ cup Roasted Garlic puree (page 410)
2 tablespoons chipotle peppers in adobo sauce
2 tablespoons balsamic vinegar; for a slightly less sweet sauce, use red wine vinegar
1 tablespoon fresh lime juice
1 teaspoon fine sea salt

1. In a food processor fitted with a metal blade, combine all ingredients and add ⅓ cup hot water. Process until smooth. Cover and refrigerate until serving.

Nutrition Facts

Serving Size: 2 tablespoons
Servings: 18

AMOUNT PER SERVING
Calories: 31
Calories from Fat: 0

	AMOUNT PER SERVING	% DAILY VALUE
Total Fat:	0 g	0%
Saturated Fat:	0 g	0%
Trans Fat:	0 g	
Cholesterol:	0 mg	0%
Sodium:	142 mg	6%
Total Carbohydrate:	7 g	2%
Dietary Fiber:	1 g	4%
Sugars:	3 g	
Protein:	1 g	2%

GOOD SOURCE OF: vitamin C

Edamole

A dip made from edamame (green soybeans), peas, silken tofu, and fresh herbs may not sound like a tailgate party's delight, but trust us: this creative spin on guacamole is a winner. Put out a bowl of this creamy green dip surrounded by carrot and cucumber sticks, red bell pepper wedges, endive leaves, and sugar snap peas, and let the compliments roll in. This dip can be made 1–2 days in advance and refrigerated until needed.

Serves: 8
   Serving Size: ¼ cup
   Prep Time: 10 minutes
   Cook Time: N/A
   Ready Time: 10 minutes

   1½ cups frozen shelled edamame (green soybeans)
   1 cup frozen peas
   ¾ cup silken tofu
   ¼ cup chopped cilantro or fresh mint
   2 tablespoons fresh lime juice
   ½ tablespoon fine sea salt or to taste
   ½ teaspoon minced garlic
   ½ teaspoon ground cumin
   ¼ teaspoon ground coriander
   3 dashes green hot sauce (optional)

1. Place a vegetable steamer basket in a saucepan and add water to just below bottom of steamer basket. Over high heat, bring water to a boil. Place edamame in steamer basket, cover, and let steam for 2 minutes. Add peas. Continue steaming for about 3 more minutes, until both edamame and peas are tender and bright green.
2. Remove steamer basket from saucepan. Transfer edamame and peas to a strainer and rinse with cold water. Let drain, then pat dry with a paper towel to remove excess moisture.
3. In a food processor fitted with a metal blade, combine edamame, peas, tofu, cilantro or mint, lime juice, 2 tablespoons water, salt,

garlic, cumin, coriander, and hot sauce, if using. Pulse until ingredients form a smooth, thick paste, scraping down the sides of the bowl with a rubber spatula.

4. Taste for seasoning and add more salt, spices, lime juice, or hot sauce, as needed. Serve as a dip with an assortment of raw vegetables or nonfat whole-grain crackers, or use as a sandwich spread.

Chef's Notes

Steaming the edamame and peas brightens their flavor, but if you are short on time, you can skip steps 1 and 2. Thaw edamame and peas and begin with step 3.

Nutrition Facts

Serving Size: ¼ cup
Servings: 8

AMOUNT PER SERVING
Calories: 64
Calories from Fat: 18

	AMOUNT PER SERVING	% DAILY VALUE
Total Fat:	2 g	3%
Saturated Fat:	0 g	0%
Trans Fat:	0 g	
Cholesterol:	0 mg	0%
Sodium:	174 mg	7%
Total Carbohydrate:	7 g	2%
Dietary Fiber:	3 g	12%
Sugars:	2 g	
Protein:	5 g	10%

GOOD SOURCE OF: vitamin A, fiber

Roasted Garlic

Roasted garlic cloves pack a big flavor punch without the "bite" of raw garlic. They are easy to make at home, with no added oil. To make this recipe even easier, you can start with pre-peeled garlic cloves from the supermarket. The puree can be frozen in ice cube trays and stored in the freezer until needed.

Serves: 13

Serving Size: 1 tablespoon
Prep Time: 15 minutes
Cook Time: 1 hour
Ready Time: 1 hour 15 minutes

1½ cups peeled garlic cloves (8 ounces)

1. Preheat oven to 375°F.
2. Spread garlic cloves in a baking pan. Cut any large cloves in half to ensure even cooking. Add ⅓ cup water. Cover garlic loosely with parchment paper.
3. Roast garlic until largest cloves are soft enough to mash easily, and cloves have a light yellow to golden color. Start checking after 35 minutes; continue roasting garlic up to 15 more minutes if necessary, being careful not to let the cloves brown or burn. Add more water if the bottom of the pan is too dry. Ultimately, all the water will evaporate by the time the cloves appear golden brown.
4. Remove the garlic from the oven. Let cool, then refrigerate until needed.
5. To make roasted garlic puree, mash cloves thoroughly with a fork or blend in a food processor, adding up to 2 tablespoons of water as necessary to make a smooth puree. This recipe will make ⅔ cup puree.

Chef's Notes

For long storage, freeze roasted garlic puree in ice cube trays until solid. Pack the cubes in freezer bags. Keep frozen until needed.

Nutrition Facts

Serving Size: 1 tablespoon
Servings: 13

AMOUNT PER SERVING
Calories: 28
Calories from Fat: 0

	AMOUNT PER SERVING	% DAILY VALUE
Total Fat:	0 g	0%
Saturated Fat:	0 g	0%
Trans Fat:	0 g	
Cholesterol:	0 mg	0%
Sodium:	4 mg	0%
Total Carbohydrate:	6 g	2%
Dietary Fiber:	0 g	0%
Sugars:	0 g	
Protein:	1 g	2%

GOOD SOURCE OF: vitamin B_6

Hummus

Hummus is a delicious, nutritious way to add heart-healthy plant protein and cholesterol-reducing fiber to your diet. We've updated this Ornish Kitchen hummus with fresh and fragrant green herbs, lowering the fat and calories by leaving out the usual high-fat tahini (sesame seed paste) and olive oil. Serve this creamy hummus as a dip with whole-grain pita chips and fresh vegetables, or use as a base for a sandwich or wrap.

Serves: 10
Serving Size: ¼ cup
Prep Time: 5 minutes
Cook Time: N/A
Ready Time: 5 minutes

3 cups cooked or 2 cans (15 ounces each) no-salt-added chickpeas, rinsed and drained
1½ tablespoons lemon juice
2 teaspoons ground cumin
1½ teaspoons ground coriander
1 teaspoon minced garlic
½ teaspoon fine sea salt
¼ teaspoon freshly ground pepper
2 tablespoons chopped fresh herbs, such as mint, cilantro, or rosemary (optional) (see Chef's Notes)
Paprika, for garnish

1. Place chickpeas, ½ cup water, lemon juice, cumin, coriander, garlic, salt, and pepper in a food processor fitted with a metal blade. Process until smooth and creamy, adding more water as needed to achieve desired consistency.
2. Add fresh herbs, if using. Pulse briefly to incorporate; herbs should speckle the mixture rather than turn it completely green.
3. Spoon hummus into a serving bowl. Sprinkle with paprika before serving.

Chef's Notes

In addition to trying different herbs, you can add infused salts, such as truffle salt, or sauces, such as sriracha, to create different types of hummus.

Nutrition Facts

Serving Size: ¼ cup
Servings: 10

AMOUNT PER SERVING
Calories: 83
Calories from Fat: 9

	AMOUNT PER SERVING	% DAILY VALUE
Total Fat:	1 g	2%
Saturated Fat:	0 g	0%
Trans Fat:	0 g	
Cholesterol:	0 mg	0%
Sodium:	136 mg	6%
Total Carbohydrate:	14 g	5%
Dietary Fiber:	3 g	12%
Sugars:	1 g	
Protein:	4 g	8%

Red Enchilada Sauce

Many commercial enchilada sauces include added oils. Instead, you can make your own using flavorful, mild New Mexico chiles. Look for dried chiles in the Latino/Hispanic foods section of your supermarket.

Serves: 4

Serving Size: ¾ cup
Prep Time: 10 minutes
Cook Time: 25 minutes
Ready Time: 35 minutes

2 ounces dried New Mexico chiles (about 10 peppers), stems and seeds removed
1½ cups chopped onion
2 medium garlic cloves, sliced
¼ teaspoon fine sea salt
1 tablespoon lime juice
1 tablespoon pure maple syrup

1. Combine dried chiles, onions, garlic, 3½ cups water, and salt in a medium saucepan over high heat. Bring to a boil. Reduce heat and simmer, stirring occasionally, until onions and chiles are soft, about 25 minutes. Remove from heat.
2. Working in batches as needed, pour mixture into a blender. Add lime juice and maple syrup. Starting on lowest speed, puree mixture until smooth. Enchilada sauce can be prepared up to 14 days in advance. Let cool, transfer to a covered container, and store in the refrigerator until needed.

Nutrition Facts

Serving Size: ¾ cup
Servings: 4

AMOUNT PER SERVING
Calories: 356
Calories from Fat: 54

	AMOUNT PER SERVING	% DAILY VALUE
Total Fat:	0 g	0%
Saturated Fat:	0 g	0%
Trans Fat:	0 g	
Cholesterol:	0 mg	0%
Sodium:	164 mg	7%
Total Carbohydrate:	17 g	6%
Dietary Fiber:	3 g	12%
Sugars:	10 g	
Protein:	5 g	10%

EXCELLENT SOURCE OF: fiber, vitamin A, vitamin B_6, vitamin C

GOOD SOURCE OF: folate, iron, calcium, potassium

Appendix A

Two Weeks of Recommended Packaged Foods

If it seems a little overwhelming to make big changes in your way of eating, here is a listing of two weeks' worth of commercially available breakfasts, lunches, dinners, and snacks that fit our guidelines, as well as frozen entrées you can order online or find in many stores. (We don't have any financial relationships with these vendors; this is just presented for your convenience.)

If you eat just these foods for just a week or so, because the underlying biological mechanisms we've been discussing are so dynamic, you're likely to feel so much better, so quickly, you'll be that much more motivated to learn how to shop and cook meals on your own. At that point, you can include these prepared meals on a less frequent basis, perhaps just after a long day of work or a busy weekend.

They'll show you that foods can be familiar, delicious, *and* health-promoting. And you'll make the connection between what you eat and how you feel because it comes from your own experience: "When I eat this, I feel really good; when I eat that, not so good." This helps make it sustainable.

At the time this book was written, all of these foods were available on Amazon.com, and many can be found at other online sites, including Target.com, Vitacost.com, Walmart.com, WholeFoods.com,

GroceryGateway.com, FreshDirect.com, Google Express (express .google.com), and others.

A lot of these can be found in your local supermarket, and most grocery stores will special-order them for you, especially if you let them know that you'll be purchasing them on a regular basis.

Some of these foods are higher in fat or sugar than others, but think in terms of the total amount you're consuming in a given day or over several days rather than in each food item.

Also, if you follow the entire two-week plan, you'll find that some of these days have calorie totals that may fall lower than your individual needs. If you're trying to lose weight, this is a good thing; if not, make your portion sizes a little larger or add some items on your own that fit within our nutritional guidelines.

Appendix B gives you a long list of commercially available foods available in most supermarkets that you can use to stock your pantry and freezer.

DAY 1 FOOD ITEM	BRAND	CALORIES	FAT	SFA	CHOL	SODIUM	CARBS	FIBER	SUGAR	PROTEIN	SERVING SIZE
BREAKFAST											
Oatmeal	Nature's Path	190	1	0.5	0	0	34	6	1	8	1 packet
Soy milk	Silk	80	4	0.5	0	75	4	0	1	7	1 cup
Blueberries	Whole Foods	84	0	0	0	1	21	4	15	1	1 cup
Flax meal	Spectrum Essentials	35	3	0	0	2	2	1.5	0	1.5	1 T
LUNCH											
Gluten Free Beans & Rice Burrito	Amy's	240	6	0.5	0	430	38	5	3	7	1 burrito
Leafy greens	Organic Girl	20	0	0	0	95	3	2	0	2	3 cups
Shredded carrots	365 Organic	15	0	0	0	30	4	1	2	0.5	¾ cup
Green peas	365 Organic	70	0	0	0	0	4	4	4	5	⅔ cup
Walden Farm salad dressing	Walden Farm	0	0	0	0	200	0	0	0	0	2 T
DINNER											
Sweet & Sour Asian Noodle Bowl—Light & Lean	Amy's	250	3	0	0	610	16	3	10	10	1 bowl
Broccoli slaw	365 Organic	15	0	0	0	15	3	1	1	1	½ cup
Leafy greens	Organic Girl	20	0	0	0	95	3	2	0	2	3 cups
Skinny Girl Fat Free Salad Dressings	Skinny Girl	10	0	0	0	90	1	0	0	0	2 T
Walden Farm salad dressing	Walden Farm	0	0	0	0	200	0	0	0	0	2 T
SNACKS											
Fuji apple	Whole Foods	90	0	0	0	0	25	4	18	0.5	1 medium
Petite carrots	365 Organic	21	0	0	0	47	1	1	3	0	6 baby carrots
TJ Black Bean Dip	Trader Joe's	35	0	0	0	210	8	2	1	2	2 T
Whole Grain Wasa Cracker	Wasa	40	0	0	0	50	10	2	0	1	1 cracker
Dry roasted edamame	Seapoint	130	4.5	0.5	0	130	9	7	1	14	¼ cup
TOTAL		1,345	22	2	0	2,277	186	46	60	64	

DAY 2 FOOD ITEM	BRAND	CALORIES	FAT	SFA	CHOL	SODIUM	CARBS	FIBER	SUGAR	PROTEIN	SERVING SIZE
BREAKFAST											
Tofu Scramble in a Pocket Sandwich	Amy's	180	6	0	0	490	23	0	2	11	1 entrée
Blueberries	Whole Foods	84	0	0	0	1	21	4	15	1	1 cup
Flax meal	Spectrum Essentials	35	3	0	0	2	2	1.5	0	1.5	1 T
LUNCH											
Leafy greens	Organic Girl	20	0	0	0	95	3	2	0	2	3 cups
Carrots	365 Organic	21	0	0	0	47	1	1	3	0	6 baby carrots
Green peas	365 Organic	70	0	0	0	0	4	4	4	5	⅓ cup
Skinny Girl Fat Free Salad Dressings	Skinny Girl	10	0	0	0	90	1	0	0	0	2 T
Quarter Pound Veggie Burger	Amy's	210	3.5	0.5	0	600	24	6	6	20	1 burger
Whole-grain bun	Orowheat	170	2.5	0.5		360	32	7	3	7	1 bun
DINNER											
Spaghetti Italiano (Light & Lean)	Amy's	240	5	0.5	0	590	38	5	6	11	1 entrée
Leafy greens	Organic Girl	20	0	0	0	95	3	2	0	2	3 cups
Skinny Girl Fat Free Salad Dressings	Skinny Girl	10	0	0	0	90	1	0	0	0	2 T
Broccoli slaw	365 Organic	15	0	0	0	15	3	1	1	1	½ cup
SNACKS											
Edamame	Cascadian Farms	120	5	0	0	45	9	4	2	10	½ cup
Fuji apple	Whole Foods	90	0	0	0	0	25	4	18	0.5	1 medium
TOTAL		1,220	24	1.5	0	2,348	190	41	57	70	

DAY 3 FOOD ITEM	BRAND	CALORIES	FAT	SFA	CHOL	SODIUM	CARBS	FIBER	SUGAR	PROTEIN	SERVING SIZE
BREAKFAST											
Oatmeal	Nature's Path	190	1	0	0	0	34	6	1	8	1 packet
Soy milk	Silk	80	4	0.5	0	75	4	2	1	7	1 cup
Blueberries	Whole Foods	84	0	0	0	1	21	4	15	1	1 cup
LUNCH											
Lentil Vegetable Soup—Light Sodium	Amy's	320	8	1	0	680	48	16	10	14	1 can
Leafy greens	Organic Girl	20	0	0	0	95	3	2	0	2	3 cups
Broccoli slaw	365 Organic	15	0	0	0	15	3	1	1	1	½ cup
Walden Farm salad dressing	Walden Farm	0	0	0	0	200	0	0	0	0	2 T
Dave's 21 Whole Grain & Seeds Bread	Dave's Killer Bread	120	2	0	0	180	22	5	5	5	1 slice
Orange	Whole Foods	62	0	0	0	0	15	3	12	1	1
DINNER											
Black Bean & Vegetable Enchilada	Amy's	160	6	0.5	0	390	22	4	2	5	1 enchilada
Leafy greens	Organic Girl	20	0	0	0	95	3	2	0	2	3 cups
Walden Farm salad dressing	Walden Farm	0	0	0	0	200	0	0	0	0	2 T
SNACKS											
Edamame	Cascadian Farms	240	10	0	0	90	18	8	4	10	1 cup
Fuji apple	Whole Foods	90	0	0	0	0	25	4	18	0.5	1 medium
TOTAL		1,412	27	2	0	2,241	231	61	71	66	

DAY 4 FOOD ITEM	BRAND	CALORIES	FAT	SFA	CHOL	SODIUM	CARBS	FIBER	SUGAR	PROTEIN	SERVING SIZE
BREAKFAST											
Nature's Path Cereal Optimum Breakfast	Nature's Path	200	3	0	0	230	38	9	9	9	¾ cup
Soy milk	Silk	80	4	0.5	0	75	4	2	1	7	1 cup
Strawberries	Whole Foods	49	0.5	0	0	2	2	3	7	1	1 cup
LUNCH											
Anasazi Burrito	Sweet Earth	340	5	0	0	640	58	6	4	18	1 burrito (198 g)
Leafy greens	Organic Girl	20	0	0	0	95	3	2	0	2	3 cups
Walden Farm salad dressing	Walden Farm	0	0	0	0	200	0	0	0	0	2 T
Shredded carrots	365 Organic	15	0	0	0	30	4	1	2	0.5	¾ cup
DINNER											
Teriyaki Bowl	Amy's	290	4.5	0.5	0	780	52	6	15	12	1 entrée (269 g)
Leafy greens	Organic Girl	20	0	0	0	95	3	2	0	2	3 cups
Carrots	365 Organic	21	0	0	0	47	1	1	3	0	6 baby carrots
Green peas	365 Organic	70	0	0	0	0	4	4	4	5	⅔ cup
Walden Farm salad dressing	Walden Farm	0	0	0	0	200	0	0	0	0	2 T
SNACKS											
Dry roasted edamame	Seapoint	130	4.5	0.5	0	130	9	7	1	14	¼ cup
Apple	Whole Foods	93	0	0	0	2	25	4	19	0.5	1
Orange	Whole Foods	62	0	0	0	0	15	3	12	1	1
TOTAL		1,390	22	1	0	2,526	218	50	77	72	

DAY 5 FOOD ITEM	BRAND	CALORIES	FAT	SFA	CHOL	SODIUM	CARBS	FIBER	SUGAR	PROTEIN	SERVING SIZE
BREAKFAST											
Oatmeal	Nature's Path	190	1	0	0	0	34	6	1	8	1 packet
Soy milk	Silk	80	4	0.5	0	75	4	2	1	7	1 cup
Blueberries	Whole Foods	84	0	0	0	1	21	4	15	1	1 cup
Flax meal	Spectrum Essentials	70	6	0.5	0	5	4	3	0	3	2 T
LUNCH											
Organic Minestrone Soup	Amy's	90	1.5	0	0	580	17	3	5	3	1 cup (245 g)
Leafy greens	Organic Girl	20	0	0	0	95	3	2	0	2	3 cups
Carrots	365 Organic	21	0	0	0	47	1	1	3	0	6 baby carrots
Green peas	365 Organic	70	0	0	0	0	4	4	4	5	⅔ cup
Walden Farm salad dressing	Walden Farm	0	0	0	0	200	0	0	0	0	2 T
Wasa Crispbread, multi-grain	Wasa	80	0	0	0	100	20	4	0	2	
DINNER											
Indian Mattar Tofu	Amy's	280	8	1	0	680	40	5	5	12	1 entrée
Leafy greens	Organic Girl	20	0	0	0	95	3	2	0	2	3 cups
Walden Farm salad dressing	Walden Farm	0	0	0	0	200	0	0	0	0	2 T
Pear	Whole Foods	120	0	0	0	0	29	6	18	1	1
SNACKS											
Edamame	Cascadian Farms	180	7	0	0	15	13	4	3	15	1 cup
Apple	Whole Foods	90	0	0	0	0	25	4	18	0.5	1 med
TOTALS		1,395	27	2	0	2,092	197	40	58	62	

DAY 6 FOOD ITEM	BRAND	CALORIES	FAT	SFA	CHOL	SODIUM	CARBS	FIBER	SUGAR	PROTEIN	SERVING SIZE
BREAKFAST											
Nature's Path Cereal Optimum Breakfast	Nature's Path	200	2	0	0	230	38	9	9	9	¾ cup
Soy milk	Silk	80	4	0.5	0	75	4	2	1	7	1 cup
Flax meal	Spectrum Essentials	35	3	0	0	0	2	1.5	0	1.5	1 T
Strawberries	Whole Foods	49	0.5	0	0	2	2	3	7	1	1 cup
LUNCH											
Leafy greens	Organic Girl	20	0	0	0	95	3	2	0	2	3 cups
Walden Farm salad dressing	Walden Farm	0	0	0	0	200	0	0	0	0	2 T
Broccoli slaw	365 Organic	15	0	0	0	15	3	1	1	1	½ cup
Whole-grain bun	Orowheat	170	2.5	0	0	360	32	7	3	7	1 bun
Quarter Pounder Veggie Burger	Amy's	210	3.5	0.5	0	600	24	6	6	20	1 burger
Orange	Whole Foods	62	0	0	0	0	15	3	12	1	1
DINNER											
Leafy greens	Organic Girl	20	0	0	0	95	3	2	0	2	3 cups
Skinny Girl Fat Free Salad Dressings	Skinny Girl	10	0	0	0	90	1	0	0	0	2 T
Roasted Vegetable Pizza	Amy's	280	9	1.5	0	540	42	3	5	7	⅓ pizza (113 g)
Garbanzo beans	365 Organic	120	2	0	0	85	20	6	1	6	½ cup
Broccoli slaw	365 Organic	15	0	0	0	15	3	1	1	1	½ cup
SNACKS											
Fuji apple	Whole Foods	90	0	0	0	0	25	4	18	0.5	1 med
Petite carrots	365 Organic	21	0	0	0	47	1	1	3	0	6 baby carrots
TJ Black Bean Dip	Trader Joe's	70	0	0	0	420	16	4	2	4	¼ cup
Wasa Crispbread, multi-grain	Wasa	80	0	0	0	100	20	4	0	1	2 crackers
TOTAL		1,547	26	2.5	0	2,969	253	59	69	71	

DAY 7 FOOD ITEM	BRAND	CALORIES	FAT	SFA	CHOL	SODIUM	CARBS	FIBER	SUGAR	PROTEIN	SERVING SIZE
BREAKFAST											
Breakfast Burrito	Amy's	270	8	1	0	540	38	6	3	12	1 burrito
Strawberries	Whole Foods	49	0.5	0	0	2	2	3	7	1	1 cup
Soy milk	Silk	80	4	0.5	0	75	4	0	1	7	1 cup
LUNCH											
Brown Rice & Lentils	Tasty Bite	240	5	2	0	780	64	10	0	12	full pack, 2 servings
Shredded carrots	365 Organic	15	0	0	0	30	4	1	2	0.5	¾ cup
Leafy greens	Organic Girl	20	0	0	0	95	3	2	0	2	3 cups
Walden Farm salad dressing	Walden Farm	0	0	0	0	200	0	0	0	0	2 T
DINNER											
Sweet Potato Quinoa Bowl	Kashi	270	6	1	0	280	48	12	11	9	1 entrée
Leafy greens	Organic Girl	20	0	0	0	95	3	2	0	2	3 cups
Broccoli slaw	365 Organic	15	0	0	0	15	3	1	1	1	½ cup
Walden Farm salad dressing	Walden Farm	0	0	0	0	200	0	0	0	0	2 T
SNACKS											
Dry roasted edamame	Seapoint	130	4.5	0.5	0	130	9	7	1	14	¼ cup
Apple	Whole Foods	93	0	0	0	2	25	4	19	0.5	1
Orange	Whole Foods	62	0	0	0	0	15	3	12	1	1
TOTALS		1,264	28	5	0	2,444	218	51	57	62	

DAY 8 FOOD ITEM	BRAND	CALORIES	FAT	SFA	CHOL	SODIUM	CARBS	FIBER	SUGAR	PROTEIN	SERVING SIZE
BREAKFAST											
Kind raspberry granola	Kind	190	3	0	0	60	37	3	5	4	½ cup
Soy milk	Silk	80	4	0.5	0	75	4	2	1	7	1 cup
Blackberries	Whole Foods	62	0	0	0	1	15	8	7	2	1 cup
LUNCH											
Light & Lean Quinoa & Black Beans with Butternut Squash & Chard	Amy's	240	5	0.5	0	440	38	11	6	10	1 bowl
Leafy greens	Organic Girl	20	0	0	0	95	3	2	0	2	3 cups
Carrots	365 Organic	21	0	0	0	47	1	1	3	0	6 baby carrots
Green peas	365 Organic	70	0	0	0	0	4	4	4	5	⅔ cup
Skinny Girl Fat Free Salad Dressings	Skinny Girl	10	0	0	0	90	1	0	0	0	2 T
DINNER											
Sweet Potato Quinoa Bowl	Kashi	270	6	1	0	280	48	12	11	9	1 entrée
Orange	Whole Foods	62	0	0	0	0	15	3	12	1	1
SNACKS											
Dry roasted edamame	Whole Foods	260	9	1	0	260	18	14	2	28	½ cup
Apple	Whole Foods	93	0	0	0	2	25	4	19	0.5	1
TOTALS		1,378	27	3	0	2,444	218	51	57	69	

DAY 9 FOOD ITEM	BRAND	CALORIES	FAT	SFA	CHOL	SODIUM	CARBS	FIBER	SUGAR	PROTEIN	SERVING SIZE
BREAKFAST											
Oatmeal	Nature's Path	190	1	0.5	0	0	34	6	1	8	1 packet
Soy milk	Silk	80	4	0.5	0	75	4	2	1	7	1 cup
Blueberries	Whole Foods	84	0	0	0	1	21	4	15	1	1 cup
Flax meal	Spectrum Essentials	70	6	0.5	0	5	4	3	0	3	2 T
LUNCH											
Organic Low-fat Black Bean Chili	Amy's	200	3	0	0	680	31	13	3	13	1 cup
Quinoa with Vegetables	365	140	2	0	0	10	27	3	2	5	1 serving
Leafy greens	Organic Girl	20	0	0	0	95	3	2	0	2	3 cups
Broccoli slaw	365 Organic	15	0	0	0	15	3	1	1	1	½ cup
Grape tomatoes	Organic Greenhouse	15	0	0	0	10	3	1	2	1	8
Skinny Girl Fat Free Salad Dressings	Skinny Girl	10	0	0	0	90	1	0	0	0	2 T
DINNER											
Meatless Veggie Meatballs	Amy's	200	5	0.5	0	550	24	3	3	14	8 (85 g)
Whole grain pasta	Barilla	180	1.5	0	0	0	39	7	1	8	2 oz
Pasta sauce, tomato basil	Classico	60	2	0	0	430	8	2	4	2	½ cup
Leafy greens	Organic Girl	20	0	0	0	95	3	2	0	2	3 cups
Skinny Girl Fat Free Salad Dressings	Skinny Girl	10	0	0	0	90	1	0	0	0	2 T
Shredded carrots	365 Organic	15	0	0	0	30	4	1	2	0.5	¾ cup
SNACKS											
Fuji apple	Whole Foods	90	0	0	0	0	25	4	18	0.5	1 medium
Petite carrots	365 Organic	21	0	0	0	47	1	1	3	0	6 baby carrots
TJ Black Bean Dip	Trader Joe's	35	0	0	0	210	8	2	1	2	2 T
Brown rice cake	Lundberg	140	1	0	0	0	28	2	0	2	2 rice cakes
TOTAL		1,517	25	2	0	2,346	270	76	57	72	

DAY 10 FOOD ITEM	BRAND	CALORIES	FAT	SFA	CHOL	SODIUM	CARBS	FIBER	SUGAR	PROTEIN	SERVING SIZE
BREAKFAST											
Arrowhead Spelt Flakes	Arrowhead Mills	100	1	0	0	100	23	3	2	3	1 cup
Soy milk	Silk	80	4	0.5	0	75	4	2	1	7	1 cup
Flax meal	Spectrum Essentials	70	6	0.5	0	5	4	3	0	3	2 T
Strawberries	Whole Foods	49	0.5	0	0	2	2	3	7	1	1 cup
LUNCH											
Leafy greens	Organic Girl	20	0	0	0	95	3	2	0	2	3 cups
Skinny Girl Fat Free Salad Dressings	Skinny Girl	10	0	0	0	90	1	0	0	0	2 T
Carrots	365 Organic	21	0	0	0	47	1	1	3	0	6 baby carrots
Whole-grain bun	Orowheat	170	2.5	0	0	360	32	7	3	7	1 bun
Quarter Pounder Veggie Burger	Amy's	210	3.5	0.5	0	600	24	6	6	20	1 burger
DINNER											
Leafy greens	Organic Girl	20	0	0	0	95	3	2	0	2	3 cups
Skinny Girl Fat Free Salad Dressings	Skinny Girl	10	0	0	0	90	1	0	0	0	2 T
Broccoli slaw	365 Organic	15	0	0	0	15	3	1	1	1	½ cup
Spanish Rice & Beans Enchiladas	Amy's	330	8	1	0	740	53	9	4	9	1 meal
Pear	Whole Foods	120	0	0	0	0	29	6	18	1	1 medium
SNACKS											
Fuji apple	Whole Foods	90	0	0	0	0	25	4	18	0.5	1 medium
Petite carrots	365 Organic	21	0	0	0	47	1	1	3	0	6 baby carrots
TJ Black Bean Dip	Trader Joe's	35	0	0	0	210	8	2	1	2	2 T
Brown rice cake	Lundberg	140	2	0	0	0	28	2	0	2	2 rice cakes
Pear	Whole Foods	70	0	0	0	0	17	3	14	2	1 large
TOTALS		1,481	26	2	0	2,471	239	54	79	60	

DAY 11 FOOD ITEM	BRAND	CALORIES	FAT	SFA	CHOL	SODIUM	CARBS	FIBER	SUGAR	PROTEIN	SERVING SIZE
BREAKFAST											
Soy milk	Silk	80	4	0.5	0	75	4	2	1	7	1 cup
Oatmeal	Nature's Path	190	1	0.5	0	0	34	6	1	8	1 packet
Strawberries	Whole Foods	49	0.5	0	0	2	2	3	7	1	1 cup
LUNCH											
Leafy greens	Organic Girl	20	0	0	0	95	3	2	0	2	3 cups
Walden Farm salad dressing	Walden Farm	10	0	0	0	90	0	0	0	0	2 T
Broccoli slaw	365 Organic	15	0	0	0	15	3	1	1	1	½ cup
Whole Grain Medley: Brown & Wild Rice	Uncle Ben	210	2.5	0	0	660	38	3	1	6	1 cup
Indian Jodhpur Lentils	Tasty Bite	260	6	0	0	820	32	8	10	12	1 pack (2 servings)
Orange	Whole Foods	62	0	0	0	0	15	3	12	1	1
DINNER											
Leafy greens	Organic Girl	20	0	0	0	95	3	2	0	2	3 cups
Skinny Girl Fat Free Salad Dressings	Skinny Girl	10	0	0	0	90	1	0	0	0	2 T
Shredded carrots	365 Organic	0	0	0	0	30	4	1	2	0.5	¾ cup
Mattar tofu	Amy's	280	8	1	0	680	40	5	5	12	1 entrée
SNACKS											
Dry roasted edamame	Seapoint	130	4.5	0.5	0	130	9	7	1	14	¼ cup
Apple	Whole Foods	93	0	0	0	2	25	4	19	0.5	1
TOTALS		1,429	26	2	0	2,784	198	47	61	67	

DAY 12 FOOD ITEM	BRAND	CALORIES	FAT	SFA	CHOL	SODIUM	CARBS	FIBER	SUGAR	PROTEIN	SERVING SIZE
BREAKFAST											
Kind raspberry granola	Kind	190	3	0	0	60	37	3	5	4	½ cup
Soy milk	Silk	80	4	0.5	0	75	4	2	1	7	1 cup
Blackberries	Whole Foods	62	0	0	0	1	15	8	7	2	1 cup
LUNCH											
Leafy greens	Organic Girl	20	0	0	0	95	3	2	0	2	3 cups
Shredded carrots	365 Organic	0	0	0	0	30	4	1	2	0.5	¾ cup
Green peas	365 Organic	70	0	0	0	0	4	4	4	5	⅔ cup
Skinny Girl Fat Free Salad Dressings	Skinny Girl	10	0	0	0	90	1	0	0	0	2 T
Light & Lean Spaghetti Italiano Bowl	Amy's	240	5	0.5	0	590	38	5	6	11	1 bowl
DINNER											
Sweet Potato Quinoa Bowl	Kashi	270	6	1	0	280	48	12	11	9	1 entrée
Strawberries	Whole Foods	49	0.5	0	0	2	1.7	3	7	1	1 cup
SNACKS											
Fuji apple	Whole Foods	90	0	0	0	0	25	4	18	0.5	1 medium
Petite carrots	365 Organic	21	0	0	0	47	1	1	3	0	6 baby carrots
TJ Black Bean Dip	Trader Joe's	35	0	0	0	210	8	2	1	2	2 T
Brown rice cake	Lundberg	70	0.5	0.5	0	0	14	1	0	1	1 rice cake
Edamame	Cascadian Farms	120	5	0	0	45	9	4	2	10	½ cup
TOTALS		1,391	24	3	0	2,175	213	57	65	78	

DAY 13 FOOD ITEM	BRAND	CALORIES	FAT	SFA	CHOL	SODIUM	CARBS	FIBER	SUGAR	PROTEIN	SERVING SIZE
BREAKFAST											
Arrowhead Spelt Flakes	Arrowhead Mills	100	1	0	0	100	23	3	2	3	1 cup
Soy milk	Silk	80	4	0.5	0	75	4	2	1	7	1 cup
Strawberries	Whole Foods	49	0.5	0	0	2	2	3	7	1	1 cup
LUNCH											
Leafy greens	Organic Girl	20	0	0	0	95	3	2	0	2	3 cups
Carrots	365 Organic	21	0	0	0	47	1	1	3	0	6 baby carrots
Green peas	365 Organic	70	0	0	0	0	4	4	4	5	⅔ cup
Skinny Girl Fat Free Salad Dressings	Skinny Girl	10	0	0	0	90	1	0	0	0	2 T
Teriyaki Bowl	Amy's	290	4.5	0.5	0	780	52	6	15	12	1 bowl
DINNER											
Leafy greens	Organic Girl	20	0	0	0	95	3	2	0	2	3 cups
Skinny Girl Fat Free Salad Dressings	Skinny Girl	10	0	0	0	90	1	0	0	0	2 T
Broccoli slaw	365 Organic	15	0	0	0	15	3	1	1	1	½ cup
Chimichurri Quinoa Bowl	Kashi	240	7	1	0	330	41	12	5	10	1 entrée
SNACKS											
Edamame	Cascadian Farms	240	10	0	0	90	18	8	4	20	1 cup
Fuji apple	Whole Foods	90	0	0	0	0	25	4	18	0.5	1 medium
TOTALS		1,255	27	2	0	1,809	181	48	60	63	

DAY 14 FOOD ITEM	BRAND	CALORIES	FAT	SFA	CHOL	SODIUM	CARBS	FIBER	SUGAR	PROTEIN	SERVING SIZE
BREAKFAST											
Oatmeal	Nature's Path	190	1	0.5	0	0	34	6	1	8	1 packet
Soy milk	Silk	80	4	0.5	0	75	4	2	1	7	1 cup
Blueberries	Whole Foods	84	0	0	0	0	21	4	15	1	1 cup
Flax meal	Spectrum Essentials	35	3	0	0	2	24	2	0	2	1 T
LUNCH											
Leafy greens	Organic Girl	20	0	0	0	95	3	2	0	2	3 cups
Skinny Girl Fat Free Salad Dressings	Skinny Girl	10	0	0	0	90	1	0	0	0	2 T
Organic Hearty Spanish Rice & Red Bean Soup	Amy's	140	2	0	0	690	24	5	5	5	2 servings
Dave's 21 Whole Grain & Seeds Bread	Dave's Killer Bread	120	2	0	0	180	22	5	5	5	2 slices
PB Fit	PB2	50	1	0	0	115	4	2	2	6	2 T
DINNER											
Leafy greens	Organic Girl	20	0	0	0	95	3	2	0	2	3 cups
Skinny Girl Fat Free Salad Dressings	Skinny Girl	10	0	0	0	90	1	0	0	0	2 T
Shredded carrots	365 Organic	15	0	0	0	30	4	1	2	0.5	¾ cup
Roasted Veggie Pizza	Amy's	280	9	1.5	0	540	42	3	5	7	⅓ pizza
Fuji apple	Whole Foods	90	0	0	0	0	25	4	18	0.5	1 medium
SNACKS											
Orange	Whole Foods	62	0	0	0	0	15	3	12	1	1
Petite carrots	365 Organic	21	0	0	0	47	1	1	3	0	6 baby carrots
TJ Black Bean Dip	Trader Joe's	35	0	0	0	210	8	2	1	2	2 T
Brown rice cake	Lundberg	70	0.5	0.5	0	0	14	1	0	1	1 rice cake
Dry roasted edamame	Seapoint	130	4.5	0.5	0	130	9	7	1	14	¼ cup
TOTALS		1,462	27	3	0	2,389	259	52	71	64	

Appendix B

Stocking Your Kitchen for Success

Having a well-stocked kitchen is your culinary toolbox for healthy eating and cooking. It's beneficial to maintain a solid stock of the basics, such as whole grains, fresh vegetables, fruit, beans and lentils, and soy foods (tofu, tempeh, miso). Buying a few convenient packaged foods such as peeled garlic, low-sodium vegetable broth, and pre-cut mixes of celery, onions, and carrots are all great shortcuts to quick and easy cooking, and add flavor to most any dish.

Keeping your refrigerator stocked with simple staples like unsweetened organic soy milk, fat-free salad dressings, fresh ginger, and some precooked foods like beans, baked tofu, and tempeh, and whole grains such as cooked brown rice and quinoa, make it easy to toss together a delicious meal in minutes.

Other canned or boxed foods that are good to have available for quick and easy meals are canned or boxed tomato products such as marinara sauce, salsa, or diced fire-roasted tomatoes. Many of these have a long shelf life, so it's easy to keep your pantry full of healthy choices.

However, we recognize that you just might not have the time to navigate food labels in order to get started restocking your kitchen. If this sounds like you, please read on! In addition to the two weeks of packaged meals listed above, here is an extensive list of packaged foods that are available at most grocery stores, making it easy for you to get started eating well right away. Availability of products may vary based on changes in the market. Plant-based foods are on the rise with a large variety of new products being added.

Stocking Your Refrigerator

Stocking your refrigerator with fresh and healthy food will allow you the convenience of having what you need at your fingertips to make a variety of delicious, health-promoting meals and quick and easy healthy snacks.

Having prepped fresh produce on hand, such as chopped cauliflower, broccoli, leafy greens, green beans, and sliced and shredded carrots, makes it easy to make healthy choices, even when you are in a hurry to eat. Precooked beans and lentils are also great to have on hand.

Other simple staples, like nonfat salad dressings and sauces and precooked brown rice and quinoa, make it easy to toss together a delicious meal in minutes.

Fresh Produce
- All fruits and vegetables
- Edamame

Soy Milk (Unsweetened)
- *Silk:* Organic Unsweetened
- *Westsoy:* Organic Unsweetened, Organic Plus, Low-fat, Nonfat, Soy Slender
- *Soy Dream:* Enriched Original
- *Edensoy:* Organic Original, Organic Unsweetened, Extra Original
- *Earth Balance:* Organic Original
- *Pacific Organic:* Original Unsweetened

Rice Milk (Unsweetened)
- *Rice Dream:* Enriched Original, Unsweetened, Sprouted, Enriched Rice and Quinoa
- *365:* Organic Original, Organic Unsweetened

Oat Milk (Unsweetened)
- *Pacific*

Flax Milk
- *Good Karma Foods:* Flax and Protein Original

Low-Fat Almond Milk (Unsweetened)
- *Silk, Eden:* Almond Dream
- *Califia Farms*
- *Blue Diamond:* Almond Breeze

Nonfat Nondairy Soy Creamers
- *Silk, Wildwood, Califia Farms, Trader Joe's*

Nondairy Cheeses
- *Go Veggie:* Vegan American, Vegan Cheddar, Vegan Pepper Jack, Vegan Mozzarella, Vegan

Tofu (Organic; Non-GMO)
- *Nasoya:* Organic firm, organic extra firm, organic silken, organic sprouted super firm, organic super firm and sprouted cubed, teriyaki and chipotle baked
- *Wildwood:* Organic silken, soft, firm, extra firm, super firm, high protein super firm; variety of baked tofu such as teriyaki, savory, sriracha
- *Westsoy:* Organic, soft, firm, extra firm; a variety of baked such as Mexican Jalapeño, Asian Teriyaki, Italian Garlic Herb, Zesty Lemon Pepper, Roma Tomato Basil
- *Soy Boy:* Organic firm and extra firm, Tofu Lin, Italian, Caribbean, Smoked
- *Morinaga:* nigari, puree, silken soft, firm, lite, and extra firm
- *365 Organic:* Organic firm and extra firm
- *O Organics:* soft, firm, and extra firm
- *House Foods Organic:* Organic soft, extra soft, medium, firm, extra firm, super firm, cubed; variety of baked tofus such as spicy garlic, teriyaki, umami, savory orange
- *Hodo*
- *Sol Cuisine:* organic firm, sprouted organic extra firm

- *Woodstock Organic:* firm and extra firm
- *Sprouts:* Organic firm, extra firm, medium and soft, high protein, baked varieties

Tempeh (Organic; Non-GMO)
- *Lightlife:* Flax, Soy, Three Grain, Garden Vegetable, Wild Rice, Smoky Tempeh Strips, Fakin' Bacon Tempeh Strips
- *Westsoy:* Five Grain, Original
- *Trader Joe's:* Organic 3 Grain Tempeh
- *Tofurkey:* Organic 5 Grain, soy cake, and garlic
- *SoyBoy:* Organic Soy Tempeh and 5 Grain Tempeh

Seitan
- *Upton's Naturals:* Traditional, Ground, Italian, Chorizo, Bacon
- *Westsoy:* Seitan Strips, Cubed, Ground, Chicken-Style
- *Primal Strips:* Meatless Vegan Jerky; Thai Peanut, Mesquite Lime, Teriyaki, Hickory Smoked, Texas BBQ

Veggie Burgers and Dogs
- *Gardenburger:* Veggie Medley, Black Bean Chipotle, Portabella
- *Boca Burger:* Non-GMO Vegan, Non-GMO All American, Original Vegan
- *Amy's:* Bistro Veggie Burger
- *Tofurky:* Mighty Mushroom Veggie Burger
- *Lightlife:* Smart Dogs, Tofu Pups
- *Yves:* Veggie Hot Dogs
- *365 Whole Foods:* Veggie Dogs

TVP (Textured Vegetable Protein)
- *Bob's Red Mill*

Spreads and Dips
- *Wild Garden:* Hummus
- *Oasis Mediterranean Cuisine:* Hummus
- *Trader Joe's:* Eggplant Spread, Roasted Red Pepper Spread, Fat Free Smoky Black Bean Dip, Fat Free Spicy Pinto Bean Dip
- *Bearitos:* Bean Dip, Black Bean Dip

- *Guiltless Gourmet:* Mild Black Bean Dip, Spicy Black Bean Dip
- *365:* Chile Black Bean Salsa

Dressings

- *Trader Joe's:* Fat Free Balsamic Vinaigrette Dressing, No Oil Dill and Garlic Dressing, Fat Free Italian
- *Spectrum Naturals:* Fat Free Sweet Onion and Garlic
- *Walden Farms Fat Free Dressings:* Creamy Chipotle, Zesty Italian, Asian, Slaw, Honey Dijon, Thousand Island
- *Whole Foods Market:* Health Starts Here Oil-Free
- *Cindy's Kitchen:* Vegan Caesar Dressing, Fig Balsamic Dressing, Fat Free Balsamic Vinaigrette, Oil Free Pomegranate Vinaigrette, Fat Free Sun-Dried Tomato, Oil Free Carrot and Ginger, Oil Free Tamari Miso, Oil Free Tangerine, Sweet Chili and Lime, Oil Free Tomato Basil
- *Kozlowski Farms:* Fat Free Honey Mustard, Fat Free Raspberry Poppy Seed, Roasted Garlic, Fat Free Zesty Herb
- *Hain:* fat-free dressings
- *Bragg:* Fat Free Hawaiian Dressing and Marinade

Stocking Your Freezer

A freezer full of frozen produce is a great help. Most frozen fruits and vegetables are promptly blanched, boiled, or steamed and then frozen within hours of being picked. This process helps lock in both fresh taste and nutritional value. Frozen produce is also available year-round, and in most cases is less expensive than fresh. Frozen vegetables can be quickly steamed or added to a stir-fry, soup, whole grains, whole-grain pasta, plant-based casserole, or lasagna. Include a variety of frozen vegetables and starchy vegetables, such as cut spinach, broccoli, cauliflower, mixed vegetables, pearl onions, corn, green peas, and chopped winter squash such as butternut.

Keep your freezer stocked with some heart-healthy plant proteins for quick and easy well-balanced meals or a healthy high-protein snack. Some great protein choices that freeze and reheat well are edamame, black-eyed peas, and lentils. These can be either store-bought or homemade. Cooking and freezing big batches of beans can be a great time and money saver.

Frozen veggie burger and ground vegan crumbles are excellent to make a quick high-protein pasta sauce or vegan lasagna, tacos, or chili. Frozen chicken-less strips or patties are a quick way to add protein to a salad, pasta dish, or stir-fry.

Also, keeping some precooked whole grains in the freezer, like quinoa or brown rice, provides yet another quick approach to a healthy balanced meal.

Frozen Vegetables (100% Vegetables, No Added Fat/Oils or Sauces)

- *Cascadian Farms, Earthbound, Kroger, Birds Eye, Green Giant, Great Value, 365, Lakeside:* A variety of frozen vegetables are available such as: edamame, asparagus, broccoli florets and cuts, cut spinach, green beans, winter squash, kale, sweet corn, sweet peas, Swiss chard, peas and carrots, peas, various blends (Garden Vegetable Medley, California-Style Blend, Chinese-Style Stir-fry Blend, Gardener's Blend, Thai-Style Stir-fry Blend, Country-Style Potatoes)
- *Alexia:* Hash Browns (without added fat/oil), sweet corn, green peas, carrots, Vegetable Medley

Frozen Fruit (100% Fruit)

- *Cascadian Farms, Earthbound, Kroger, Birds Eye, 365, Green Giant, Market Pantry, Welches, Dole, Great Value:* A variety of frozen fruit are available such as blackberries, blueberries, raspberries, strawberries, sliced peaches, pineapple, banana, tropical fruit blends, and mixed fruit

Frozen Packaged Foods

- *Rising Moon:* Organic Manicotti with Marinara & Organic Soy Filling, Butternut Squash Ravioli, Slim Trim Soy Lasagna
- *Amy's:* Light & Lean Sweet & Sour Asian Noodle

Breakfast and Meat Analogs

- *Lightlife:* Gimme Lean Sausage, Smart Bacon
- *Morningstar:* Soy Sausage Links, Soy Sausage Patties, Soy Grillers

- *365:* Meatless Breakfast Patties
- *Quorn:* Breakfast Sausage Patties

Veggie Grounds
- *Trader Joe's:* Beef-less Ground Beef
- *Lightlife:* Original, Mexican
- *Boca Burger:* Veggie Ground Crumbles
- *Quorn:* Grounds

Analog Chicken Strips
- *Beyond Meat:* Grilled Chicken, Southwest Chicken Strips
- *Lightlife:* Smart Strips Chick'n, Smart Tenders Lemon Pepper Chick'n, Smart Tenders Savory Chick'n
- *Trader Joe's:* Chicken-less Strips
- *Quorn:* Vegan Chick'n Tenders, Vegan Naked Chick'n Cutlets, Vegan Spicy Chick'n Patty, Vegan Breaded Chick'n Cutlet

Other Meat Analogs
- *Lightlife:* Gimme Lean Beef, Smart Buffalo Wings, Smart Honey BBQ Wings, Smart Cutlets Original, Smart Cutlets Classic Marinara, Smart Strips Steak Style, Smart Deli Bologna, Smart Deli Ham, Smart Deli Pepperoni, Smart Deli Turkey
- *Yves Veggie Cuisine:* Veggie Ham, Veggie Turkey, Veggie Salami, Veggie Pepperoni, Veggie Bacon, Veggie Breakfast Patties, Veggie Ground

Stocking Your Pantry

A well-stocked pantry is an essential part of your culinary toolbox. Try to keep a variety of dried beans, lentils, and peas along with a collection of your favorite canned beans (no salt added) on hand, as well as a variety of whole grains, flours, pastas, and breads. Low-fat, low-sodium, plant-based soups and stocks and other canned or boxed foods such as marinara sauce, salsa, or fire-roasted tomatoes are all good to have available to toss into a soup, stew, salad, or sauce. All of these have a long shelf life, so they're practical to keep in your pantry.

Whole Grains

- Amaranth, barley, buckwheat, bulgur, corn (popcorn kernels, polenta), einkorn, farro, kamut, millet, oats, quinoa, rice (wild, brown, black, red, purple), rye, sorghum, spelt, teff, triticale, wheat

Whole-Grain Pasta

- *Barilla Plus*
- *Jovial*
- *DeLallo*
- *Trader Joe's*
- *Westbrae*
- *Dreamfields*
- *365*
- *Gia Russa*

Precooked Polenta

- *San Gennaro:* Traditional, Sun-Dried Tomato Garlic, Southern Style Grits, Basil Garlic
- *Food Merchant:* Traditional Italian, Organic Quinoa Polenta, Basil Garlic, Sun-Dried Tomato, Green Chili & Cilantro

Gluten-Free Pasta

- *Tolerant Organic:* Black Bean Penne, Red or Green Lentil Pasta
- *Tinkyada:* Brown Rice Pasta
- *Lundberg:* Brown Rice Pasta
- *Jovial:* Brown Rice Pasta
- *Annie's:* Brown Rice Pasta
- *Westbrae:* Corn Angel Hair
- *Explore Asian:* Black Bean Pasta

Whole Grain Breads

- *Alvarado Bakery:* Sprouted Wheat Multi-Grain, Fundamental Fiber, Sprouted No Salt, Low Glycemic Bread, Sprouted Barely, Sprouted Sourdough French, Sprouted Wheat Cinnamon Raisin, Sprouted Wheat California Style Original
- *Alpine Valley Organic Bakery:* 12 Grains & Seeds, Multi Grain with Omega-3, Honey Sprout
- *Archer Farms:* 100% Whole Wheat, 100% Whole Wheat Honey

- *Arnold:* 100% Whole Wheat, 100% Whole Wheat Country, 100% Whole Grain, Barely Light 100% Whole Wheat, Stone Ground 100% Whole Wheat
- *Aunt Millie's:* 100% Whole Wheat
- *Brownberry:* 100% Whole Wheat, 100% Whole Grain
- *Country Hearth:* 100% Whole Wheat
- *Trader Joe's:* Multigrain English Muffins, Whole Wheat Lavash Bread
- *Food for Life:* (Ezekiel) 7 Sprouted, Cinnamon Raisin, Low Sodium, Brown Rice
- *Oroweat:* 100% Whole Wheat
- *Pepperidge Farm:* 100% Whole Wheat
- *Nature's Harvest:* 100% Stone Ground Whole Wheat
- *Nature's Own:* 100% Whole Wheat
- *Roman Meal:* 100% Whole Wheat, 100% Whole Grain

Whole-Grain English Muffins
- *Thomas':* Sprouted Whole Grain English Muffins
- *Food for Life:* (Ezekiel) Multigrain English Muffins

Whole-Grain Pita and Pocket Breads, Flatbreads
- *Trader Joe's:* Whole-Grain Pita Pockets, Whole Wheat Middle Eastern Flatbread, Whole Grain Naan
- *Brownberry:* 100% Whole Wheat Pocket Thins
- *Food for Life:* (Ezekiel) Whole Grain Pocket Bread

Whole Grain Bread Thins
- *Arnold:* 100% Whole Wheat, Flax & Fiber
- *Archer Farms:* Whole Wheat Sandwich Flats
- *Brownberry:* 100% Whole Wheat Sandwich Thins

Whole Grain Buns
- *Alvarado Bakery, Food for Life* (Ezekiel), *Brownberry, Trader Joe's*

Tortillas
- *Food for Life:* (Ezekiel) Whole Wheat Tortillas, Sprouted Whole Grain, Sprouted Whole Grain Taco Size, Sprouted Corn, Brown Rice, Exotic Black Rice

- *La Tortilla Factory:* Low Carb, High Fiber, Whole Wheat, Organic, Non-GMO Yellow Corn, Corn Tortillas
- *Engine 2*
- *Mission:* Corn
- *Mi Rancho:* Corn

Whole-Wheat Pizza Dough
- *Whole Foods*

Gluten-Free Breads
- *Udi's:* Whole Grain
- *Trader Joe's:* Gluten Free Whole Grain Bread
- *Food for Life:* Bhutanese Red Rice Bread, Brown Rice Bread, Exotic Black Rice Bread, Rice Millet Bread, Yeast Free Brown Rice Bread, Yeast Free Multi Seed Rice Bread, Sprouted For Life Gluten Free Almond Bread, Sprouted For Life Gluten Free Original 3 Seed Bread, Gluten Free Tortillas, Brown Rice Tortillas, Gluten Free English Muffins or Buns, Gluten Free Brown Rice English Muffins, Gluten Free Multi-Seed English Muffin

Whole-Grain Hot Cereals
- *Arrowhead Mills:* Instant Oatmeal (Maple Apple Spice, Original Plain), Bear Mush, Bits O Barley, Oat Bran, Oat Flakes, Old Fashion Oatmeal, Rice and Shine, 7 Grain, Steel Cut Oats, Wheat Free 7 Grain
- *Bob's Red Mill:* Steel Cut Oats, Barley Grits/Meal, Barley Rolled Flakes, Cracked Rye, Cracked Wheat, Creamy Brown Rice Farina, Oat Bran, Organic Creamy Buckwheat Cereal, Organic Kamut Cereal, Organic Rolled Oats, Scottish Oatmeal, Wheat Bran
- *Country Choice Naturals:* Multigrain Cereal, Old Fashioned Oats, Quick Oats, Regular Flavor Instant Oatmeal, Steel Cut Oatmeal
- *Lundberg Family Farms:* Hot 'n Creamy Rice Cereal Original
- *McCann's:* Irish Oatbran, Irish Oatmeal
- *Nature's Path:* Oatmeal Original, Optimum Cranberry Ginger
- *Quaker Oats:* Quaker Oats, Quaker Oat Bran, Quaker Quick Oats
- *The Silver Palate:* Thick and Rough Oatmeal

- *US Mills: Erewhon:* Apple Cinnamon Oatmeal, Barley Plus, Oat Bran with Toasted Wheat Germ, Oatmeal with Added Oat Bran
- *Amy's:* Multi-Grain Hot Cereal Bowl, Cream of Rice Hot Cereal Bowl

Whole-Grain Cold Cereals

- *Arrowhead Mills:* Amaranth Flakes, Wheat Flakes, Bran Flakes, Corn Flakes, Kamut Flakes, Spelt Flakes, Multigrain Flakes, Puffed Wheat, Puffed Rice, Puffed Millet, Puffed Corn, Puffed Kamut, Nature O's, Shredded Wheat
- *Barbara's Bakery:* Breakfast O's, Brown Rice Crisps, Corn Flakes, Shredded Wheat, Shredded Spoonfuls, Shredded Oats, Shredded Oats Cinnamon Crunch, Ultima Original, Ultima Pomegranate
- *Cascadian Farm:* Purely O's, Honey Nut O's, Raisin Bran, Multi-Grain Squares, Wheat Crunch
- *General Mills:* Cheerios
- *Health Valley:* Real Oat Bran Almond Crunch, Organic Blue Corn Flakes, Organic Oat Bran Flakes, Organic Oat Bran Flakes with Raisins, Organic Fiber 7 Flakes, Organic Amaranth Flakes

Soups

- *Health Valley:* Vegetable Broth, Organic Split Pea Soup, Fat Free Soups, 14 Garden Vegetable Soup, Vegetable Barley, Corn and Vegetable, 5 Bean Vegetable, Tomato Vegetable, Split Pea and Carrots, Lentil and Carrots, Black Bean and Vegetable, Fat-Free Carotene Soups, Italian Plus, Super Broccoli, Organic Tomato Soup
- *Imagine:* Tomato, Red Pepper, Organic Moroccan Chickpea & Carrot, Organic White Bean & Kale, Organic Italian Vegetables & Beans, Organic Savory Black Bean
- *Pacific:* Tomato, Organic Spicy Black Bean and Kale
- *Muir Glen:* Organic Tomato Soup, Organic Homestyle Split Pea
- *Amy's:* organic fat free and low-fat soups, Organic Black Bean Chili
- *Westbrae Natural Foods:* Great Plains Savory Bean, Santa Fe Vegetable, Louisiana Bean Stew, Alabama Black Bean Gumbo, Old World Split Pea, Spicy Southwest Vegetable, Mediterranean Lentil

Plain Canned Beans and Lentils
- Black beans, black-eyed peas, black soybeans, butter beans, cannellini, garbanzo, great northern, kidney, navy, pinto, small red

Flavored Canned Beans and Lentils, Mixed Beans and Rice
- *Trader Joe's:* Cuban Style Black Beans, Organic Baked Beans, Steamed Lentils
- *Amy's:* Organic Vegetarian Beans, Chili
- *Eden:* Brown Rice & Chickpeas, Brown Rice & Kidney Beans, Brown Rice & Lentils, Brown Rice & Pinto Beans, Curried Rice & Lentils, Moroccan Rice & Garbanzo Beans, Spanish Rice & Pinto Beans, Mexican Rice & Black Beans, Caribbean Rice & Black Beans, Cajun Rice & Small Red Beans, Spanish Rice & Pinto Beans, Black Bean & Quinoa Chili, Great Northern Beans & Barely Chili, Kidney Bean & Kamut Chili, Pinto Bean & Spelt Chili

Canned, Boxed, and Bottled Vegetable Products

Canned Pumpkin
- *Farmers Market:* cans have BPA-free liner

Capers
- *Star, Roland, Mezzetta, Safeway*

Roasted Red Peppers (in Water)
- *Mezzetta, DeLallo*

Fire-Roasted Green Chiles
- *Hatch, Ortega, La Costena, La Victoria, Trader Joe's*

Chipotles in Adobo Sauce
- *La Costena, Embasa, Goya, San Marcos, La Moreno*

Pickles
- *Ricks Picks:* Phat Beets, Sweet & Sassy Mix, Handy Corn, Pepi Pep Peps, K.O. Pickles, Spicy Pickles, Windy City Wasabeans, Kool Gherks

Dry Soup Mixes
- *Right Foods, McDougall:* Low Sodium Split Pea Soup, Lentil Couscous, White Bean & Pasta Soup, Black Bean & Rice Soup
- *Nile Spice:* Lentil, Black Bean, Split Pea, Chili 'n Beans
- *Eden Foods:* Ramen-Buckwheat, Whole Wheat
- *Spice Hunter:* Moroccan Couscous, Mediterranean Minestrone, French Lentil, Spicy Thai, Curry Lentil, Spicy Black Bean, Miso Udon, Spring Onion, Split Pea, Hot & Sour, Mandarin Noodle
- *Westbrae Natural Foods:* Whole Wheat Ramen, Instant Miso Soup

Sauces
- Soy sauce: *Eden, Kikkoman, San-J International*
- Tamari: *Kikkoman, San-J*
- Teriyaki: *OrganicVille Skye, Annie's, One Bite*
- Korean: *OrganicVille Skye, Braggs Amino Acids*
- Sweet chili sauce: *Trader Joe's, OrganicVille Skye, Cindy's Kitchen, Thai Kitchen*
- BBQ: *Annie's, Trader Joe's, Austins, Podah's*
- Cocktail sauce: *Trader Joe's, Bellas*
- Steak sauce: *Lea & Perrins*
- Vegan Worcestershire: *Annie's Naturals, Edward & Sons, Wizard Organic*
- Mustard sauce: *Earth & Vine*
- Hoisin: *Edward & Sons*
- Ginger and Tamari: *Edward & Sons*
- Miso: *Organic Gourmet, Miso Master Organic Chickpea Miso*
- Balsamic glaze: *OrganicVille Skye, Trader Giotto's, Gia Russa*
- Chutney: *Trader Joe's, Stonewall, Wild Thyme Farms, Sukki*

Miso Paste
- Soy miso (red, barley, brown rice, white): *South River, Westbrae Natural, Miso Master Organic*
- Chickpea miso: *South River, Miso Master Organic*
- Adzuki bean miso: *South River*

Hot Sauces
- *Cholula, Melinda's Hot Sauces*
- Sriracha: *OrganicVille Skye*

- Enchilada sauce: *OrganicVille Skye, Trader Joe's, Parrot, El Pato*
- Tomatillo sauce: *Frontera, White Girl*

Salsa (Brands without Added Oil or Fats)
- *Amy's, Trader Joe's, 365, Frontera, Pace, Muir Glen, Newman's Own, White Girl*

Tomato Sauces and Products

Pasta Sauce
- *Muir Glen:* (nonfat) Portobello Mushroom; (low-fat) Cabernet Marinara, Chunky Tomato Fire Roasted, Garden Vegetable, Garlic Roasted, Italian Herb, Tomato Basil
- *Newman's:* Cabernet Marinara, Fire Roasted Tomato and Garlic, Fra Diavolo, Garden Peppers, Marinara, Marinara with Mushrooms, Roasted Garlic, Sockarooni, Sweet Onion and Roasted Garlic, Tomato and Basil Bombolina
- *Dave's:* Organic Red Heirloom, Organic Spicy Heirloom
- *Prego:* (nonfat) Light Smart Traditional; (low-fat) Traditional, Marinara, Tomato Basil Garlic, Fresh Mushroom, Roasted Garlic and Herb, Chunky Garden Tomato, Onion and Garlic, Heart Smart, Heart Smart Mushroom, Heart Smart Roasted Red Pepper and Garlic, Veggie Smart, Veggie Smart Chunky and Savory
- *Pomi:* Marinara

Pizza Sauce
- *Muir Glen, Trader Joe's, Pomi*

Canned, Diced, and Chopped Tomatoes
- *Muir Glen, Hunt's, 365, Contadina, Del Monte, Pomi*

Stocks and Broths
- Vegetable: *Imagine, Pacific*
- Mushroom: *Pacific*
- Low Sodium No-Chicken Broth: *Imagine*

Sweeteners
- Stevia powder: *Sweet Leaf, 365, Nunaturals, Pyure*
- Stevia liquid: *NOW, Sweet Leaf, Omica Organics*
- Agave: *Madhava, Wholesome Sweeteners*
- Molasses: *Wholesome Sweeteners*
- Maple Syrup: *Rapunzel, Pure Organics, Springtree*
- Honey: *Ambrosia, Wholesome Sweetener, Clarks,* local honey brands
- Barley malt: *Eden*
- Date sugar: *Bob's Red Mill, Chatfields, NOW*

Thickeners
- Kuzu: *Eden*
- Agar: *Eden, Rapunzel, Bob's Red Mill*
- Xanthan gum: *Bob's Red Mill, NOW*
- Cornstarch: *Rapunzel, Rumford, Clabber Girl, Bob's Red Mill*
- Sweet rice flour: *Koda Farms, Mochiko Blue Star*

Cocoa Powder (Unsweetened)
- *Green & Black's:* 100% Organic Cocoa Powder (alkalized)
- *Hershey's:* Natural (non-alkalized), Special Dark (half alkalized, half natural)
- *Chatfield's:* Natural (non-alkalized)
- *Dagoba:* Certified Organic (non-alkalized)
- *Scharffenberger:* Natural (non-alkalized)

Carob Powder
- *Chatfields:* All Natural Carob Powder
- *Bob's Red Mill:* Toasted, Ground Carob Powder

Condiments
- Mustard (Dijon, brown, or yellow): *Eden,* most brands (read label)
- Ketchup: *Muir Glen, Heinz,* most brands (read label)
- Fat-free mayonnaise: *Nasoya, Kraft's Miracle Whip*

Vinegars
- Balsamic (white or red): *Trader Joe's, Alessi, Colavita, Lucini, Fini, Archer Farms, Star, Roland, Bionature*

- Champagne: *Rapunzel, Star, Regina, Spectrum*
- Red wine: *Alessi, Napa Valley Naturals*
- Mirin

Seasoned rice vinegar
- Brown rice: *Spectrum, Marukan, Eden*
- Apple cider: *Braggs*

Spices
Here are some recommended spices to have in stock:
- Sweet: allspice, cinnamon, nutmeg, apple pie spice, pumpkin pie spice, vanilla bean
- Hot/heat: cayenne, chipotle, red pepper flakes, chili powder, black pepper, Cajun spice, paprika (sweet, hot, smoked)
- Italian: Basil, oregano, garlic, thyme, rosemary
- Asian: Chinese five-spice
- Mexican: cilantro, coriander
- Indian: turmeric, curry powders, garam masala, ginger
- Savory: bay leaf, onion powder, caraway, celery, chive, dill, lemon pepper, sage, cumin, cloves

Seasonings and Rubs
- Nutritional yeast: *Bob's Red Mill, Braggs*
- *Bearitos:* Simply Organic Taco Seasoning
- *Simply Organics:* (packet mixes) Southwest Taco, Sloppy Joe Seasoning, Vegetarian Chili, Chipotle Black Bean Dip, Chili Seasoning, Italian Dressing
- *Mrs. Dash:* Seasoning Blends
- Vanilla extract: *Rapunzel, Nielsen-Massey, Penzey's, Frontier, Golden Gate*

Protein Powders
- *Oriya Organics: 100% Plant Protein, Superfood Protein Medley*
- *Vega:* Clean Protein Chocolate & Vanilla, Vega One: Protein & Greens, Tango, Bodacious Berry
- *UB Super:* Plant Based Protein Superfood Nutritional Shake and Smoothie
- *Growing Naturals:* Raw Pea Protein: Vanilla, Chocolate, and

Original; Brown Rice Protein: Vanilla Blast, Strawberry Burst, Chocolate Power, Original
- *Trader Joe's:* Vanilla Soy
- *NutriBiotic:* Rice Protein Powder
- *Jarrow Formulas:* Brown Rice Protein Vanilla, Berry Chocolate, Ultra Smooth Brown Rice Protein: Vanilla, Chocolate, Berry
- *Amazing Grass:* Amazing Meal, Pomegranate Mango

Snacks

Equipping your pantry with appetizing, healthy meal options and grab-and-go snacks can make the difference between making a good choice or not. Here are just a few ideas. (It's important to read the label for serving sizes and limit portions to 3 grams or less of fat per serving.)

Crackers and Chips
- *Ryvita:* Crispbread, Mediterranean Herbs Rye, Hint of Chili Rye, Dark Rye, Original, Sweet Onion, Cracked Pepper, Golden Rye, Whole Grain Cracker Bread
- *Manischewitz:* Whole Wheat Matzos
- *Streit's:* Whole Wheat Matzos
- *Wasa:* Crispbread, Fiber, Light-Rye, Multi-Grain, Hearty
- *365:* Baked Woven Wheat
- *Lundberg:* Brown Rice Cakes, Tamari Seaweed Rice Cakes, Wild Rice Cakes
- *Koyo:* Dulse Rice Cakes, Hijiki Rice Cakes, Nori Rice Cakes, Plain Rice Cakes
- *Guiltless Gourmet:* Baked Tortilla Chips: Yellow Corn, Blue Corn, Chili Lime
- *Beanitos Baked Skinny Dippers:* Black Bean Chips, White Bean Chips

Bars
These items are low in fat but are limited or not encouraged because they are high in added sugar.
- *Trader Joe's:* cereal bars
- *Newman's Own:* Fig Newmans

- *Barbara's:* Fig Newtons
- *Nature's Path:* Organic Crispy Rice Bars, Harvest Berry Chewy
- *Enjoy Life:* Chewy Bar: Carmel Apple, Mixed Berry
- *Cascadian Farms:* Chewy Granola Bars: Harvest Berry, Oatmeal Raisin
- *NuGo Fiber d'Lish:* Apple Cobbler, Orange Cranberry, Cinnamon Raisin, Blueberry Cobbler
- *NuGo:* Gluten Free Vegan Bar: Carrot Cake

Dry-Roasted Edamame
- *Seapoint Farms*

Hot Beverages

Lastly, you may want to include in your pantry a selection of herbal and green teas or caffeine-free alternatives to coffee. Tea helps protect your GI tract from cancer. Coffee, in moderation, has health benefits as well. Limit caffeine consumption if it makes you feel anxious or causes palpitations.

Hot Beverages
- Grain Beverages: *Kaffree Roma, Pero, Postum, Inka, Coree, Karee, Raja, Cafix, Teeccino, Bambu*
- Herbal teas (all brands)
- Green tea (a sample of brands): *Yogi, Tetley, Teavana, Tazo, Lipton, Twinings, Bigelow, Organic India, Tea Garden, Celestial Seasonings Authentic, Stash*
- Decaffeinated coffees and teas: choose the CO_2 method of decaffeinating

Cold Beverages and Water Enhancers
- *Hint Beverages:* all flavors
- *Stur Water Enhancer:* all fruit flavors, all coconut water flavors
- *Madhava Agave Five Drink Mix:* Blissful Berry, Coconut Quench, Raspberry Refresh
- *Sweet Leaf Water Drops:* all flavors

Notes

Chapter 1

8   **only 5 percent of patients account for 50–80 percent:** Conwell LJ, Cohen JW. Statistical Brief #73. Rockville, MD: Agency for Healthcare Quality and Research; 2005.

8   **In a demonstration project, Mutual of Omaha:** Ornish D. Avoiding revascularization with lifestyle changes: the Multicenter Lifestyle Demonstration Project. *Am J Cardiol.* 1998;82:72T–76T.

13   **Our earlier book, *The Spectrum*:** Ornish D. *The Spectrum.* New York: Ballantine Books; 2008.

14   **Dr. Michael P. O'Leary writes that erections "serve as a barometer":** Skerrett PJ. Erectile dysfunction often a warning sign of heart disease. Harvard Health Blog. 2011 Oct 24. https://www.health.harvard.edu/blog/erectile-dysfunction-often-a-warning-sign-of-heart-disease-201110243648.

14   **Erectile dysfunction affects at least 18 million men:** Selvin E, Burnett AL, Platz EA. Prevalence and risk factors for erectile dysfunction in the US. *Am J Med.* 2007 Feb;120(2):151–157.

14   **even a single meal high in animal protein and fat:** Benson TW, Weintraub NL, Kim HW. A single high-fat meal provokes pathological erythrocyte remodeling and increases myeloperoxidase levels:

implications for acute coronary syndrome. *Lab Invest.* 2018 Mar 23. doi: 10.1038/s41374-018-0038-3.

14   *The Game Changers:* http://gamechangersmovie.com.

Chapter 2

18   **people who are lonely and depressed are three to ten times:** Ornish D. *Love and Survival: The Scientific Basis for the Healing Power of Intimacy.* New York: HarperCollins; 1998.

19   **Those with four healthy lifestyle factors:** Ford ES, Bergmann MM, Kröger J, Schienkiewitz A, Weikert C, Boeing H. Healthy living is the best revenge: findings from the European Prospective Investigation into Cancer and Nutrition—Potsdam study. *Arch Intern Med.* 2009 Aug 10;169(15):1355–1362. doi: 10.1001/archinternmed.2009.237.

19   **the majority of Americans have type 2 diabetes or pre-diabetes:** Menke A, Casagrande S, Geiss L, Cowie CC. Prevalence of and trends in diabetes among adults in the United States, 1988–2012. *JAMA.* 2015 Sep 8;314(10):1021–1029. doi: 10.1001/jama.2015.10029.

19   **lived an average of *twelve to fourteen years longer:*** Li Y, Pan A, Wang DD, Liu X, Dhana K, Franco OH, Kaptoge S, Di Angelantonio E, Stampfer M, Willett WC, Hu FB. Impact of healthy lifestyle factors on life expectancies in the US population. *Circulation.* 2018 Apr 30. doi: 10.1161/CIRCULATIONAHA.117.032047. [Epub ahead of print]

22   **In contrast, chronic inflammation . . . plays an important role:** Hunter P. The inflammation theory of disease. *EMBO Rep.* 2012 Nov;13(11):968–970. Bosma-den Boer MM, van Wetten ML, Pruimboom L. Chronic inflammatory diseases are stimulated by current lifestyle: how diet, stress levels and medication prevent our body from recovering. *Nutr Metab* (Lond). 2012 Apr 17;9(1):32. doi: 10.1186/1743-7075-9-32.

22   **Chronic inflammation injures the lining of your arteries:** Paoletti R, Poli A, Cignarella A. The emerging link between nutrition, inflammation and atherosclerosis. *Expert Rev Cardiovasc Ther.* 2006;

4:385–393. Harrington RA. Targeting inflammation in coronary artery disease. *N Engl J Med.* 2017;377:1197–1198.

23 **Some researchers believe that an inflammatory microenvironment:** Mantovani A, Allavena P, Sica A, Balkwill F. Cancer-related inflammation. *Nature.* 2008 Jul 24;454(7203):436–444.

23 **Smoking also promotes lung cancer:** Takahashi H, Ogata H, Nishigaki R, Broide DH, Karin M. Tobacco smoke promotes lung tumorigenesis by triggering IKKbeta- and JNK1-dependent inflammation. *Cancer Cell.* 2010 Jan 19;17(1):89–97.

23 **A sedentary lifestyle increases inflammation, whereas exercise:** Ihalainen JK, Schumann M, Eklund D, et al. Combined aerobic and resistance training decreases inflammation markers in healthy men. *Scand J Med Sci Sports.* 2018 Jan;28(1):40–47. doi: 10.1111/sms.12906. Epub 2017 Jun 13.

23 **Only twenty minutes of walking:** Dimitrova S, Hultenga E, Honga S. Inflammation and exercise: inhibition of monocytic intracellular TNF production by acute exercise via β2-adrenergic activation. *Brain, Behavior and Immunity.* 2017 Mar;61:60–68.

23 **A typical American diet is high in animal protein:** Levine ME, Suarez JA, Brandhorst S, et al. Low protein intake is associated with a major reduction in IGF-1, cancer, and overall mortality in the 65 and younger but not older population. *Cell Metab.* 2014 Mar 4;19(3):407–417. doi: 10.1016/j.cmet.2014.02.006.

23 **reduce levels of a growth factor called IGF-1:** Levine ME, Suarez JA, Brandhorst S, et al. Low protein intake is associated with a major reduction in IGF-1, cancer, and overall mortality in the 65 and younger but not older population. *Cell Metab.* 2014 Mar 4;19(3):407–417. doi: 10.1016/j.cmet.2014.02.006.

23 **lower IGF-1 levels are linked to longer life span:** Couzin-Franke J. Diet studies challenge thinking on proteins versus carbs. *Science.* 2014 Mar 7;343:1068.

23 **In a study of over 6,000 people:** Levine ME, Suarez JA, Brandhorst S, et al. Low protein intake is associated with a major reduction in IGF-1, cancer, and overall mortality in the 65 and younger but not older

population. *Cell Metab.* 2014 Mar 4;19(3):407–417. doi: 10.1016/j
.cmet.2014.02.006.

24 **In this study, 100 patients with coronary heart disease:** Shah B,
Ganguzza L, Slater J, Newman JD, Allen N, Fisher E, et al. The effect of
a vegan versus AHA Diet in coronary artery disease (EVADE CAD)
trial: study design and rationale. *Contemporary Clinical Trials Communications.* 2017;8:90–98.

24 **Naturally occurring sugars, when found:** Joseph SV, Edirisinghe I, Burton-Freeman BM, et al. Fruit polyphenols: a review of anti-
inflammatory effects in humans. *Crit Rev Food Sci Nutr.* 2016;56(3):
419–444. doi: 10.1080/10408398.2013.767221.

24 **However, added sugar, high-fructose corn syrup:** Buyken AE,
Flood V, Empson M, et al. Carbohydrate nutrition and inflammatory
disease mortality in older adults. *Am J Clin Nutr.* 2010 Sep;92(3):634–643.
doi: 10.3945/ajcn.2010.29390. Epub 2010 Jun 23.

24 **In one study, for example, consuming just one can:** Dickinson S, Hancock DP, Petocz P, Ceriello A, Brand-Miller J. High-glycemic
index carbohydrate increases nuclear factor-kappaB activation in mononuclear cells of young, lean healthy subjects. *Am J Clin Nutr.* 2008
May;87(5):1188–1193.

24 **consuming just one can of soda:** Aeberli I, Gerber PA, Hochuli
M, et al. Low to moderate sugar-sweetened beverage consumption impairs glucose and lipid metabolism and promotes inflammation in
healthy young men: a randomized controlled trial. *Am J Clin Nutr.* 2011
Aug;94(2):479–485. doi: 10.3945/ajcn.111.013540. Epub 2011 Jun 15.

25 **Another study found that microscopic toxins causing chronic
inflammation:** Erridge C. The capacity of foodstuffs to induce innate
immune activation of human monocytes in vitro is dependent on food
content of stimulants of Toll-like receptors 2 and 4. *Br J Nutrition.* 2011
Jan;105(1):15–23.

25 **New research is showing that reducing chronic inflammation
with drugs:** Kneisel K. Atherosclerosis consensus paper highlights
CANTOS data. *Medpage Today.* 2018 May 15. https://www.medpage
today.com/cardiology/atherosclerosis/72875. Ridker PM, Everett BM,

Thuren T, et al. Antiinflammatory therapy with canakinumab for atherosclerotic disease. *N Engl J Med.* 2017 Sep 21;377(12)1119–1131. doi: 10.1056/NEJMoa 1707914. Epub 2017 Aug 27.

25   Chronic emotional stress also causes chronic: Rohleder N. Stimulation of systemic low-grade inflammation by psychosocial stress. *Psychosom Med.* 2014 Apr;76(3):181–189.

25   Chronic emotional stress is a common risk factor: Liu YZ, Wang YX, Jiang CL. Inflammation: the common pathway of stress-related diseases. *Front Hum Neurosci.* 2017;11:316.

26   The researchers found that perceived chronic stress or depression: Tawakol A, Ishai A, Takx RA, et al. Relation between resting amygdalar activity and cardiovascular events: a longitudinal and cohort study. *Lancet.* 2017 Feb 25;389(10071):834–845. doi: 10.1016/S0140-6736(16)31714-7. Epub 2017 Jan 12.

27   We found that over 500 genes were favorably changed: Ornish D, Magbanua MJM, Weidner G, Weinberg V, Kemp C, Green C, et al. Changes in prostate gene expression in men undergoing an intensive nutrition and lifestyle intervention. *Proc Nat Acad Sci U S A.* 2008; 105:8369–8374.

27   oncogenes that promote prostate cancer: Liu J, Yang G, Thompson-Lanza JA, Glassman A, Hayes K, Patterson A, Marquez RT, Auersperg N, Yu Y, Hahn WC, Mills GB, Bast RC Jr. A genetically defined model for human ovarian cancer. *Cancer Res.* 2004 Mar 1;64(5):1655–1663.

27   In another study: Ellsworth DL, Croft DT Jr, Weyandt J, et al. Intensive cardiovascular risk reduction induces sustainable changes in expression of genes and pathways important to vascular function. *Circ Cardiovasc Genet.* 2014 Apr;7(2):151–160. doi: 10.1161/CIRCGENETICS.113.000121. Epub 2014 Feb 21.

27   After twelve weeks, these lifestyle medicine changes: Ellsworth DL, Croft DT Jr, Weyandt J, et al. Intensive cardiovascular risk reduction induces sustainable changes in expression of genes and pathways important to vascular function. *Circ Cardiovasc Genet.* 2014 Apr;7(2): 151–160. doi: 10.1161/CIRCGENETICS.113.000121. Epub 2014 Feb 21.

27   **Think of sirtuins as anti-aging genes:** Guarente L. Sirtuins, aging, and medicine. *N Engl J Med.* 2011;364:2235–2244.

28   **AGEs crosslink proteins together:** Di Pino A, Currenti W, Urbano F, et al. High intake of dietary advanced glycation end-products is associated with increased arterial stiffness and inflammation in subjects with type 2 diabetes. *Nutr Metab Cardiovasc Dis.* 2017 Nov; 27(11):978–984. doi: 10.1016/j.numecd.2017.06.014. Epub 2017 Jul 8.

28   **In the brain, AGE molecules may contribute:** Luevano-Contreras C, Chapman-Novakofski K. Dietary advanced glycation end products and aging. *Nutrients.* 2010;2:1247–1265. doi: 10.3390/nu2121247.

28   **Both the type of food and the way it's cooked:** Uribarri J, Woodruff S, Goodman S, et al. Advanced glycation end products in foods and a practical guide to their reduction in the diet. *J Am Diet Assoc.* 2010 June;110(6):911–916.e12. doi: 10.1016/j.jada.2010.03.018.

28   **a soy burger cooked in a microwave has only 20 AGE units:** Ulrich P, Cerami A. Protein glycation, diabetes, and aging. *Recent Prog Horm Res.* 2001;56:1–21.

29   **In anti-aging research, caloric restriction:** van Niekerk G, du Toit A, Loos B, Engelbrecht AM. Nutrient excess and autophagic deficiency: explaining metabolic diseases in obesity. *Metabolism.* 2018 May;82:14–21. doi: 10.1016/j.metabol.2017.12.007. Epub 2017 Dec 28.

29   **Also, sugar causes your body to produce more insulin:** Jabr F. How sugar and fat trick the brain into wanting more food. *Scientific American.* 2016 Jan 1. http://www.scientificamerican.com/article/how -sugar-and-fat-trick-the-brain-into-wanting-more-food.

30   **"Longevity and health were optimized":** Solon-Biet SM, McMahon AC, Ballard JW, et al. The ratio of macronutrients, not caloric intake, dictates cardiometabolic health, aging, and longevity in ad libitum-fed mice. *Cell Metab.* 2014 Mar 4;19(3):418–430. doi: 10.1016 /j.cmet.2014.02.009.

30   **lowering TOR extends life:** Harrison DE, Strong R, Sharp ZD, et al. Rapamycin fed late in life extends lifespan in genetically heterogeneous mice. *Nature.* 2009;460(7253):392–395. doi: 10.1038/nature 08221.

30   **downregulates TOR, prolonging life:** Solon-Biet SM, McMahon AC, Ballard, JW, et al. Ibid.

30   **"speeding car without brakes":** Blagosklonny MV. TOR-driven aging: speeding car without brakes. *Cell Cycle.* 2009;8:(24):4055–4059. doi: 10.4161/cc.8.24.10310.

31   **In modern times, public health advances:** Blagosklonny MV, Hall MN. Growth and aging: a common molecular mechanism. *Aging.* 2009;1:357–362.

31   **limiting intake of animal protein downregulates TOR:** McCarty MF. mTORC1 activity as a determinant of cancer risk— rationalizing the cancer-preventive effects of adiponectin, metformin, rapamycin, and low-protein vegan diets. *Med Hypotheses.* 2011 Oct;77(4):642–648. doi: 10.1016/j.mehy.2011.07.004.

31   **Plants . . . inhibit TOR:** Verburgh K. Nutrigerontology: why we need a new scientific discipline to develop diets and guidelines to reduce the risk of aging-related diseases. *Aging Cell.* 2015;14:17–24.

31   **Substances called flavonols:** Jung CH, Kim H, Ahn J, et al. Fisetin regulates obesity by targeting mTORC1 signaling. *J Nutr Biochem.* 2013 Aug;24(8):1547–1554. doi: 10.1016/j.jnutbio.2013.01.003. Epub 2013 Mar 18.

31   **They also enhance autophagy:** Jung CH, Kim H, Ahn J, et al. Fisetin regulates obesity by targeting mTORC1 signaling. *J Nutr Biochem.* 2013 Aug;24(8):1547–1554. doi: 10.1016/j.jnutbio.2013.01.003. Epub 2013 Mar 18. Hasima N, Ozpolat B. Regulation of autophagy by polyphenolic compounds as a potential therapeutic strategy for cancer. *Cell Death Dis.* 2014 Nov 6;5:e1509. doi: 10.1038/cddis.2014.467.

32   **They wondered if putting these mice on a high-fat:** Kolata G. High-fat diet may fuel spread of prostate cancer. *New York Times.* 2018 Jan 16. Chen M, Zhang J, Sampieri K, et al. An aberrant SREBP-dependent lipogenic program promotes metastatic prostate cancer. *Nat Genet.* 2018 Feb;50(2):206–218. doi: 10.1038/s41588-017-0027-2. Epub 2018 Jan 15.

32   **"Neither genotype pattern":** Gardner CD, Trepanowski JF, Del Gobbo LC, et al. Effect of low-fat vs low-carbohydrate diet on 12-month weight loss in overweight adults and the association with genotype pattern or insulin secretion: the DIETFITS randomized clinical trial. *JAMA*. 2018 Feb 20;319(7):667–679. doi: 10.1001/jama.2018.0245.

32   In our study of almost 3,000 people: Silberman A, Banthia R, Estay IS, Kemp C, Studley J, Hareras D, Ornish D. The effectiveness and efficacy of an intensive cardiac rehabilitation program in 24 sites. *Am J Health Promot.* 2010;24(4):260–266.

33   "This was not a result of either his lifestyle or his diet": CNN. Bill Clinton Hospitalized. 2010 Feb 11. http://archives.cnn.com /TRANSCRIPTS/1002/11/ec.01.html.

33   He's remained on it since then: Conason J. Bill Clinton explains why he became a vegan. *AARP The Magazine.* 2013 Aug–Sep; https://www.aarp.org/health/healthy-living/info-08-2013/bill-clinton -vegan.html.

33   Japanese people living in Japan had a fraction: Buettner D. *The Blue Zones: Lessons for Living Longer From the People Who've Lived the Longest.* Washington DC: *National Geographic;* 2010.

33   However, those Japanese who moved: Benfante R. Studies of cardiovascular disease and cause-specific mortality trends in Japanese-American men living in Hawaii and risk factor comparisons with other Japanese populations in the Pacific region: a review. *Hum Biol.* 1992 Dec;64(6):791–805.

34   Coronary artery disease mortality was *sixteen times*: Campbell TC, Parpia B, Chen J. Diet, lifestyle, and the etiology of coronary artery disease: the Cornell China study. *Am J Cardiol.* 1998;82:187–267.

34   we measured . . . a 30 percent increase in telomerase: Ornish D, Lin J, Daubenmier J, Weidner G, Epel E, Kemp C, Magbanua MJM, Marlin R, Yglecias L, Carroll P, Blackburn E. Increased telomerase activity and comprehensive lifestyle changes. *Lancet Oncol.* 2008;9:1048–1057.

35   telomere length actually *increased* by 10 percent: Ornish D, Lin J, Chan JM, Epel E, Kemp C, Weidner G, Marlin R, Frenda SJ, Magbanua MJM, Daubenmier J, Estay I, Hills NK, Chainani-Wu N, Caroll PR, Blackburn EH. Effect of comprehensive lifestyle changes on telomerase activity and telomere length in men with biopsy-proven low-risk prostate cancer: 5-year follow-up of a descriptive pilot study. *Lancet Oncol.* 2013 Oct;14(11):1112–1120. doi: 10.1016/S1470–2045(13) 70366–8. Epub 2013 Sep 17.

35 **Some of our best friends are germs:** Pollan M. Some of my best friends are germs. *New York Times.* 2013 May 15.

35 **They have co-evolved with us over millennia:** Kolata G. In good health? Thank your 100 trillion bacteria. *New York Times.* 2012 Jun 13.

36 **Your microbiome contains more than:** Komaroff AL. The microbiome and risk for atherosclerosis. *JAMA.* 2018 Jun 19;319(23):2381–2382. doi: 10.1001/jama.2018.5240.

36 **We are now conducting research with Dr. Rob Knight:** KnightLab, University of California. https://knightlab.ucsd.edu/word press/?page_id=47.

36 **interact with our microbiome in healing ways:** Tremaroli V, Bäckhed F. Functional interactions between the gut microbiota and host metabolism. *Nature.* 2012;489:242.

36 **One study compared the microbiome:** Franco-de-Moraes AC, de Almeida-Pititto B, da Rocha Fernandes G, et al. Worse inflammatory profile in omnivores than in vegetarians associates with the gut microbiota composition. *Diabetol Metab Syndr.* 2017 Aug 15;9:62. doi: 10.1186/s13098-017-0261-x. eCollection 2017.

37 **Just a single weeklong course of antibiotics:** Zaura E, Brandt BW, Teixeira de Mattos MJ, et al. Same exposure but two radically different responses to antibiotics: resilience of the salivary microbiome versus long-term microbial shifts in feces. *mBio.* 2015;6(6):e01693–01715. doi: 10.1128/mBio.01693-15. Beck J. Taking antibiotics can change the gut microbiome for up to a year. *Atlantic.* 2015 Nov 16.

37 **Almost 80 percent of antibiotics sold in this country:** Cohan WD. Antibiotics in meat could be damaging our guts. *New York Times.* 2018 May 25.

37 **The Centers for Disease Control and Prevention:** CDC. Protecting the food supply. 2018 Jan 31. https://www.cdc.gov/drug resistance/protecting_food-supply.html.

37   **In 2013, researchers showed that people living near pig farms:** Guglielmi G. Are antibiotics turning livestock into superbug factories? *Science.* 2017 Sep 28.

37   **"One of the public food safety issues":** Harden GH, Office of Inspector General, United States Department of Agriculture. FSIS National Residue Program for Cattle. *Audit Report.* 24601-08-KC. 2010 Mar.

38   **high-fat diets . . . alter the microbes in your gut:** Murphy EA, Velasquez KT, Herbert KM. Influence of high-fat-diet on gut microbiota: a driving force for chronic disease risk. *Curr Opin Clin Nutr Metab Care.* 2015 Sep;18(5):515–520.

38   **When we eat a lot of sugar, harmful bacteria thrive:** Kruis W, Forstmaier G, Scheurlen C, and Stellaard F. Effect of diets low and high in refined sugars on gut transit, bile acid metabolism, and bacterial fermentation. *Gut.* 1991 Apr;32(4):367–371.

38   **Microbes leaking through the gut into the bloodstream:** Gregory JC, Buffa JA, Org E, et al. Transmission of atherosclerosis susceptibility with gut microbial transplantation. *J Biol Chem.* 2015 Feb 27;290(9):5647–5660. He J, Guo H, Zheng W, Yao W. Effects of stress on the mucus-microbial interactions in the gut. *Curr Protein Pept Sci.* 2018 May 14. doi: 10.2174/1389203719666180514152406.

39   **In one study, six weeks of moderate exercise:** Allen JM, Mailing LJ, Niemiro GM, et al. Exercise alters gut microbiota composition and function in lean and obese humans. *Med Sci Sports Exerc.* 2018 Apr;50(4):747–757.

39:   **bolster our metabolism:** Reynolds G. Exercise alters our microbiome. Is that one reason it's so good for us? *New York Times.* 2018 Jan 3.

39   **Emotional stress changes the relative proportion of microbes:** Bailey MT, Dowd SE, Galley JD, et al. Exposure to a social stressor alters the structure of the intestinal microbiota: implications for stressor-induced immunomodulation. *Brain Behav Immun.* 2011 Mar; 25(3):397–407.

39   **Also, inflammation increases depression:** Kaplan BJ, Rucklidge JJ, Romijn A, McLeod K. The emerging field of nutritional mental health: inflammation, the microbiome, oxidative stress, and mitochondrial function. *Clinical Psychological Science.* 2015. doi: 10.1177 /2167702614555413.

39   help restore a healthy balance in your microbiome: Househam AM, Peterson CT, Mills PJ, Chopra D. The effects of stress and meditation on the immune system, human microbiota, and epigenetics. *Adv Mind Body Med.* 2017 Fall;31(4):10–25.

39   Some clinical studies have shown that probiotics: Mancuso C, Santangelo R. Alzheimer's disease and gut microbiota modifications. *Pharmacol Res.* 2018 Mar;129:329–336. doi: 10.1016/j.phrs.2017.12.009. Epub 2017 Dec 9.

40   When your DNA is damaged, it can lead to many types of cancer: Halliwell B. Oxidative stress and cancer: have we moved forward? *Biochem J.* 2007;401(1):1–11. doi: 10.1042/BJ20061131. PMID 17150040. Buttke TM, Sandstrom PA. Oxidative stress as a mediator of apoptosis. *Immunol Today.* 1994 Jan;15(1):7–10.

40   When your arteries are damaged, it can lead: Singh N, Dhalla AK, Seneviratne C, Singal PK. Oxidative stress and heart failure. *Mol Cell Biochem.* 1995 Jun;147(1):77–81. doi: 10.1007/BF00944786. Rautiainen S, Larsson S, Virtamo J, Wolk A. Total antioxidant capacity of diet and risk of stroke: a population-based prospective cohort of women. *Stroke.* 2012 Feb;43(2):335–340. doi: 10.1161/STROKEAHA.111.635557.

40   When your cell membranes are damaged: Gems D, Partridge L. Stress-response hormesis and aging: "that which does not kill us makes us stronger." *Cell Metab.* 2008 Mar;7(3):200–203. doi: 10.1016 /j.cmet.2008.01.001. Best BP. Nuclear DNA damage as a direct cause of aging. *Rejuvenation Res.* 2009;12(3):199–208. doi: 10.1089/rej.2009 .0847. PMID 19594328.

40   When the cells in your pancreas are damaged: Cohen G, Riahi Y, Sunda V, Deplano S, Chatgilialoglu C, Ferreri C, Kaiser N, Sasson S. Signaling properties of 4-hydroxyalkenals formed by lipid peroxidation in diabetes. *Free Radic Biol Med.* 2013;65:978–987. doi: 10.1016/j.freeradbiomed.2013.08.163.

41   When the cells in your brain are damaged: Patel VP, Chu CT. Nuclear transport, oxidative stress, and neurodegeneration. *Int J Clin Exp Pathol.* 2011;4(3):215–229.

41   **When proteins in your body are damaged:** Hoffmann MH, Griffiths HR. The dual role of ROS in autoimmune and inflammatory diseases: evidence from preclinical models. *Free Radic Biol Med.* 2018 Mar 15. doi: 10.1016/j.freeradbiomed.2018.03.016. Epub ahead of print.

41   **data from eight countries showed:** Grant WB. The role of meat in the expression of rheumatoid arthritis. *Br J Nutr.* 2000 Nov;84(5):589–595.

41   **Methionine is one of the essential amino acids:** Cavuoto P, Fenech MF. A review of methionine dependency and the role of methionine restriction in cancer growth control and life-span extension. *Cancer Treat Rev.* 2012 Oct;38(6):726–736. doi: 10.1016/j.ctrv.2012.01.004. Epub 2012 Feb 17.

41   **This provides another reason why:** Cavuoto P, Fenech MF. A review of methionine dependency and the role of methionine restriction in cancer growth control and life-span extension. *Cancer Treat Rev.* 2012 Oct;38(6):726–36. doi: 10.1016/j.ctrv.2012.01.004. Epub 2012 Feb 17.

41   **"Comparing the mean value":** Carlsen MH, Halvorsen BL, Holte K, Bøhn SK, Dragland S, Sampson L, Willey C, Senoo H, Umezono Y, Sanada C, Barikmo I, Berhe N, Willett WC, Phillips KM, Jacobs DR Jr, Blomhoff R. The total antioxidant content of more than 3100 foods, beverages, spices, herbs and supplements used worldwide. *Nutr J.* 2010 Jan 22;9:3. doi: 10.1186/1475-2891-9-3.

42   **There are anti-angiogenesis drugs like Avastin:** Kolata G, Pollack A. Costly cancer drug offers hope, but also a dilemma. *New York Times.* 2008 Jul 6.

42   **My colleagues and I conducted a randomized controlled trial of men:** Ornish DM, Weidner G, Fair WR, et al. Intensive lifestyle changes may affect the progression of prostate cancer. *J Urol.* 2005;174:1065–1070.

42   **In collaboration with Dr. Will Li:** Ornish D, Li W, Klement GL, et al. Diet and lifestyle interventions influence angiogenesis biomarkers and outcomes in men with prostate cancer. *Lancet Oncol.* 2018. Under editorial review.

43   **Angiogenesis also enhances chronic inflammation:** Jackson JR, Seed MP, Kircher CH, Willoughby DA, Winkler JD. The codependence of angiogenesis and chronic inflammation. *FASEB J.* 1997 May;11(6):457–465.

43   Most of the foods that beneficially affect angiogenesis: Li WW, Li VW, Hutnik M, Chiou AS. Tumor angiogenesis as a target for dietary cancer prevention. *J Oncol.* 2012;2012:879623.

43   Even a single meal high in animal protein and fat: Vogel RA, Corretti MC, Plotnick GD. Effect of a single high-fat meal on endothelial function in healthy subjects. *Am J Cardiol.* 1997 Feb 1;79(3):350–354.

43   In another study comparing diets: Miller M, Beach V, Sorkin JD. Comparative effects of three popular diets on lipids, endothelial function, and C-reactive protein during weight maintenance. *J Am Diet Assoc.* 2009;109:713–717.

43   A 2018 study documented that a single high-fat meal: Benson TW, Weintraub NL, Kim HW. A single high-fat meal provokes pathological erythrocyte remodeling and increases myeloperoxidase levels: implications for acute coronary syndrome. *Lab Invest.* 2018 Mar 23. doi: 10.1038/s41374-018-0038-3. Epub ahead of print.

44   You can actually grow so many new brain neurons: Pereira AC, Huddleston DE, Brickman AM, et al. An in vivo correlate of exercise-induced neurogenesis in the adult dentate gyrus. *Proc Natl Acad Sci U S A.* 2007 Mar 27;104(13):5638–5643. Epub 2007 Mar 20.

44   Roman gladiators: Curry G. The gladiator diet. *Archaeology Archive.* 2008 Nov–Dec;61(6).

44   Your eyes get more blood flow: Kommana SS, Padgaonkar P, Mendez N, et al. Fundus autofluorescence captured with a nonmydriatic retinal camera in vegetarians versus nonvegetarians. *J Diabetes Sci Technol.* 2015 Sep 9;10(1):151–156. doi: 10.1177/1932296815599003.

44   Your ears get more blood flow: Curhan SG, Wang M, Eavey RD, et al. Adherence to healthful dietary patterns is associated with lower risk of hearing loss in women. *J Nutr.* 2018 May 11. doi: 10.1093/jn/nxy058. Epub ahead of print.

45   When your heart doesn't receive enough blood flow: Ornish DM, Scherwitz LW, Doody RS, Kesten D, McLanahan SM, Brown SE,

DePuey G, Sonnemaker R, Haynes C, Lester J, McAllister GK, Hall RJ, Burdine JA, Gotto AM. Effects of stress management training and dietary changes in treating ischemic heart disease. *JAMA*. 1983;249: 54–59.

45   In our research studies, people with severe heart disease: Ornish DM, Scherwitz LW, Doody RS, Kesten D, McLanahan SM, Brown SE, DePuey G, Sonnemaker R, Haynes C, Lester J, McAllister GK, Hall RJ, Burdine JA, Gotto AM. Effects of stress management training and dietary changes in treating ischemic heart disease. *JAMA*. 1983;249:54–59.

45   the Queen's Guards: Quinn D. London's guards are falling down! *People*. 2017 Jun 17. http://people.com/royals/queens-guard -faints-at-trooping-the-colour-2017.

45   Spending a lot of time sitting: Kumar A, Prasad M, Kathuria P. Sitting occupations are an independent risk factor for ischemic stroke in North Indian population. *Int J Neurosci*. 2014 Oct;124(10):748–754. doi: 10.3109/00207454.2013.879130. Epub 2014 Feb 7.

45   Sitting for more than eight hours a day: Biswas A, Oh PI, Faulkner GE, Bajaj RR, Silver MA, Mitchell MS, Alter DA. Sedentary time and its association with risk for disease incidence, mortality, and hospitalization in adults: a systematic review and meta-analysis. *Ann Intern Med*. 2015 Jan 20;162(2):123–132. doi: 10.7326/M14-1651.

46   The combination of both sitting more than six hours: Patel AV, Bernstein L, Deka A, et al. Leisure time spent sitting in relation to total mortality in a prospective cohort of US adults. *Am J Epidemiol*. 2010 Aug 15;172(4):419–429, https://doi.org/10.1093/aje/kwq155.

46   Researchers recently found that sitting: Carter SE, Draijer R, Holder SM, et al. Regular walking breaks prevent the decline in cerebral blood flow associated with prolonged sitting. *J Appl Physiol* (1985). 2018 Jun 7. doi: 10.1152/japplphysiol.00310.2018.

46   Studies show that both are important: Duvivier BMFM, Bolijn JE, Koster A, et al. Reducing sitting time versus adding exercise: differential effects on biomarkers of endothelial dysfunction and metabolic risk. *Scientific Reports*. 2018;8:8657.

46 **One study found that the more breaks you take:** Carson V, Wong SL, Winkler E, et al. Patterns of sedentary time and cardiometabolic risk among Canadian adults. *Prev Med.* 2014 Aug;65:23–27.

47 **One large study of almost 30,000 men:** Leitzmann MF, Platz EA, Stampfer MJ, Willett WC, Giovannucci E. Ejaculation frequency and subsequent risk of prostate cancer. *JAMA.* 2004 Apr 7;291(13):1578–1586.

47 **A follow-up study:** Rider JR, Wilson KM, Sinnott JA, Kelly RS, Mucci LA, Giovannucci EL. Ejaculation frequency and risk of prostate cancer: updated results with an additional decade of follow-up. *Eur Urol.* 2016 Dec;70(6):974–982.

48 **carcinogens contained in it:** Cummings JH, Engineer A. Denis Burkitt and the origins of the dietary fibre hypothesis. *Nutrition Research Review.* 2018;31:1–15.

Chapter 3

50 **His LDL cholesterol fell by almost 50 percent:** Williams KA, Cardiobuzz: vegan diet, healthy heart? *Medpage Today.* 2014 July 21. http://www.medpagetoday.com/Blogs/CardioBuzz/46860.

50 **others were turned away at the door:** Ward T. Dean Ornish in Defense of the Dietary Fat—Heart Disease Link. *Medscape Cardiology,* May 12, 2016; Ward T. Dean Ornish on Love and Connection (the Touchy-Feely Stuff). *Medscape Cardiology.* 2016 May 12.

50 **I am one of the founders of the American:** lifestylemedicine.org.

51 **Advisory Group on Prevention:** Advisory Group on Prevention, Health Promotion, and Integrative and Public Health. Fulfilling the legacy. Washington DC: US Dept. of Health and Human Services; 2016. https://www.surgeongeneral.gov/priorities/prevention/advisorygrp/2016-12-20-fulfilling-the-legacy-report.pdf.

51 ***Lancet Oncology* "Moonshot" Commission:** Future cancer research priorities in the USA: a Lancet Oncology Commission. *Lancet*

Oncol. 2017 Nov;18(11):e653–e706. doi: 10.1016/S1470–2045(17) 30698-8. Epub 2017 Oct 31.

52   **more than one doctor a day kills themself:** Andrew LB. Physician suicide. *Medscape.* 2017 Jun 12.

52   **the word "nutrition" is completely absent:** Devries S, Dalen J, Eisenberg DM, Maizes V, Ornish D, Prasad A, Sierpina V, Weil AT, Willett W. A deficiency of nutrition education in medical training. *Am J Med.* 2014 Sep;127(9):804–806.

52   **Lifestyle medicine is better than angioplasties and stents:** Stergiopoulos K, Brown DL. Initial coronary stent implantation with medical therapy vs medical therapy alone for stable coronary artery disease: meta-analysis of randomized controlled trials. *Arch Intern Med.* 2012 Feb 27;172(4):312–319. Boden WE, O'Rourke RA, Teo KK, et al. COURAGE Trial Research Group. Optimal medical therapy with or without PCI for stable coronary disease. *N Engl J Med.* 2007;356(15):1503–1516.

53   **did not reduce angina more than doing nothing:** Al-Lamee R, Thompson D, Dehbi H-M, et al. Percutaneous coronary intervention in stable angina (ORBITA): a double-blind, randomized controlled trial. *Lancet.* 2017; published online Nov 2. http://dx.doi org/10.1016/S0140-6736(17)32714-9.

53   **"All cardiology guidelines should be revised":** Brown DL, Redberg RF. Last nail in the coffin for PCI in stable angina? *Lancet.* 2017 Nov 2. http://dx.doi.org/10.1016/S0140-6736(17)32757-5.

54   **there was still no reduction in heart attacks or premature deaths:** Xaplanteris P, Fournier S, Pijls NHJ, et al. Five-year outcomes with PCI guided by fractional flow reserve. *N Engl J Med.* 2018 May 22. doi: 10.1056/NEJMoa1803538.

54   **Within a month, there was significant:** Ornish DM, Gotto AM, Miller RR, et al. Effects of a vegetarian diet and selected yoga techniques in the treatment of coronary heart disease. *Clinical Research.* 1979;27:720A.

54   **in the ability of the heart to pump:** Ornish DM, Scherwitz LW, Doody RS, Kesten D, McLanahan SM, Brown SE, DePuey G, Sonnemaker R, Haynes C, Lester J, McAllister GK, Hall RJ, Burdine JA, Gotto AM. Effects of stress management training and dietary changes in treating ischemic heart disease. *JAMA.* 1983;249:54–59.

54   Within one year, even severely clogged: Ornish DM, Brown SE, Scherwitz LW, et al. Can lifestyle changes reverse coronary atherosclerosis? The Lifestyle Heart Trial. *Lancet.* 1990;336:129–133. Reprinted in *Yearbook of Medicine and Yearbook of Cardiology* (New York: C.V. Mosby; 1991).

54   There was even more reversal after five years: Ornish D, Scherwitz L, Billings J, Brown SE, et al. Intensive lifestyle changes for reversal of coronary heart disease: five-year follow-up of the Lifestyle Heart Trial. *JAMA.* 1998;280:2001–2007.

54   Cardiac PET (positron emission tomography) scans: Gould KL, Ornish D, Scherwitz L, Stuart Y, Buchi M, Billings J, Armstrong W, Ports T, Scherwitz L. Changes in myocardial perfusion abnormalities by positron emission tomography after long-term, intense risk factor modification. *JAMA.* 1995;274:894–901.

55   In a study of over 23,000 European men and women: Ford ES, Bergmann MM, Kröger J, Schienkiewitz A, Weikert C, Boeing H. Healthy living is the best revenge: findings from the European Prospective Investigation into Cancer and Nutrition—Potsdam study. *Arch Intern Med.* 2009 Aug 10;169(15):1355–1362. doi: 10.1001/archinternmed.2009.237.

55   In the Diabetes Prevention Program: Diabetes Prevention Program Research Group. Reduction in the incidence of type 2 diabetes with lifestyle intervention or metformin. *N Engl J Med.* 2002 Feb 7;346(6).

55   In the Finnish Diabetes Prevention Study Group: Tuomilehto J, Lindström J, Eriksson JG, Valle TT, Hämäläinen H, Ilanne-Parikka P, Keinänen-Kiukaanniemi S, Laakso M, Louheranta A, Rastas M, Salminen V, Uusitupa M, Finnish Diabetes Prevention Study Group. Prevention of type 2 diabetes mellitus by changes in lifestyle among subjects with impaired glucose tolerance. *N Engl J Med.* 2001 May 3;344(18):1343–1350.

55   **A study of over 200,000 men and women:** Satija A, Bhupathi-raju SN, Rimm EB, et al. Plant-based dietary patterns and incidence of type 2 diabetes in US men and women: results from three prospective cohort studies. *PLoS Med.* 2016 Jun 14;13(6):e1002039. doi: 10.1371 /journal.pmed.1002039. eCollection 2016 Jun.

55   **A review article from the Mayo Clinic:** Montori VM, Fernández-Balsells M. Glycemic control in type 2 diabetes: time for an evidence-based about-face? *Ann Intern Med.* 2009;150:803–808.

56   **A meta-analysis . . . thirteen randomized controlled trials:** Boussageon R, Saadatian-Elahi M, Bergeonneau C, et al. Effect of intensive glucose lowering treatment on all cause mortality, cardiovascular death, and microvascular events in type 2 diabetes: meta-analysis of randomised controlled trials. *BMJ.* 2011;343:d4169. doi: https://doi .org/10.1136/bmj.d4169.

56   **A systematic review of studies from the Therapeutics Initiative:** Therapeutics Initiative. Is the current "glucocentric" approach to management of type 2 diabetes misguided? *Therapeutics Letter.* 2016 Nov–Dec;103:1–2.

56   **Data from two large randomized controlled trials:** The AC-CORD Study Group. Long-term effects of intensive glucose lowering on cardiovascular outcomes. *N Engl J Med.* 2011;364:818–828. The NAVI-GATOR Study Group. *N Engl J Med.* 2010 Apr 22;362(16):1463–1476.

56   **Another study found that a different drug (empagliflozin):** Zinman B, Wanner C, Lachin JM, Fitchett D, Bluhmki E, Hantel S, Mattheus M, Devins T, Johansen OE, Woerle HJ, Broedl UC, Inzucchi SE; EMPA-REG OUTCOME Investigators. Empagliflozin, cardiovascular outcomes, and mortality in type 2 diabetes. *N Engl J Med.* 2015 Nov 26;373(22):2117–2128. doi: 10.1056/NEJMoa1504720. Epub 2015 Sep 17.

56   **In our research, we were able to document reductions in their blood sugar:** Silberman A, Banthia R, Estay IS, Kemp C, Studley J, Hareras D, Ornish D. The effectiveness and efficacy of an intensive cardiac rehabilitation program in 24 sites. *Am J Health Promot.* 2010; 24(4):260–266.

57   **Similarly, a large randomized controlled trial found:** The Look AHEAD Research Group. Cardiovascular effects of intensive lifestyle intervention in type 2 diabetes. *N Engl J Med.* 2013;369:145–154. doi: 10.1056/NEJMoa1212914.

57   **One study showed that statin treatment:** Cederberg H, Stančáková A, Yaluri N, Modi S, Kuusisto J, Laakso M. Increased risk of diabetes with statin treatment is associated with impaired insulin sensitivity and insulin secretion: a 6 year follow-up study of the METSIM cohort. *Diabetologia.* 2015 May;58(5):1109–1117.

57   **Approximately one-third of men:** Bell KJ, Del Mar C, Wright G, Dickinson J, Glasziou P. Prevalence of incidental prostate cancer: a systematic review of autopsy studies. *Int J Cancer.* 2015 Oct 1;137(7):1749–1757.

58   **men diagnosed with early-stage prostate cancer who did nothing:** ProtecT Study Group. 10-Year outcomes after monitoring, surgery, or radiotherapy for localized prostate cancer. *N Engl J Med.* 2016;375:1415–1424.

58   **Similar results were found in an earlier study:** Wilt TJ, Brawer MK, Jones KM, Barry MJ, Aronson WJ, Fox S, Gingrich JR, Wei JT, Gilhooly P, Grob BM, Nsouli I, Iyer P, Cartagena R, Snider G, Roehrborn C, Sharifi R, Blank W, Pandya P, Andriole GL, Culkin D, Wheeler T. Prostate Cancer Intervention versus Observation Trial (PIVOT) Study Group. Radical prostatectomy versus observation for localized prostate cancer. *N Engl J Med.* 2012 Jul 19;367(3):203–213.

58   **Few things are more distressing and humiliating:** Resnick MJ, Koyama T, Fan KH, et al. Long-term functional outcomes after treatment for localized prostate cancer. *N Engl J Med.* 2013;368:436–445.

58   **Memorial Sloan-Kettering Cancer Center:** Ornish DM, Weidner G, Fair WR, Marlin R, Pettengill EB, Raisin CJ, Dunn-Emke S, Crutchfield L, Jacobs NF, Barnard RJ, Aronson WJ, McCormac P, McKnight DJ, Fein JD, Dnistrian AM, Weinstein J, Ngo TH, Mendell NR, Carroll PR. Intensive lifestyle changes may affect the progression of prostate cancer. *J Urol.* 2005;174:1065–1070.

58   **There is a relatively small subset of men:** Schröder FH, Hugosson J, Roobol MJ, Tammela TL, et al. Screening and prostate-cancer mortality in a randomized European study. *N Engl J Med.* 2009 Mar 26;360(13):1320–1328. doi: 10.1056/NEJMoa0810084. Epub 2009 Mar 18.

58   **have rapidly rising prostate-specific** Cooperberg MR, Brooks JD, Faino AV, Newcomb LF, Kearns JT, Carroll PR, et al. Refined analysis of prostate-specific antigen kinetics to predict prostate cancer active surveillance outcomes. *Eur Urol.* 2018 Aug;74(2):211–217. doi: 10.1016 /j.eururo.2018.01.017. Epub 2018 Feb 9.

59   **men who were diagnosed with prostate cancer who ate:** Yang M, Kenfield SA, Van Blarigan EL, Batista JL, Sesso HD, Ma J, Stampfer MJ, Chavarro JE. Dietary patterns after prostate cancer diagnosis in relation to disease-specific and total mortality. *Cancer Prev Res (Phila).* 2015 Jun. doi: 10.1158/1940–6207.

59   **Although we have not yet conducted:** Coffey D. Similarities of prostate and breast cancer: evolution, diet, and estrogens. *Urology.* 2001 Apr;57(4 Suppl 1):31–38.

59   **women who reduced their dietary fat intake:** Chlebowski RT, Blackburn GL, Thomson CA, et al. Dietary fat reduction and breast cancer outcome: interim efficacy results from the Women's Intervention Nutrition Study. *J Natl Cancer Inst.* 2006 Dec 20;98(24):1767–1776.

Chapter 4

61   **A consensus is emerging:** Oldways Common Ground website. https://oldwayspt.org/programs/oldways-common-ground/oldways -common-ground.

62   **paraphrasing Michael Pollan:** Pollan M. *In Defense of Food.* New York: Penguin; 2008.

62   **increasing evidence that it may be better to avoid dairy and eggs:** Aune D, Navarro Rosenblatt DA, Chan DS. Dairy products, calcium, and prostate cancer risk: a systematic review and meta-analysis of cohort studies. *Am J Clin Nutr.* 2015 Jan;101(1):87–117. doi: 10.3945/ajcn.113.067157. Epub 2014 Nov 19.

63   Too much protein leads to increased risks: Delimaris I. Adverse effects associated with protein intake above the recommended dietary allowance for adults. *ISRN Nutr.* 2013 Jul 18;2013:126929. doi: 10.5402/2013/126929.

63   In 2016 the USDA dietary guidelines stated: O'Connor A. New dietary guidelines urge less sugar for all and less protein for boys and men. *New York Times.* 2016 Jan 7.

63   For most people, it's only 0.36 grams: National Research Council. Recommended Dietary Allowances. 10th ed. Washington DC: National Academies Press; 1989.

65   strongman Patrik Baboumian . . . Dotsie Bausch: http://gamechangersmovie.com.

65   Ötillö Swimrun World Championship: Lelinwalla M. The world's fittest vegan is a 51-year-old ultra-endurance athlete. *Men's Health.* 2018 Mar 19.

66   the pages of the *Journal of the American Medical Association***:** Atkins RC, Ornish D, Wadden T. Low-carb, low-fat diet gurus face off. Interview by Joan Stephenson. *JAMA.* 2003 Apr 9;289(14):1767–1768, 1773.

66   An optimal way of eating: Ornish DM, Scherwitz LW, Doody RS, Kesten D, McLanahan SM, Brown SE, DePuey G, Sonnemaker R, Haynes C, Lester J, McAllister GK, Hall RJ, Burdine JA, Gotto AM. Effects of stress management training and dietary changes in treating ischemic heart disease. *JAMA.* 1983;249:54–59. Ornish DM, Brown SE, Scherwitz LW, et al. Can lifestyle changes reverse coronary atherosclerosis? The Lifestyle Heart Trial. *Lancet.* 1990;336:129–133. (Reprinted in *Yearbook of Medicine and Yearbook of Cardiology.* New York: C.V. Mosby; 1991.) Gould KL, Ornish D, Kirkeeide R, Brown S, et al. Improved stenosis geometry by quantitative coronary arteriography after vigorous risk factor modification. *Am J Cardiol.* 1992;69:845–853. Gould KL, Ornish D, Scherwitz L, Stuart Y, Buchi M, Billings J, Armstrong W, Ports T, Scherwitz L. Changes in myocardial perfusion abnormalities by positron emission tomography after long-term, intense risk factor modification. *JAMA*. 1995;274:894–901. Ornish D, Scherwitz L, Billings J, Brown SE, Gould KL, Merritt TA, Sparler S, Armstrong WT, Ports TA, Kirkeeide RL, Hogeboom C, Brand RJ. Intensive lifestyle changes for reversal of coronary heart disease: five-year follow-up of the Lifestyle Heart Trial. *JAMA*. 1998;280:2001–2007. Freeman AM, Morris PB, Barnard N, Esselstyn CB, Ros E, Agatston A, Devries S, O'Keefe J, Miller M, Ornish D, Williams K, Kris-Etherton P. Trending cardiovascular nutrition controversies. *J Am Coll Cardiol*. 2017 Mar 7;69(9):1172–1187. doi:10.1016/j.jacc.2016.10.086. Esselstyn CB Jr. Updating a 12-year experience with arrest and reversal therapy for coronary heart disease (an overdue requiem for palliative cardiology). *Am J Cardiol*. 1999 Aug 1;84(3):339–341, A8. Silberman A, Banthia R, Estay IS, Kemp C, Studley J, Hareras D, Ornish D. The effectiveness and efficacy of an intensive cardiac rehabilitation program in 24 sites. *Am J Health Promot*. 2010;24(4):260–266. Ornish D, Lin J, Daubenmier J, Weidner G, Epel E, Kemp C, Magbanua MJM, Marlin R, Yglecias L, Carroll P, Blackburn E. Increased telomerase activity and comprehensive lifestyle changes: a pilot study. *Lancet Oncol*. 2008;9:1048–1057. Ornish D, Lin J, Chan JM, Epel E, Kemp C, Weidner G, Marlin R, Frenda SJ, Magbanua MJM, Daubenmier J, Estay I, Hills NK, Chainani-Wu N, Caroll PR, Blackburn EH. Effect of comprehensive lifestyle changes on telomerase activity and telomere length in men with biopsy-proven low-risk prostate cancer. *Lancet Oncol*. 2013 Oct;14(11):1112–1120. doi: 10.1016/S1470-2045(13)70366-8. Epub 2013 Sep 17. PMID: 24051140. Ornish DM, Weidner G, Fair WR, Marlin R, Pettengill EB, Raisin CJ, Dunn-Emke S, Crutchfield L, Jacobs NF, Barnard RJ, Aronson WJ, McCormac P, McKnight DJ, Fein JD, Dnistrian AM, Weinstein J, Ngo TH, Mendell NR, Carroll PR. Intensive lifestyle changes may affect the progression of prostate cancer. *J Urol*. 2005;174:1065–1070.

66   a Harvard Study of heart attack survivors: Li S, Flint A, Pai JK, et al. Low carbohydrate diet from plant or animal sources and mortality among myocardial infarction survivors. *J Am Heart Assoc*. 2014 Sep 22;3(5):e001169. doi: 10.1161/JAHA.114.001169.

66   in a study of over 130,000 men and women: Song M, Fung TT, Hu FB, et al. Association of animal and plant protein intake with all-cause and cause-specific mortality. *JAMA Intern Med*. 2016;176(10):1453–1463.

67 **In almost 30,000 postmenopausal women:** Keleman LE, et al. Associations of dietary protein with disease and mortality in a prospective study of postmenopausal women. *Am J Epidemiol.* 2005;161:239–249.

67 **In other studies, diets high in animal protein:** Barbour MF, et al. Mostly meat, high protein diet linked to heart failure in older women. American Heart Association Annual Scientific Sessions. 2016 Nov 14. Virtanen HEK, Voutilainen S, Koskinen TT, Mursu J, Tuomainen TP, Virtanen JK. Intake of different dietary proteins and risk of heart failure in men: the Kuopio Ischaemic Heart Disease Risk Factor Study. *Circ Heart Fail.* 2018 Jun;11(6):e004531. doi: 10.1161/CIRCHEARTFAIL URE.117.004531.

67 **in a study of over 6,000 people:** Levine ME, Suarez JA, Brandhorst S, et al. Low protein intake is associated with a major reduction in IGF-1, cancer, and overall mortality in the 65 and younger but not older population. *Cell Metab.* 2014 Mar 4;19(3):407–417. doi: 10.1016/j .cmet.2014.02.006.

67 **An article in the *New England Journal of Medicine:*** Smith SR. A look at the low-carbohydrate diet. *N Engl J Med.* 2009 Dec 3;361(23):2286–2288. doi: 10.1056/NEJMcibr0908756.

69 **meat actually *increases* insulin levels in your blood:** Roden M, Price TB, Perseghin G, et al. Mechanism of free fatty acid–induced insulin resistance in humans. *J Clin Invest.* 1996 Jun 15;97(12):2859–2865. Tucker LA, LeCheminant JD, Bailey BW, et al. Meat intake and insulin resistance in women without type 2 diabetes. *J Diabetes Res.* 2015;2015: 174742.

69 **So does fat:** Muoio DM. Revisiting the connection between intramyocellular lipids and insulin resistance: a long and winding road. *Diabetologia.* 2012 Oct;55(10):2551–2554. doi: 10.1007/s00125-012-2597-y. Epub 2012 Jun 3. Krssak M, Falk Petersen K, Dresner A, et al. Intramyocellular lipid concentrations are correlated with insulin sensitivity in humans: a 1H NMR spectroscopy study. *Diabetologia.* 1999 Jan;42(1):113–116.

69 **diabetes increases as the frequency of meat consumption increases:** Snowdon DA, Phillips RL. Does a vegetarian diet reduce the occurrence of diabetes? *Am J Public Health.* 1985;75:507–512.

69   **In contrast, insulin levels are lower:** Roberts CK, Vaziri ND, Barnard RJ. Effect of diet and exercise intervention on blood pressure, insulin, oxidative stress, and nitric oxide availability. *Circulation.* 2002; 106:2530–2532.

69   **A study of 37,000 men:** Pan A, Sun Q, Bernstein AM, et al. Red meat consumption and risk of type 2 diabetes: 3 cohorts of US adults and an updated meta-analysis. *Am J Clin Nutr.* 2011;94(4):1088–1096.

69   **This study also found that consumption of both processed:** Pan A, Sun Q, Bernstein AM, et al. Red meat consumption and mortality: results from 2 prospective cohort studies. *Arch Intern Med.* doi:10.1001/archinternmed.2011.2287. Epub 2012 Mar 12. Ornish D. Holy cow! What's good for you is good for our planet. *Arch Intern Med.* 2012 Apr 9;172(7):563–564. doi: 10.1001/archinternmed.2012.174. Epub 2012 Mar 12.

69   **Again, it's not low-fat versus low-carb:** Ward T. Dean Ornish in defense of the dietary fat–heart disease link. *Medscape.* 2016 May 12. https://www.medscape.com/viewarticle/862903.

69   **As a result, your body increases the uptake of fat:** Kern PA, Ong JM, Saffari B, Carty J. The effects of weight loss on the activity and expression of adipose-tissue lipoprotein lipase in very obese humans. *N Engl J Med.* 1990;322(15):1053–1059.

69   **patients in our Lifestyle Heart Trial lost:** Ornish D, Scherwitz L, Billings J, et al. Intensive lifestyle changes for reversal of coronary heart disease: five-year follow-up of the Lifestyle Heart Trial. *JAMA.* 1998;280:2001–2007.

70   **When your insulin levels rise, your liver:** Dietschy JM, Brown MS. Effect of alterations of the specific activity of the intracellular acetyl CoA pool on apparent rates of hepatic cholesterogenesis. *J Lipid Res.* 1974;15:508–516.

70   **insulin enhances the growth and proliferation of arterial smooth muscle cells:** Stout RW. Insulin-stimulated lipogenesis in arterial tissue in relation to diabetes and atheroma. *Lancet* 1968;2:702–703. Sato Y, Shiraishi S, Oshida Y, Ishiguro T, Sakamoto N. Experimental atherosclerosis-like lesions induced by hyperinsulinism in Wistar rats. *Diabetes.* 1989;38:91–96.

70   Other studies have confirmed: Fabry P, Tepperman J. Meal frequency—a possible factor in human pathology. *Am J Clin Nutr.* 1970;23:1059–1068.

70   Another study found higher blood flow: Miller M, Beach V, Sorkin JD, et al. Comparative effects of three popular diets on lipids, endothelial function, and C-reactive protein during weight maintenance. *J Am Diet Assoc.* 2009;109:713–717. Fleming R. The effect of high-, moderate-, and low-fat diets on weight loss and cardiovascular disease risk factors. *Prev Cardiol.* 2002 Summer;5(3):110–118. Erratum in: *Prev Cardiol.* 2002 Fall;5(4):203.

70   In one study, scientists found that rats: Murray AJ, Knight NS, Cochlin LE, et al. Deterioration of physical performance and cognitive function in rats with short-term high-fat feeding. *FASEB J.* 2009 Dec;23(12):4353–60. doi: 10.1096/fj.09-139691. Epub 2009 Aug 10; Edwards LM, Murray AJ, Holloway CJ, et al. Short-term consumption of a high-fat diet impairs whole-body efficiency and cognitive function in sedentary men. *FASEB J.* 2011 Mar;25(3):1088–1096. doi: 10.1096/fj.10-171983. Epub 2010 Nov 24.

71   "Calorie for Calorie": Hall KD, Bemis T, Brychta R, et al. Calorie for calorie, dietary fat restriction results in more body fat loss than carbohydrate restriction in people with obesity. *Cell Metab.* 2015 Sep 1;22(3):427–436. doi: 10.1016/j.cmet.2015.07.021. Epub 2015 Aug 13.

71   The PURE study made headlines: Dehghan M, Mente A, Zhang X, et al. Associations of fats and carbohydrate intake with cardiovascular disease and mortality in 18 countries from five continents (PURE): a prospective cohort study. *Lancet.* 2017 Nov 4;390(10107):2050–2062. doi: 10.1016/S0140-6736(17)32252-3. Epub 2017 Aug 29; Katz D. Why Mainstream Reporting on the PURE Study Is Getting It Horribly Wrong. https://foodrevolution.org/blog/food-and-health/pure-study-reporting/.

72   There is also a lot of misinformation: De Souza RJ, et al. Intake of saturated and trans unsaturated fatty acids and risk of all cause mortality, cardiovascular disease, and type 2 diabetes, systematic review and meta-analysis of observational studies. *BMJ.* 2015; 351:h3978. https://doi.org/10.1136/bmj.h3978.

73   **It turns out that in every decade since 1950:** United States Department of Agriculture. Agriculture Fact Book 2001–2002. http://www.usda.gov/factbook/2002factbook.pdf.

73   **Those who had an overall decrease in total fat intake:** Blankenhorn DH, Johnson RL, Mack WJ, et al. The influence of diet on the appearance of new lesions in human coronary arteries. *JAMA.* 1990; 263:1646–1652.

73   **My colleagues and I found a similar relationship:** Ornish DM, Brown SE, Scherwitz LW, et al. Can lifestyle changes reverse coronary atherosclerosis? The Lifestyle Heart Trial. *Lancet.* 1990;336:129–133. (Reprinted in *Yearbook of Medicine and Yearbook of Cardiology.* New York: C.V. Mosby; 1991.) Ornish D, Scherwitz L, Billings J, et al. Intensive lifestyle changes for reversal of coronary heart disease: five-year follow-up of the Lifestyle Heart Trial. *JAMA.* 1998;280:2001–2007.

73   **A high-fat diet increases the likelihood of prostate cancer spreading:** Chen M, Zhang J, Sampieri K, et al. An aberrant SREBP-dependent lipogenic program promotes metastatic prostate cancer. *Nat Genet.* 2018 Feb;50(2):206–218. doi: 10.1038/s41588-017-0027-2. Epub 2018 Jan 15.

74   **In 2013, a study was published:** Estruch R, Ros E, Salas-Salvadó J, et al. Primary prevention of cardiovascular disease with a Mediterranean diet. *N Engl J Med.* 2013 Apr 4;368(14):1279–1290. doi: 10.1056/NEJMoa1200303. Epub 2013 Feb 25.

74   **This was likely because the Mediterranean diet:** Skerrett PJ, Hennekens CH. Consumption of fish and fish oils and decreased risk of stroke. *Prev Cardiol.* 2003 Winter;6(1):38–41.

74   **This is why for more than twenty-five years:** O'Connor A. Fish oil drug may reduce heart attack and stroke rate for some. *New York Times.* 2018 Sep 25.

74   **Because of methodological irregularities and errors:** Retraction and republication: primary prevention of cardiovascular disease with a Mediterranean diet. *N Engl J Med.* 2013;368:1279–1290.

74 **To repeat: a Mediterranean diet is better:** Ornish D. Primary prevention of cardiovascular disease with a Mediterranean diet. *N Engl J Med.* 2013 Aug 15;369(7):675–676. doi: 10.1056/NEJMc1306659.

75 **In 2014, NASA issued a report:** NASA. West Antarctic glacier loss appears unstoppable. Press release. 2015 May 12. https://www.jpl.nasa.gov/news/news.php?release=2014-148.

75 **In 2018, scientists learned that Antarctica's ice sheet:** The IMBIE Team. Mass balance of the Antarctic ice sheet from 1992 to 2017. *Nature.* 2018;558:219–222. https://www.nature.com/articles/s41586-018-0179-y.

75 **"Health is inextricably linked to climate change":** Patz JA, et al. Climate change: challenges and opportunities for global health. *JAMA.* 2014;312(15):1565–1580. doi: 10.1001/jama.2014.13186.

75 **A major UN report:** Gillis J. U.N. panel issues its starkest warning yet on global warming. *New York Times.* 2014 Nov 2.

75 **animal agribusiness generates more greenhouse gases:** Goodland R. FAO yields to meat industry pressure on climate change. *New York Times.* 2012 Jul 11.

76 **The United States maintains more than 9 billion head:** Pimentel D, Pimentel M. Sustainability of meat-based and plant-based diets and the environment. *Am J Clin Nutr.* 2003 Sep 1;78(3):660S–663S. https://doi.org/10.1093/ajcn/78.3.660S.

76 **more than half of U.S. grain and nearly 40 percent:** Cornell University. U.S. could feed 800 million people with grain that livestock eat, Cornell ecologist advises animal scientists. ScienceDaily. 1997 Aug 12. <www.sciencedaily.com/releases/1997/08/970812003512.htm>.

76 **there is enough food to feed everyone on the planet:** Sundaram JK, Elver H. The world produces enough food to feed everyone. So why do people go hungry? World Economic Forum, June 11, 2016. https://www.weforum.org/agenda/2016/07/the-world-produces-enough-food-to-feed-everyone-so-why-do-people-go-hungry. Buff E. Can we solve world hunger and feed 9 billion people just by eating less meat? One Green Planet. 2017 May 20. http://www.onegreenplanet.org/environment/world-hunger-population-growth-ditching-meat.

80   **it's worth noting that even one glass of wine per day:** Lowry SJ, Kapphahn K, Chlebowski R, Li CI. Alcohol use and breast cancer survival among participants in the Women's Health Initiative. *Cancer Epidemiol Biomarkers Prev.* 2016;25(8):1268. doi: 10.1158/1055-9965. EPI-16-0151.

80   **The widely held view of the health:** GBD 2016 Alcohol Collaborators. Alcohol use and burden for 195 countries and territories, 1990–2016: a systematic analysis for the Global Burden of Disease Study 2016. *Lancet.* 2018 Sep 22;392(10152):1015–1035. doi: 10.1016/S0140-6736(18)31310-2. Epub 2018 Aug 23.

81   **According to USDA dietary guidelines:** USDA. Dietary guidelines 2015–2020. Appendix 2. Estimated calorie needs per day, by age, sex, and physical activity level. https://health.gov/dietaryguidelines /2015/guidelines/appendix-2.

82   **Some people claim that saturated fats are not harmful, but evidence shows:** Jakobsen MU, O'Reilly EJ, Heitmann BL, et al. Major types of dietary fat and risk of coronary heart disease: a pooled analysis of 11 cohort studies. *Am J Clin Nutr.* 2009 May;89(5):1425–1432. doi: 10.3945/ajcn.2008.27124. Epub 2009 Feb 11.

83   **including the Adventist Study:** Fraser GE, Sabaté J, Beeson WL, Strahan TM. A possible protective effect of nut consumption on risk of coronary heart disease. The Adventist Health Study. *Arch Intern Med.* 1992 Jul;152(7):1416–1424.

83   **One reason is that omega-3 fatty acids:** Albert CM, Gaziano JM, Willett WC, Manson JE. Nut consumption and decreased risk of sudden cardiac death in the Physicians' Health Study. *Arch Intern Med.* 2002 Jun 24;162(12):1382–1387.

83   **Also, consuming nuts in small quantities reduces:** de Souza RGM, Schincaglia RM, Pimentel GD, Mota JF. Nuts and human health outcomes: a systematic review. *Nutrients.* 2017 Dec 2;9(12). doi: 10.3390 /nu9121311.

90   **When people eat in front of a TV:** Tumin R, Anderson SE. Television, home-cooked meals, and family meal frequency: associations with adult obesity. *J Acad Nutr Diet.* 2017 Jun;117(6):937–945. doi: 10.1016/j.jand.2017.01.009. Epub 2017 Feb 24.

Chapter 5

102 **cut premature death rates by 20–30 percent:** Blair SN, Kohl HW, Paffenbarger RS, et al. Physical fitness and all-cause mortality. A prospective study of healthy men and women. *JAMA*. 1989 Nov 3;262(17):2395–2401.

102 **Another study found that walking thirty minutes:** Arem H, Moore SC, Patel, A, et al. Leisure time physical activity and mortality: a detailed pooled analysis of the dose-response relationship. *JAMA Intern Med*. 2015 Jun;175(6):959–967. doi: 10.1001/jamainternmed.2015.0533.

102 **Just twenty-five minutes of brisk walking:** Brisk daily walks can increase lifespan, research says. *Guardian*. 2015 Aug 30. https:// www.theguardian.com/society/2015/aug/30/brisk-daily-walks-reduce -ageing-increase-life-span-research.

102 **In the Women's Health Study:** Lee IM, Rexrode KM, Cook NR, Manson JE, Buring JE. Physical activity and coronary heart disease in women: is "no pain, no gain" passé? *JAMA*. 2001;285(11):1447–1454.

102 **In one study of over 55,000 adults:** Lee DC, Pate RR, Lavie CJ, et al. Leisure-time running reduces all-cause and cardiovascular mortality risk. *J Am Coll Cardiol*. 2014 Aug 5;64(5):472–481. doi: 10.1016 /j.jacc.2014.04.058.

103 **For every hour you spend running, you gain:** Lee DC, Brellenthin AG, Thompson PD, et al. Running as a key lifestyle medicine for longevity. *Prog Cardiovasc Dis*. 2017 Jun–Jul;60(1):45–55. doi: 10.1016 /j.pcad.2017.03.005. Epub 2017 Mar 30.

103 **While seven-minute high-intensity workouts appeal:** Hardesty P. Is high intensity interval exercise safe for heart patients? https:// www.ornish.com/zine/is-high-intensity-interval-exercise-safe-for-a -person-with-cardiovascular-disease.

103 **In one study, adults with high physical activity:** Tucker LA, et al. Physical activity and telomere length in U.S. men and women: an NHANES investigation. *Prev Medicine*. 2017;100:145. doi: 10.1016 /j.ypmed.2017.04.027.

103   **In another study, scientists studied men and women:** Duggal NA, Pollock RD, Lazarus NR, et al. Major features of immunesenescence, including reduced thymic output, are ameliorated by high levels of physical activity in adulthood. *Aging Cell.* 2018 Apr;17(2). doi: 10.1111/acel.12750. Epub 2018 Mar 8.

104   **Chronic emotional stress can shorten telomeres:** Puterman E, Lin J, Blackburn E, O'Donovan A, Adler N, Epel E. The power of exercise: buffering the effect of chronic stress on telomere length. *PLoS ONE.* 2010;5(5).

104   **A new study tested the effect:** Puterman E, et al. Aerobic exercise lengthens telomeres and reduces stress in family caregivers: a randomized controlled trial. *Psychoneuroendocrinology,* in press, 2018.

104   **Postmenopausal women who exercised:** Beate I, et al. Telomere length and long-term endurance exercise: does exercise training affect biological age? a pilot study. *PLoS ONE.* 2012;7(12).

104   **Researchers found that twins who were active:** Cherkas LF, et al. The association between physical activity in leisure time and leukocyte telomere length. *Arch Int Med.* 2008;168(2).

104   **It didn't take much—just ten minutes a week:** Zhang Z, Chen W. A systematic review of the relationship between physical activity and happiness. *J Happiness Stud.* 2018. https://doi.org/10.1007/s10902-018-9976-0.

105   **those with the lowest fitness were 76 percent more likely:** Schuch FB, Vancampfort D, Sui X, et al. Are lower levels of cardiorespiratory fitness associated with incident depression? A systematic review of prospective cohort studies. *Prev Med.* 2016 Dec;93:159–165. doi: 10.1016/j.ypmed.2016.10.011. Epub 2016 Oct 17.

105   **"exercise had a large and significant effect on depression":** Schuch FB, Vancampfort D, Richards J, et al. Exercise as a treatment for depression: a meta-analysis adjusting for publication bias. *J Psychiatr Res.* 2016 Jun;77:42–51. doi: 10.1016/j.jpsychires.2016.02.023. Epub 2016 Mar 4.

105   **Even a single bout of exercise:** Schuch FB, Deslandes AC, Stubbs B, et al. Neurobiological effects of exercise on major depressive disorder: a systematic review. *Neurosci Biobehav Rev.* 2016 Feb;61:1–11. doi: 10.1016/j.neubiorev.2015.11.012. Epub 2015 Dec 2.

105 **Strength training also reduces and helps prevent depression:** Reynolds G. Weight training may help to ease or prevent depression. *New York Times.* 2018 Jun 6.

105 **"an alternative and/or adjuvant therapy":** Gordon BR, McDowell CP, Hallgren M, et al. Association of efficacy of resistance exercise training with depressive symptoms. *JAMA Psychiatry.* 2018; 75(6):566–576. doi:10.1001/jamapsychiatry.2018.0572.

106 **Exercise makes you smarter:** Van Praag H. Exercise and the brain: something to chew on. *Trends Neurosci.* 2009 May;32(5):283–290.

106 **Children who exercise in school:** Sibley BA, Etnier JL. The relationship between physical activity and cognition in children: a meta-analysis. *Pediatric Exercise Science.* 2003;15:243–256.

106 **Similar results were obtained in young adults:** Pereira AC, Huddleston DE, Brickman AM, et al. An in vivo correlate of exercise-induced neurogenesis in the adult dentate gyrus. *Proc Natl Acad Sci U S A.* 2007 Mar 27;104(13):5638–5643.

106 **Those who are physically active between ages fifteen:** Dik M, Deeg DJ, Visser M, Jonker C. Early life physical activity and cognition at old age. *J Clin Exp Neuropsychol.* 2003 Aug; 25(5):643–653.

106 **overall physical activity improves cognitive function:** Kramer AF, Hahn S, Cohen NJ, et al. Ageing, fitness and neurocognitive function. *Nature.* 1999 Jul 29;400(6743):418–419.

106 **People who are fit are more likely to remember:** Reynolds G. How exercise can help you recall words. *New York Times.* 2018 May 15.

106 **Part of the reason for this:** He C, Sumpter R Jr, Levine B. Exercise induces autophagy in peripheral tissues and in the brain. *Autophagy.* 2012 Oct;8(10):1548–1551. doi: 10.4161/auto.21327. Epub 2012 Aug 15; Reynolds G. Exercise as housecleaning for the body. *New York Times.* 2012 Feb 1.

106 **Fathers who exercise:** Benito E, Kerimoglu C, Ramachandran B, et al. RNA-dependent intergenerational inheritance of enhanced synaptic plasticity after environmental enrichment. *Cell Rep.* 2018 Apr 10;23(2):546–554. doi: 10.1016/j.celrep.2018.03.059.

106   **In one study, people who were standing:** Rosenbaum D, Mama Y, Algom D. Stand by your stroop: standing up enhances selective attention and cognitive control. *Psychological Science.* 2017;28:1864.

107   **a randomized controlled trial of 120 older adults:** Erickson KI, Voss MW, Prakash RS, et al. Exercise training increases size of hippocampus and improves memory. *Proc Natl Acad Sci U S A.* 2011 Feb 15;108(7):3017–3022. doi: 10.1073/pnas.1015950108. Epub 2011 Jan 31.

107   **In contrast, the brains in the comparison group:** Erickson KI, Voss MW, Prakash RS, et al. Exercise training increases size of hippocampus and improves memory. *Proc Natl Acad Sci U S A.* 2011 Feb 15;108(7):3017–3022. doi: 10.1073/pnas.1015950108. Epub 2011 Jan 31.

107   **men and women with mild cognitive impairment:** Baker LD, Craft S, Jung Y, Whitlow CT. Aerobic exercise preserves brain volume and improves cognitive function. Presented at Radiological Society of North America annual scientific sessions. 2016 Nov 30. https://press.rsna.org/timssnet/media/pressreleases/14_pr_target.cfm?ID=1921.

107   **After six months, those doing moderate aerobic exercise:** Colcombe SJ, Erickson K, Scalf PE, Kim JS, et al. Aerobic exercise training increases brain volume in aging humans. *J Gerontol A Biol Sci Med Sci.* 2006 Nov;61(11):1166–1170.

107   **Exercise causes new neurons to be born:** Miller RM, Marriott D, Trotter J, et al. Running exercise mitigates the negative consequences of chronic stress on dorsal hippocampal long-term potentiation in male mice. *Neurobiol Learn Mem.* 2018 Mar;149:28–38. doi: 10.1016/j.nlm.2018.01.008. Epub 2018 Feb 9.

107   **One of the mediators of this is a protein:** Flatow I. Growing a bigger brain is a walk in the park. *Talk of the Nation.* National Public Radio. 2011 Feb. 4.

107   **"It's not just a matter of slowing down":** Carmichael M. Can exercise make you smarter? *Newsweek.* 2007 Mar 26.

Chapter 6

135 It has a direct effect on our health: Editor. Focus on stress. *Nature Neuroscience.* 2015;18:1343.

135 When it's chronic, stress can increase inflammation: Sorrells SF, Caso JR, Munhoz CD, Sapolsky RM. The stressed CNS. *Neuron.* 2009 Oct 15;64(1):33–39. doi: 10.1016/j.neuron.2009.09.032.

135 people who are HIV positive and depressed: Mayne TJ, Vittinghoff E, Chesney MA, Barrett DC, Coates TJ. Depressive affect and survival among gay and bisexual men infected with HIV. *Arch Intern Med.* 1996 Oct 28;156(19):2233–2238.

136 It shortens telomeres: Stein JY, Levin Y, Uziel O, Abumock H, Solomon Z. Traumatic stress and cellular senescence: the role of war-captivity and homecoming stressors in later life telomere length. *J Affect Disord.* 2018 May 30;238:129–135. doi: 10.1016/j.jad.2018.05.037.

136 adversely affects how your genes are expressed: Dirven BCJ, Homberg JR, Kozicz T, Henckens MJAG. Epigenetic programming of the neuroendocrine stress response by adult life stress. *J Mol Endocrinol.* 2017 Jul;59(1):R11–R31. doi: 10.1530/JME-17-0019. Epub 2017 Apr 11.

136 can have a harmful impact on the balance: Cussotto S, Sandhu KV, Dinan TG, Cryan JF. The neuroendocrinology of the microbiota-gut-brain axis: a behavioural perspective. *Front Neuroendocrinol.* 2018 May 14. doi: 10.1016/j.yfrne.2018.04.002.

136 Chronic emotional stress increases oxidative stress: Saretzki G. Extra-telomeric functions of human telomerase: cancer, mitochondria and oxidative stress. *Curr Pharm Des.* 2014;20(41):6386–6403. Saretzki G. Telomerase, mitochondria and oxidative stress. *Exp Gerontol.* 2009 Aug; 44(8):485–492. doi: 10.1016/j.exger.2009.05.004. Epub 2009 May 18.

136 negative effects on cellular metabolism and apoptosis: Picard M, McEwen B. Psychological stress and mitochondria: a systematic review. *Psychosom Med.* 2018 Feb–Mar;80(2):141–153.

136 angiogenesis: Kim YW, Byzova TV. Oxidative stress in angiogenesis and vascular disease. *Blood.* 2014 Jan 30;123(5):625–631.

136   **It causes blockages to build up faster:** Williams SCP. How stress can clog your arteries. *Science.* 2014 Jun 22. http://www.science mag.org/news/2014/06/how-stress-can-clog-your-arteries.

136   **Elizabeth Blackburn studied caregivers:** Epel ES, Blackburn EH, Lin J, et al. Accelerated telomere shortening in response to life stress. *Proc Natl Acad Sci U S A.* 2004;101(49):17312–17315. Epub 2004 Dec 1.

137   **Interestingly, the stress-is-enhancing mindset:** Crum AJ, Salovey P, Achor S. Rethinking stress: the role of mindsets in determining the stress response. *J Personality Social Psychol.* 2013;104(4):716–733.

139   **A study from Microsoft:** McSpadden K. You now have a shorter attention span than a goldfish. *Time.* 2015 May 14.

140   **For example, researchers at Harvard:** Bhasin MK, Dusek JA, Chang BH, et al. Relaxation response induces temporal transcriptome changes in energy metabolism, insulin secretion and inflammatory pathways. *PLoS ONE.* 2013 May 1;8(5):e62817. doi: 10.1371/journal .pone.0062817.

140   **We can all learn to be more positive:** Brody J. Turning negative thinkers into positive ones. *New York Times.* 2017 Apr 3.

141   **"One way to think about this is that love":** O'Donnell E. Micro-utopia, anyone? Fredrickson describes nourishing power of small, positive moments. *NIH Record.* 2013 May 10;65:10.

141   **"the wherewithal to pause":** Begley S. Rewiring your emotions. *Mindful.* 2013 Jul 27.

142   **those who meditated for about thirty minutes:** Hölzel BK, Carmody J, Vangel M, et al. Mindfulness practice leads to increases in regional brain gray matter density. *Psychiatry Res.* 2011 Jan 30;191(1): 36–43.

Chapter 7

197   In 1998, I wrote a book: Ornish D. *Love and Survival: The Scientific Basis for the Healing Power of Intimacy.* New York: HarperCollins; 1998.

197   One-third of people in industrialized countries: Cacioppo JT, Cacioppo S. The growing problem of loneliness. *Lancet.* 2018 Feb 3;391(10119):426. doi: 10.1016/S0140-6736(18)30142-9.

197   Suicide rates have increased by 25 percent: U.S. suicide rates increased more than 25% since 1999, CDC says. WHO Channel 13. 2018 Jun 10. http://whotv.com/2018/06/10/u-s-suicide-rates-increased -more-than-25-since-1999-cdc-says.

197   Dr. Vivek Murthy: Murthy V. Work and the loneliness epidemic. *Harvard Business Review.* 2017 Sep 27.

197   "minister of loneliness": Yeginsu C. U.K. appoints a minister for loneliness. *New York Times.* 2018 Jan 17.

197   For example, loneliness causes chronic emotional stress: Cacioppo JT, Cacioppo S, Capitanio JP, Cole SW. The neuroendocrinology of social isolation. *Ann Rev Psychol.* 2015 Jan 3;66:733–767. Nersesian PV, Han HR, Yenokyan G, et al. Loneliness in middle age and biomarkers of systemic inflammation: findings from midlife in the United States. *Soc Sci Med.* 2018 Apr 30. pii: S0277-9536(18)30166-7.

197   Researchers have documented that loneliness also turns on: Canli T, Wen R, Wang X, et al. Differential transcriptome expression in human nucleus accumbens as a function of loneliness. *Mol Psychiatry.* 2017 Jul;22(7):1069–1078.

197   turning on genes that promote chronic inflammation: Cole SW, Hawkley LC, Arevalo JM, Sung CY, Rose RM, Cacioppo JT. Social regulation of gene expression in human leukocytes. *Genome Biol.* 2007;8(9):R189.

197   For example, social support buffers: Kanitz E, Hameister T, Tuchscherer A, et al. Social support modulates stress-related gene expression in various brain regions of piglets. *Front Behav Neurosci.* 2016 Nov 29;10:227. Ditzen B, Heinrichs M. Psychobiology of social support:

the social dimension of stress buffering. *Restor Neurol Neurosci.* 2014;32(1):149–162. doi: 10.3233/RNN-139008.

198   Studies have shown that looking a dog in the eyes: Nagasawa M, Mitsui S, En S, et al. Oxytocin-gaze positive loop and the coevolution of human-dog bonds. *Science.* 2015 Apr 17:348(6232):333–336.

198   eight weeks of meditation decreases loneliness: Creswell JD, Irwin MR, Burklund LJ, et al. Mindfulness-based stress reduction training reduces loneliness and pro-inflammatory gene expression in older adults: a small randomized controlled trial. *Brain Behav Immun.* 2012 Oct;26(7):1095–1101. doi: 10.1016/j.bbi.2012.07.006. Epub 2012 Jul 20.

199   Since 1985, the number of people saying: McPherson M, Smith-Lovin L, Brashears ME. Social isolation in America: changes in core discussion networks over two decades. *Am Sociol Rev.* 2006;71(3):353–375. doi: 10.1177/000312240607100301. http://journals .sagepub.com/doi/abs/10.1177/000312240607100301.

199   Most people usually show only the best parts: Appel H, Gerlach AL, Crusius J. The interplay between Facebook use, social comparison, envy, and depression. *Curr Opinion Psychol.* 2016;9:44–49. doi: 10.1016/j.copsyc.2015.10.006.

199   Most measures of the frequency of Facebook use: Shakya HB, Christakis NA. A new, more rigorous study confirms: the more you use Facebook, the worse you feel. *Harvard Business Review.* 2017 Apr 10. https://hbr.org/2017/04/a-new-more-rigorous-study-confirms-the-more -you-use-facebook-the-worse-you-feel. Shakya HB, Christakis NA. Association of Facebook use with compromised well-being: a longitudinal study. *Am J Epidemiol.* 2017 Feb 1;185(3):203–211. doi: 10.1093/aje/kww189.

201   the human equivalent of quantum entanglement: Kaplan S. Quantum entanglement, science's "spookiest" phenomenon, achieved in space. *Washington Post.* 2017 Jun 15.

201   Mirror neurons: Acharya S, Shukla S. Mirror neurons: enigma of the metaphysical modular brain. *J Nat Sci Biol Med.* 2012 Jul–Dec;3(2):118–124.

201　*Shoshin:* Shoshin. Wikipedia. Accessed 2018 Jul 1. https://en.wikipedia.org/wiki/Shoshin.

201　**"In the beginner's mind":** Suzuki S. *Zen Mind, Beginner's Mind.* Boston: Shambhala; 2006.

203　**Our group support sessions . . . are designed:** Billings J, Scherwitz L, Sullivan R, Ornish D. Group support therapy in the Lifestyle Heart Trial. In: Scheidt S, Allan R, eds. *Heart and Mind: The Emergence of Cardiac Psychology.* Washington DC: American Psychological Association; 1996:233–253.

203　**There is evidence from at least fifteen:** Spiegel D. Minding the body: psychotherapy and cancer survival. *Br J Health Psychol.* 2014 Sep;19(3):465–485. doi: 10.1111/bjhp.12061. Epub 2013 Aug 26.

204　**One classic randomized controlled trial:** Spiegel D, Bloom JR, Kraemer HC, Gottheil E. Effect of psychosocial treatment on survival of patients with metastatic breast cancer. *Lancet.* 1989 Oct 14;2(8668):888–891.

204　**In our research, we found that group support:** Schulz U, Pischke CR, Weidner G, Daubenmier J, Elliot-Eller M, Scherwitz L, Bullinger M, Ornish D. Social support group attendance is related to blood pressure, health behaviours, and quality of life in the Multicenter Lifestyle Demonstration Project. *Psychol Health Med.* 2008 Aug;13(4):423–437. doi: 10.1080/13548500701660442.

205　**Group support increases empathy:** Park KH, Kim DH, Kim SK, et al. The relationships between empathy, stress and social support among medical students. *Int J Med Educ.* 2015 Sep 5;6:103–108. doi: 10.5116/ijme.55e6.0d44.

214　**Matthew D. Lieberman:** Lieberman MD, Eisenberger NI, Crockett MJ, et al. Putting feelings into words: affect labeling disrupts amygdala activity in response to affective stimuli. *Psychol Sci.* 2007 May;18(5):421–428.

221　**the time required to reach conflict resolution:** Rosenberg MD. *Nonviolent Communication.* Encinatas CA: PuddleDancer Press; Chapter 7, 2015.

229   **People who smile are perceived as being more likable:** Krys K, et al. Be careful where you smile: culture shapes judgments of intelligence and honesty of smiling individuals. *J Nonverbal Behav.* 2016; 40: 101–116.

229   **people with positive emotions have more stable marriages:** Diener E, Chan MY. Happy people live longer: subjective well-being contributes to health and longevity. *Applied Psychology: Health and Well-Being.* 2011;3(1):1–43. doi: 10.1111/j.1758-0854.2010.01045.x.

229   **researchers at the Face Research Laboratory:** Conway CA, et al. Evidence for adaptive design in human gaze preference. *Proceedings of the Royal Society B.* 2008 Jan 7. doi: 10.1098/rspb.2007.1073.

230   **In his book *Laughter*:** Provine RR. *Laughter: A Scientific Investigation.* New York: Penguin Books; 2001.

230   **published in the journal *Human Nature*:** Gray AW, Parkinson B, Dunbar RI. Laughter's influence on the intimacy of self-disclosure. *Hum Nat.* 2015 Mar;26(1):28–43. doi: 10.1007/s12110-015-9225-8.

232   **Dr. Glen Affleck:** Affleck G, Tennen H, Croog S, Levine S. Causal attribution, perceived benefits, and morbidity after a heart attack: an 8-year study. *J Consult Clin Psychol.* 1987 Feb;55(1):29–35.

232   **As part of the pioneering work done by Robert Emmons:** Emmons R. *Thanks! How the New Science of Gratitude Can Make You Happier.* New York: Houghton Mifflin Harcourt; 2007.

232   **Researchers from Gonzaga University.** Bartlett MY, et al. Gratitude: prompting behaviours that build relationships. *Cogn Emot.* 2012;26(1):2-13.

232   **Gratitude can actually boost your mood:** Mills PJ, et al. The role of gratitude in spiritual well-being in asymptomatic heart failure patients. *Spirituality in Clinical Practice.* 2015;2(1):5–17.

235   **In a study published in the *American Journal of Public Health*:** Poulin MJ, Brown SL, Dillard AJ, Smith DM. Giving to others and the association between stress and mortality. *Am J Public Health.* 2013 Sep;103(9):1649–1655. doi: 10.2105/AJPH.2012.300876. Epub 2013 Jan 17.

235   **published in the journal *Psychological Science*:** Brown SL, Nesse RM, Vinokur AD, Smith DM. Providing social support may be more beneficial than receiving it: results from a prospective study of mortality. *Psychol Sci.* 2003 Jul;14(4):320–327.

235   **Stanford psychologist Sonja Lyubomirsky researches:** Lyubomirsky, S. (2013). *The Myths of Happiness: What Should Make You Happy, but Doesn't, What Shouldn't Make You Happy, but Does.* New York: Penguin Books; 2014.

236   **prescriptions for antidepressants have risen nearly 400 percent:** Szalavitz M. What does a 400% increase in antidepressant use really mean? *Time.* 2011 Oct 20. http://healthland.time.com/2011/10/20 /what-does-a-400-increase-in-antidepressant-prescribing-really-mean.

237   ***Kitchen Table Wisdom:*** Remen R. *Kitchen Table Wisdom: Stories that Heal.* 10th ed. New York: Riverhead Books; 2006.

238   **depression scores were reduced by almost 50 percent:** Silberman A, Banthia R, Estay IS, Kemp C, Studley J, Hareras D, Ornish D. The effectiveness and efficacy of an intensive cardiac rehabilitation program in 24 sites. *Am J Health Promot.* 2010;24(4):260–266.

242   **For example, a Harvard study of over 12,000 people:** Christakis NA, Fowler JH. The spread of obesity in a large social network over 32 years. *N Engl J Med.* 2007 Jul 26;357(4):370–379. Epub 2007 Jul 25.

243   **The goal of all spiritual practices:** Satchidananda S. *To Know Your Self.* New York: Doubleday; 1978.

244   **"Tell them *I am* has sent you":** Exodus 3:13.

244   **"Thou art That":** Satchidananda S. *The Yoga Sutras of Patanjali.* Buckingham VA: Integral Yoga Publications; 1990.

244   **"The kingdom of God":** Luke 17:21.

244   **"You are all Buddhas":** Mitchell S. *The Enlightened Mind.* New York: HarperCollins; 1991.

244   **"Wherever you turn is God's face":** Mitchell S. *The Enlightened Mind.* New York: HarperCollins; 1991.

244   "The true value of a human being": Mitchell S. *The Enlightened Mind*. New York: HarperCollins; 1991.

244   "an immediate, nondual insight": Shantideva. *The Way of the Bodhisattva*. Boston: Shambhala; 1997.

244   "perennial philosophy": Huxley A. *The Perennial Philosophy*. New York: Harper & Row; 1945.

244   "Love your neighbor": Leviticus 19:18.

245   "A human being is a part of the whole": Letter dated 1950 by Albert Einstein, quoted in H. Eves, *Mathematical Circles Adieu*. Boston: Prindle, Weber, & Schmidt; 1977.

245   in a study of 148 million Twitter messages: Eichstaedt JC, Schwartz HA, Kern ML, et al. Psychological language on Twitter predicts county-level heart disease mortality. *Psychol Sci.* 2015 Feb;26(2):159–169. doi: 10.1177/0956797614557867. Epub 2015 Jan 20.

245   "One of the themes": Moyers B, Lucas G. Of myth and men. *Time*. 1999 Apr 18. http://content.time.com/time/magazine/article/0,9171,23298,00.html.

Acknowledgments

This book represents the distillation of more than forty years of our scientific research studies and clinical experience. As such, to thank everyone who made this book possible would require literally hundreds of pages—including those who provided recipes, endorsements, advice, and feedback on the manuscript as well as our research and clinical colleagues, mentors, teachers, journal and media editors, those at CMS and insurance companies, friends, family, board members, and others whose generous contributions made our research possible. We remain deeply grateful beyond words to each and every person for making such a meaningful difference.

In that spirit, we express our heartfelt thanks here just to those who were directly involved in making this book possible. Deep appreciation to our wise and compassionate editor, Marnie Cochran, who held and nurtured the vision of this book for over five years. And many thanks to her colleagues at Ballantine Books/Random House—including Gina Centrello, Kara Welsh, Jennifer Hershey, Susan Corcoran, Quinne Rogers, Diane Hobbing, Joe Perez, Nancy Delia, and Hanna Gibeau. Heartfelt appreciation to Esther Newberg at ICM, and to Michael Rudell, Neil Rosini, and Eric Brown at Franklin, Weinrib, Rudell, and Vassallo—it's wonderful that we've been working together for so many decades! We are grateful to everyone who provided endorsements for our book.

Our growing children, Lucas (Luke) and Jasmine (Jazz), continue to inspire us and bring deep meaning into our lives. We begin and end each day with a gratitude meditation. As we review and remember everyone who made this book possible, our hearts are overflowing with thanks. Please accept our deep bow of loving appreciation.

Dean & Anne

Recipe Index

Subject Index

Page numbers in *italics* refer to illustrations.

Avastin, 42, 43
Avatar (movie), 199
awareness:
    body, 143, 144, 146
    eating and, 86–100, *89, 92*
    as first step in healing, 4
Ayurvedic medicine and proverb, 48, 61,
    84

Baboumian, Patrik, 65
Bausch, Dotsie, 65
Beazley, Hamilton, 233
beverages:
    stocking pantry with, 450
    see also recipes
biceps curl exercise, *130*
Blackburn, Elizabeth, 34, 136
blood flow:
    effect of exercise on, 105, 107
    effect of inflammation on, 22
    effect of lifestyle medicine on, 54, 70
    effect on sexual potency, 14, 44
    guided imagery and, 182
    stasis and, 43–48, 54
bradykinin, 22
Brahman, 244
brain:
    chronic inflammation and, 22
    effect of exercise on, 106–7
    effect of meditation on, 140–42, 171
    see also specific parts
brain-derived neurotrophin factor (BDNF),
    107
breakfast:
    recommended packaged foods,
        419–32
    see also recipes
breast cancer:
    effect of alcohol on, 80
    effect of fat consumption and, 59
    oncogenes and, 23, 27, 59
    support groups for, 204
    telomeres and, 34
    TOR levels, 30
breathing techniques, *113,* 144, 167–68
    abdominal breathing, 168–69
    alternate-nostril breathing, 169–71
    gentle stretching and, *146–47*
    meditation on breath, 174–75, *175*
    three-part breathing, 169
    tips for, 167–68
British Medical Journal, 56, 72
Brown, David L., 53
Buddha, 244

California, University of:
    at San Diego, 36
    at San Francisco (UCSF), 51, 53, 58
calorie consumption:
    alcohol and, 80
    carbohydrates vs. sugar, 70–74
    effect on microbiome, 38
    fat and, 29, 81–83
    fiber and, 24, 85
    life expectancy and, 29–30
    mindful eating and, 97–98
    in recommended packaged foods
        419–32
    types of food and, 29, 43, 70–74
    USDA dietary guidelines, 81
    see also specific recipes
"Calorie for Calorie, Dietary Fat Restriction
    Results in More Body Fat Loss than
    Carbohydrate Restriction in People
    with Obesity," 71
Cameron, James, 14
Campbell, Joseph, 227
Campbell, T. Colin, 34
cancer:
    chronic inflammation and, 23
    "Moonshot" Commission for cure for,
        51
    pesticides in food supply and, 37
    support groups for cancer patients, 204
    see also specific types
carbohydrates, good:
    vs. bad, 79
    longevity and, 30
    in recommended packaged foods,
        419–32
carbohydrates, refined, 70–73
    chronic inflammation and, 24
    effect on microbiome, 38
    oxidative stress and, 41
carbon dioxide emissions, 75
Carroll, Peter, 58, 59
catastrophic progression, 53
cell death (apoptosis), 140
Centers for Disease Control and
    Prevention (CDC):
    on food-borne illnesses, 37
    on sleep deprivation, 145
Centers for Medicare and Medicaid
    Services (CMS), 6–7, 51
chest fly exercise, *124*
chest press exercise, *114*
China and Chinese:
    diet, 34, 81
    medicine, 84
China Study, 34

cholesterol:
    data analysis of, 72
    insurance coverage for, 7
    lifestyle medicine to treat, 50
    Lipitor for, 57
    in recommended packaged foods
        419–32
Clarke, Arthur C., 16
Clinton, Bill, 6, 32–33
Clinton, Hillary, 32
cobra pose exercise, *154,* 154–55
collaterals, 53
colon cancer, 23, 27, 34, 48, 59
communication strategies, 211
co-morbidities, 18–19
compassion:
    listening with, 216–18
    for livestock, 76–77
confidentiality, 221–23
Connecticut, University of, 232
cookware, nonstick, 82
coronary heart disease:
    atherosclerosis (blockages), 22, 27, 28,
        53, 73
    erectile dysfunction and, 14
    gratitude as protective effect against, 232
    lifestyle medicine to reverse, 6–7, 52–54
    mortality rate, U.S. vs. China, 34
    as most expensive healthcare cost, 8
    patient non-compliance in taking
        prescriptions for, 12
cortisol, 137, 204, 232
C-reactive protein (CRP), 24, 70
cytokines, 25

Daily Value (DV), 85
Danzig, Mac, 65
Davidson, Richard, 141
deep relaxation:
    extended version, 187–88
    short version, 186–87
    for stress management, 145, 185–86,
        188–89
dementia:
    AGE molecules and, 28
    caregivers of patients with, 104
    cell damage and, 41
    erectile dysfunction and, 14
    inflammation and, 22
    neurogenesis and, 44
depression:
    effect of on health, 18
    effect of on sympathetic nervous system,
        25

exercise to treat, 105
    gratitude and decrease in levels of, 232
    among physicians, 52
diabetes:
    damage to pancreas and, 40
    meat consumption and 69
    prevention programs, 55, 56
    see also pre-diabetes; type 2 diabetes
Diabetes Prevention Program, 55
diet:
    Atkins, 43
    effect of, on arteries, 67, *68*
    fiber in, 48
    inflammation and, 23–24
    low-carb, high-protein, 65–67, *68,* 69–70
    Mediterranean, 74–75
    microbiome's effect on, 36–37
    religious dietary guidelines, 236
    Western, and AGE molecules, 28
    Western, and prostate cancer, 32, 59
Dietary Guidelines for Americans
    2015–2020, 85
digital detoxing, 190
dinner:
    recommended packaged foods, 419–32
    see also recipes
dioxin, 37
Dr. Ornish's Program for Reversing Heart
    Disease, 7

eating:
    Hunger-Fullness Scale, *89*
    mindful, 86–90, 96–100
    religious dietary guidelines, 236
    in restaurants, 90–91, *92,* 93–94
    while traveling, 94–96
Eat More, Weigh Less (Ornish), 29
edema, 47
Einstein, Albert, 3, 244–45
ejection fraction, 9
elastic resistance bands, 112
clectrons, 40
Emmons, Robert, 232
empagliflozin, 56
empathy, 204–7, 216–18
Empower, xv
endorphins, 229, 230
Epet, Elissa, 136
epigenetics, 106
erections and erectile dysfunction:
    blood vessel flow and, 14, 44
    effect of diet on, 15
    after surgery for prostate cancer, 58
    Viagra for, 238

European Prospective Investigation into
   Cancer and Nutrition (EPIC), 19
exercise:
   benefits of, 18, 102–7
   guidelines for, 109–10
   incentives for, 108–9
   increase in beneficial bacteria and, 39
   as part of lifestyle medicine, 6
   risks of, 103
   types of, 101
   see also Resistance Band Programs;
     specific exercises
express.google.com, 78, 418

Fair, William, 58
fasting, intermittent, 29
fat:
   calories and, 29, 81–83
   effect of alcohol on metabolism, 80 high,
     14, 38, 41, 66
   high, and AGE, 28
   high, and cancer, 59
   high, and inflammation, 21
   low-fat diets, 6, 33, 34
   misinformation regarding, 70–73
   in recommended packaged foods,
     419–32
   role of insulin in metabolism of, 69–70
   see also diet
fear:
   brain structure and, 140, 142
   as motivator for change, 12, 14, 86
   stress reduction and, 191
feelings:
   differentiating from thoughts, 211–12
   expressing authentic, 214–15
   paying attention to, 213–14
   responding with, 220–21
   sharing, to reduce stress, 189–90
fiber:
   consumption of in China vs. U.S., 34
   consumption with bad carbs, 80–81
   effect on calorie consumption, 24, 29,
     79
   effect on colon cancer, 48
   in recommended packaged foods,
     417–32
   USDA recommendations, 85
   see also recipes
fight-or-flight response, 25–26, 142
Finnish Diabetes Prevention Study Group,
   55
fish pose exercise, *165,* 165–66
flavonols, 31

foods:
   recommended packaged foods,
     417–32
   websites for ordering, 78, 417–18
   see also specific foods and restaurants
Ford, Henry, 202
forgiveness, 228, 233–34
forward stretch, *159,* 159–60
Franklin, Benjamin, 234
Fredrickson, Barbara, 140–41
free radicals, 40
freezer, stocking, 437–39
FreshDirect.com, 78, 418
front deltoid raise exercise, *129*

Game Changers, The (documentary), 14
gazing meditation, 173–74
gene expression:
   effect of lifestyle medicine on, 26–34
   effect of loneliness on, 197
   effect of meditation on, 140, 144
   effect of social support on, 197
Gingrich, Newt, 6
gladiators, 44
Gleason scores, 59
global warming, 75
glycation, 27
glycemic index, 81
God, 181, 243–44
Gonzaga University, 232
Google Express, 78, 418
gratitude, 228, 231–33
greenhouse gases, 75
GroceryGateway.com, 78, 418
group support, 202–6
guided imagery, 144, 182–85

half locust exercise, *157,* 157–58
Hall, Kevin, 70–71
hammer curl exercise, *119*
Harvard Health Professionals Follow-Up
   Study:
   on diet and type 2 diabetes, 69
   on sex and prostate cancer, 47
Harvard Nurses' Health Study, 69
Harvard University:
   study on erectile dysfunction, 14
   study on heart attack survivors, 66
   study on meditation, 140, 171
   study on obesity, 242–43
   study on stress and depression, 26
Harvard University, Medical School,
   lifestyle medical training at, 50, 51

minister of loneliness, 197
mirror neurons, 201
mitochondria, 40
mobile devices, 5, 138, 139
    see also specific mobile devices
monogamy, 200–201
Moses, 244
Moyers, Bill, 245
Muhammad, 244
Murthy, Vivek, 197
musculoskeletal injury, 103
Mutual of Omaha, 8

NASA, 75
National Institutes of Health:
    obesity study, 71
    support for Medicare coverage for
        lifestyle medicine intervention, 7
Nature, 75
neck exercises, *148*
neurofibrillary tangles (tau), 22, 39
neurogenesis, 44, 106
neuroplasticity, 140
New England Journal of Medicine, 56, 58, 67,
    74
Nf-kBf inflammatory marker, 24
nitric oxide, 43
Nonviolent Communication (Rosenberg), 221
No Regrets (Beazley), 233
norepinephrine, 39
nutrition:
    as controversial field, 61
    as elements of lifestyle medicine
        program, 143, 210
    European Prospective Investigation into
        Cancer and Nutrition (EPIC), 19
    guidelines, 79–85
    myths regarding, 63–67, 69–75
    physicians' lack of education in, 9, 52
    see also specific recipes
nuts and seeds, 83–84, 96

obesity:
    calorie restriction in, 71
    chronic inflammation of pancreas and,
        23
    co-morbidities with, 18
    Harvard study on, 242–43
    insurance coverage to reverse, 7
    role of genes in, 32
office visits, 7
Old Testament, 244
O'Leary, Michael P., 14

oncogenes, 23, 27, 59
one-arm incline press exercise, *116*
Oneness, 243–44
ornish.com, xv, 12, 223
Ornish Diet, The, 4
Ötillö Swimrun World Championship, 65
overhead triceps pull exercise, *120*
oxidative stress, 40–41
oxytocin, 198

Pace, Joseph, 14
pain:
    acute inflammation and, 21
    from arthritis, 151
    endorphins and pain reduction, 229, 230
    muscle tension and, 26, 111, 145, 185
    sleep quality and, 232
    see also angina
Paleo diet, 65–67, *68*, 69–70
pancreas:
    chronic inflammation and, 23
    diabetes and, 40
    insulin secretion by, 24, 79
pantry, stocking, 439–49
passive attention, 171
perennial philosophy, 244
pesticides, 37, 62
pets, 190, 198
phagocytosis, 22
physicians:
    depression and suicide among, 52
    lifestyle medical training for, 7–8, 50, 51
    prescribing prescriptions, 12
    time spent with patient at office visit, 7
Physicians' Health Study, 59
Planck, Max, 49
plants, 31, 62, 64, 65, 79
plaque, 22, 39, 53–54
platelet factor 4, 43
PML gene, 31
Pollan, Michael, 62
positron emission tomography (PET), 26,
    54
pre-diabetes, 19, 55, 56
    see also diabetes; type 2 diabetes
prescriptions:
    for antidepressants, 236
    non-compliance in taking, 12
Preventive Medicine Research Institute, xv,
    51
probiotics, 39, 63
*Proceedings of the National Academy of
    Sciences*, 27
prostaglandins, 22

Spitz, Aaron, 15
standing pull-down exercise, *127*
standing row exercise, *115*
Stanford University, 32, 35
Staphylococcus aureus, 37
Star Wars (movie series), 245–46
stasis, blood flow and, 43–48, 54
statins, 69
steakhouse restaurants, 93
stents, 52–54
strength training:
    examples of, 101
    to treat depression, 105
stress:
    changes in microbes and, 39
    effect of, 25–26, 104, 135–36
    hormones, 17, 25–26, 137, 142, 204,
        232–38
    oxidative, 40–41
    perception of, 136–37
    as a positive response, 142
    reduction techniques, 143–47
stress management:
    benefits of, 18
    breathing techniques, 167–71
    committing to, 194–95, *195*
    exercises, 148–66
    guided imagery, 144, 182–85
    inner peace from, *191*
    meditation, 140–42, 171–82, *175, 177,
        178, 179–81,* 181–82
    overcoming barriers to, 191–94
    as part of lifestyle medicine, 6
    techniques and, 137–38, 189–90
stretching:
    benefits of, 111
    gentle, 143–44, 145–47, *146–47*
    one of three basic types of exercise, 101
stroke:
    effect of exercise on, 102
    erectile dysfunction and, 14
    Mediterranean Diet and, 74
    as result of sedentary lifestyle, 45
sudden cardiac death:
    diet to lower, 83
    as result of exercise, 103
sugar:
    added to ingredients, 84
    bad carbs and, 79–81
    vs. carb calories, myth regarding,
        70–74
    in recommended packaged foods,
        419–32
suicide:
    among physicians, 52

rates in U.S., 197
stress and, 143
superbugs, 37
supermarkets and special orders for
    customers, 78, 418
support groups:
    for cancer patients, 204, 222
    to combat isolation and loneliness,
        203–9
    goals and structure of, 224
    participating in, 207–11, 228
    recruiting members for, 223
supporting and serving others, 228, 234–35
Suzuki, Shunryu, 201
swelling:
    acute inflammation and, 21–22
    of tissues, 47
sympathetic nervous system:
    and cancer growth, 204
    effect of loneliness on, 197
    effect of stress and depression on, 25–26,
        135, 141–43, 204
    increase of insulin levels and, 70

tau (neurofibrillary tangles), 22, 39
TED conference, 50
Teflon, 82
Teilhard de Chardin, Pierre, 243
television, 138
telomeres, 34–35
    cancer growth and, 204
    diet to lengthen, 66
    effect of exercise on, 103
    effect of stress on, 104
    twins and, 104
TheraBands, 112
therapeutic armamentarium, 35
Therapeutics Initiative, 56
Thomas, Marlo, 229
thoughts:
    vs. feelings, 211–12
    mindfulness and, 141; *see also*
        meditation
toe stretch exercise, *154*
To Kill a Mockingbird (Lee), 217
TOR (protein enzyme), 30–31
Treuherz, Claudia, 8–12
Treuherz, Robert, 8–11
triceps kickback exercise, *131*
tryptophan (amino acid), 64
twins, 104
type 2 diabetes:
    effect of telomeres on, 34
    effect on erectile dysfunction, 14

About the Authors

DEAN ORNISH, M.D., is the founder and president of the nonprofit Preventive Medicine Research Institute and clinical professor of medicine at the University of California, San Francisco, and also at the University of California, San Diego. Dr. Ornish was trained in internal medicine at the Baylor College of Medicine, Harvard Medical School, and the Massachusetts General Hospital. He earned a B.A. in humanities summa cum laude from the University of Texas in Austin, where he gave the baccalaureate address.

For over forty years, he has directed clinical research demonstrating, for the first time, that comprehensive lifestyle changes may begin to reverse even severe coronary heart disease, without drugs or surgery. Medicare created a new benefit category, "intensive cardiac rehabilitation," to provide coverage for this program.

He also directed the first randomized controlled trial demonstrating that comprehensive lifestyle changes may slow, stop, or reverse the progression of early-stage prostate cancer. His research showed that comprehensive lifestyle changes affect gene expression, "turning on" disease-preventing genes and "turning off" genes that promote cancer and heart disease, as well as the first controlled study showing that these lifestyle changes may begin to reverse cellular aging by lengthening telomeres, the ends of our chromosomes that regulate aging (in collaboration with Dr. Elizabeth Blackburn, awarded the Nobel Prize in Physiology or Medicine.

His research and writings have been published in the leading peer-reviewed medical journals, including the *Journal of the American Medical Association, Lancet,* and *New England Journal of Medicine.* His work has been featured in all major media, including cover stories in *Newsweek, Time,* and *U.S. News & World Report.*

He has received numerous awards, including the 1994 Outstanding Young Alumnus Award from the University of Texas, Austin; the National Public Health Hero Award from the University of California, Berkeley; a U.S. Surgeon General Citation; a Presidential Citation from the American Psychological Association; the Plantrician Project Luminary Award; and the inaugural Lifetime Achievement Award from the American College of Lifestyle Medicine, which deemed him the "father of lifestyle medicine."

Dr. Ornish's TED talks have been viewed by more than 6 million people. He has written a monthly column for *Time, Newsweek,* and *Reader's Digest* magazines, is a LinkedIn Influencer, was the medical editor for the *Huffington Post* (2009–2016), and co-chaired Google Health with Marissa Mayer (2007–2009).

He was appointed by President Clinton to the White House Commission on the Complementary and Alternative Medicine Policy and by President Obama to the White House Advisory Group on Prevention, Health Promotion, and Integrative and Public Health.

The "Ornish diet" has been rated "#1 for Heart Health" by *U.S. News & World Report* every year from 2011 through 2017. The author of six books, all national bestsellers, Dr. Ornish was recognized as "one of the 125 most extraordinary University of Texas alumni in the past 125 years"; by *Time* magazine as a "*Time* 100 Innovator"; by *Life* magazine as "one of the fifty most influential members of his generation"; and by *People* magazine as "one of the world's seven most powerful teachers."

ANNE ORNISH is the digital director of Ornish Lifestyle Medicine and vice president of Program Development at the nonprofit Preventive Medicine Research Institute. She received a B.A. in art history and digital art in 1997 with honors from the University of Colorado, Boulder.

She is the creator of Ornish Lifestyle Medicine's digital platform—including www.ornish.com—and Empower, a turnkey learning management system that trains healthcare professionals throughout the country. Empower also guides participants through foundational courses that support people to transform suffering into health and well-being. Empower provides best-in-class tools for sustainable behavior change and ongoing healthy living via enlivening educational and practice videos, workshops, and community support.

Her multimedia series of guided meditation practices are featured on a DVD inside Dr. Ornish's book, *The Spectrum,* and at www.ornish.com. She also produced the Ornish Program's online channel at WebMD from 1998 through 2006.

Anne has over twenty-five years of advanced training in yoga and meditation. She is a certified integrative health and spirituality practitioner through the California Pacific Medical Center in San Francisco and also received professional training in mindfulness-based stress reduction in mind-body medicine with Dr. Jon Kabat-Zinn of the University of Massachusetts School of Medicine. She was featured on the cover of *Yoga Journal.*

Dean and Anne live in the San Francisco area with Lucas (Luke, age 18) and Jasmine (Jazz, age 9).

ornish.com